ATHLETIC TRAINING

AND

CONDITIONING

O. WILLIAM DAYTON

HEAD ATHLETIC TRAINER

YALE UNIVERSITY

THE RONALD PRESS COMPANY · NEW YORK

LIBRARY OF CONGRESS CATALOG CARD NUMBER: 60–14394

PRINTED IN THE UNITED STATES OF AMERICA

Preface

This is a practical handbook for trainers, for students of athletic training, and for coaches and physical education instructors who must also perform training duties. In its coverage of athletic injuries this book is strictly confined to the duties and responsibilities of the trainer, clearly delimiting them from the actual medical diagnosis, treatment, and prognosis which are the responsibility of the physician.

A chapter is devoted to each major body area and the injuries to which it is subject, systematically taking up fractures, dislocations, sprains and strains, contusions and wounds. In this approach the book deals with the trainer's specific concerns: the circumspect initial management of an injury through ascertaining its history, inspecting and palpating it, and applying first-aid care; and the subsequent treatment, physical therapy, taping, and rehabilitation under the direction of the physician. Although the book is organized according to the principal parts of the body, the point is constantly emphasized that the trainer must always treat the athlete as a person and not as an injured part.

A knowledge of anatomy, physiology, and kinesiology is assumed, but a brief and simple review of the pertinent anatomy is provided for each body area and illustrated. Step-by-step procedures are carefully and completely outlined at the risk of perhaps seeming to be dogmatic or to simplify. In full recognition of the fact that there are many ways in which injuries may be handled successfully and that there is still much controversy over certain methods of treatment, the techniques and procedures set forth here are those which the author has used at Yale University and elsewhere during more than twenty years of experience.

Equally as important as the treatment of athletic injuries is their prevention. This involves careful medical examination of the athlete to detect susceptibility to injury, proper conditioning to prepare for competition, full protection from possible injury, cautious medical control of an injury, and its rehabilitation before permitting the athlete to participate in his sport again. In addition to several chapters on these subjects, the theme of preventing injuries is stressed throughout the book. Many of the examples are drawn from training problems encountered in football, where the range of injuries is perhaps widest, but the principles and practices set forth here apply to the trainer's responsibilities in all sports.

I am deeply indebted to the many people who with patience and guidance have helped me with this book. I wish to acknowledge my gratitude to Dr. Isao Hirata, Jr., athletic surgeon of Yale University and Assistant Chief of Surgery in the Department of University Health, who read the script and made many suggestions for its improvement; to Delaney Kiphuth and Robert Kiphuth; and to Mrs. Elsie Van Dillen who diligently typed and retyped the manuscript.

O. William Dayton

Hamden, Connecticut
July, 1960

Contents

PART I: GENERAL TRAINING CONSIDERATIONS

1 THE TRAINER AND HIS DUTIES 3

2 PHYSICAL EXAMINATION AND MEDICAL COVERAGE . . 14

3 DIET IN ATHLETICS 28

4 PHYSICAL CONDITIONING 40

5 COMMON PROBLEMS IN TRAINING 60

6 TYPES OF ATHLETIC INJURIES 104

7 PHYSICAL THERAPY 126

PART II: INJURIES OF BODY AREAS

8 HEAD AND NECK 143

9 TRUNK AND BACK 158

10 SHOULDER 190

11 ARM 225

12 ELBOW 234

13 WRIST AND HAND 245

14 UPPER AND LOWER LEG 260

15 KNEE 286

16 ANKLE AND FOOT 331

APPENDIX A 373

APPENDIX B 377

INDEX 381

Part I

General Training Considerations

Chapter 1

The Trainer and His Duties

To discuss in detail the history of the "training profession" is not the aim of this manual. However, the status of the trainer has progressed from the "rubber" stage to that of a well-qualified member of a team composed of the coach, team physician, and trainer. Years ago the trainer was the "character" who hung around the dressing rooms imparting little knowledge but making many wise cracks. The day of the pat on the back and the rub with "hot stuff" on the injured athlete is past. Today's professional is a well-trained member of the staff which is responsible for the welfare and physical health of the athlete. A thorough knowledge of anatomy, physiology, physical therapy, psychology, hygiene, taping, conditioning, prevention of injury, equipment, and the care of athletic injuries is required and must be applied with great skill to injured athletes. Many trainers have advanced academic degrees and are well qualified for the job that they are doing today.

With the help of the team physician and other members of the medical profession, the trainer provides a professional service for which there is a very definite need. His work, in conjunction with that of the team physician, is the backbone of athletic fitness. Although the team physician makes all decisions, and his decisions are final, when he and the trainer work together as a team, there is plenty for both to do without the overlapping of authority. Both members of the team are indispensable.

The trainer's functional area has generally been accredited in the objectives of the National Athletic Trainers' Association. This group, founded in June of 1950 at an organizational meeting in Kansas City, Missouri, has set as its objectives:

1. To advance, encourage, and improve the athletic training profession in all its phases and to promote a better working relationship among those persons interested in the problems of training.
2. To develop further the ability of each of its members.
3. To better serve the common interest of its members by providing means for a free exchange of ideas within the profession.
4. To enable members to become acquainted personally through casual good fellowship.

Since that very memorable day, the training profession has advanced from its primitive infancy to a mature science that requires specialized technical knowledge. The organization is proud to have in its membership many members of the medical profession who give of their time and knowledge to help foster the aims of the association.

In a recent issue of *The Journal of the National Athletic Trainers' Association* an athletic training program was outlined. The importance of this article will be revealed after reading it, so it is herewith added to this chapter.

AN ATHLETIC TRAINING PROGRAM

(This training program was fully approved at the recent national meeting and it is the sole responsibility of the membership to adapt this program wholeheartedly to make it work.)

The National Athletic Trainers' Association, in an effort to raise standards of athletic training, recently approved a program of athletic training education. To make it an acceptably workable program, the athletic trainers must receive direction, advice, guidance, and supervision from two main areas (medical, NATA) and unqualified use of existing facilities in two others (Physical Education, Physical Therapy).

Medical

The medical doctor should expect qualified assistance from the athletic trainer in the management and prevention of athletic injuries, and assume the responsibility of supervising the total prescription.

The athletic trainer should cooperate completely with the team physician or any other medical advisor assigned to the organization, and carry out the minute details of the doctor's orders.

Physical Education

The physical education department, by accepting the minimal requirements as suggested by NATA in the physical education curriculum, will help relieve an established need for competent athletic training on the high school level. The Department should be able to assure prospective employers that graduates will have adequate background in the prevention and management of athletic injuries, and qualification for a teaching license. The Department should cooperate with the existing placement agency of the University in matters of placement.

In the promotion of a more comprehensive program, the athletic trainer will act as advisor, instructor, and first-aider.

Physical Therapy

NATA should encourage the athletic trainer to continue his education by completing at least a certificate course in physical therapy at an accredited school. The qualified combination of teacher-athletic trainer-physical therapist, could assume the physical therapy duties for schools and communities in times of emergency. This could be a real service to the county medical societies in their medical attention to the smaller communities.

Activities of the profession are reflected in terms of: Areas of Service, Coordination of the Total Prescription, and the Educational Program. The success of a profession is not measured by financial standards, but rather by accomplishments in serving the needs of people.

Members of the athletic training profession should be qualified to give service in the following areas:

Athletics

The primary concern of the trainer is the management and prevention of athletic injuries. Most athletic injuries are accidents. Under the guidance of the medical profession, the athletic trainer must concern himself with the prevention of these accidents. He can do this daily with the supervision of the safety factors of all athletic fields by seeing that all undue hazards are either removed or eliminated; the care and issuing of equipment; and the supervision of all training menus. Due to the brief time element involved in athletics and the inability to completely rehabilitate injured athletes in season, the athletic trainer must be accomplished in preventive and supportive strappings.

The athletic trainer, in the management of athletic injuries, must give "on the field first-aid" and follow up and carry out in detail the medical doctor's prescription of after treatment and rehabilitation.

Physical Education

The athletic trainer should assume the responsibility for the care of injuries in physical education and intra-mural sports. Since there is a high degree of similarity of injuries in these areas to that of athletics, there appears to be some sound justification for the inclusion of all injuries in physical education, athletics, and intramural sports under the term "athletic injury."

Student Health

There is evidence that school enrollment will double in the next ten years. With expanding community hospital facilities remaining overly crowded, this would indicate that there must be qualified personnel to aid the medical doctor in caring for the health of the student, faculty, and staff. The qualified athletic trainer–physical therapist would be able to carry out the prescribed physical therapy duties for the schools.

Besides participating as a member of the athletic medical team, trainers have the unique position of being closely associated with the administrators, coaches, and players. Athletic trainers should coordinate, under medical supervision, and with the cooperation of administrators and coaches, the total prescription of training and conditioning for so long as the athlete is a responsibility of the athletic department. This responsibility includes the prevention and care of athletic injuries, and can be viewed in four phases: Prevention, First-Aid, After Treatment, and Rehabilitation of all injuries.

Prevention

The trainer acts as advisor to coaches and athletes in matters concerning the various health and conditioning problems. His advice may be sought in matters pertaining to physical examinations; diet; warm-up and calisthenics; preseasonal, seasonal, and postseasonal conditioning.

First Aid

The athletic trainer's responsibility to the athlete in the first forty-eight hours requires qualification beyond the prescribed procedures as set down for Red Cross First Aid. After careful examination, the qualified trainer should make a decision as to whether or not a player is to be removed from the playing area. If the player has an injury of any severity, the athletic trainer should obtain a detailed history of the injury and make observations of symptoms and signs of inflammation. As soon as possible, the trainer should give an initial impression as to severity so as to aid the team physician in his diagnosis. The athletic trainer should follow up the incidence of injury by the application of splints, cold, pressure, elevation, or rest as indicated. The team physician should then be notified.

After Treatment

During the convalescent period following the first forty-eight hours, the qualified athletic trainer should carry out in detail the medical orders, including the prescribed use of physical agents.

Rehabilitation

The athletic trainer should make every effort to prepare the athlete mentally and physically for his successful return to partial or full-time sports participation.

THE TRAINER'S DUTIES

The three basic categories in which the trainers' duties fall are:

1. Prevention of injury.
2. Treatment of injuries.
3. Rehabilitation of the athlete after injury.

Prevention of Injury. Much more time is spent on prevention of injury than on treatment of injuries. To prevent an injury means that there is one less case that the trainer has to treat.

First on the schedule to prevent injury is the physical examination. This must be thorough and complete. The physical examination is discussed in detail in Chapter 2.

Condition is a large factor in the prevention of injury. Injuries are inevitable where competition is keen and the sport is rough. Those that are inevitable cannot be prevented, but the majority of injuries can be prevented by making proper arrangements. A well-conditioned athlete is less susceptible to injury than the poorly conditioned athlete. Conditioning will be handled in Chapter 4, but other factors in the prevention of injuries will be listed here. By assuring prompt, intelligent, and conscientious care in injuries, the minor injury will remain a minor injury, and the athlete will not be allowed to return to activity until he is ready. Many of the so-called minor injuries have been turned into serious injuries by too early resumption of activity, and successive incidences of injury have accumulated so that the injury becomes a serious one. There are very few serious injuries in athletics today, and we believe that the scientific advancement in the management of all injuries is the sole reason for this result. The manufacturers of equipment are never satisfied with their efforts; they are continually improving protective equipment so that the incidence to injury due to faulty equipment has been eliminated. Good equipment without a proper fit is useless. Care in fitting of equipment, so that the maximum benefits may be derived, is a responsibility of the coach and trainer.

Poor equipment cannot possibly provide for well-protected athletes, but budgets are constantly staring the coach in the face and he must economize where feasible. However, the practice of buying in quantity rather than quality is not a sound principle. The idea that it is better to buy more articles of an inferior nature than a limited number of quality articles that will last longer and give better protection is a fallacy. Inferior articles have to be replaced every year, whereas the quality merchandise will last for a much longer period of time. The old adage "you get what you pay for" is very true in this case. Along this line, we have seen incidences where the school has purchased football game pants for twenty dollars. These are very colorful and fancy. On the other hand, the pants that are worn in practice are ill-fitting and lack protection. These pants cost about five dollars. In adding up the hours that each pair of pants will be used, we find that the practice pants are used about 10 hours and the game pants about 2 hours. Practices are harder than games, and therefore the best equipment should be available at these practice sessions. Fortunately these economy practices are lessening and equal qualities of equipment are used in games and practices.

Many injuries are caused by carelessness due to mechanical difficulties. Mechanical difficulties refer to holes in the turf of the practice fields, dirt on the basketball court, etc. An athlete may sprain an ankle by stepping in a hole. This injury is just as serious as the injury sustained in hard play. The athlete will lose time from playing and will suffer unnecessarily. The fields and court and other playing areas should be checked regularly and dangerous conditions, if found, should be remedied. The use of lime to mark fields should be discontinued unless lime is slaked. Chalk, flour, crushed stone, and many other products are available and will not result in the nasty burns that unslaked lime has produced.

Broken equipment should not be worn; shoes that have a cleat missing are hazardous. Rigid inspection before practice should be stressed. When an equipment man is not on duty, the athlete should be taught to report broken equipment immediately after practice so that repairs or changes can be made before the next workout.

Proper warm-up comes under the heading of injury prevention. A regular warm-up should be performed before active practice is started. Warming-up takes longer in cold weather than in warm seasons and must be as thorough on practice days as on game days. To do a few push-ups and a few arm-swinging exercises is not enough; a full routine is necessary, starting with the head and progressing to all the areas of the body.

Protective strappings, etc., play a very important part in the prevention of injury, as does the wearing of "special pads" to protect a previously injured area against further injury. Strapping a weak or unstable part of the body will increase the athlete's ability to resist injury. Various types of strappings and other protectors will be taken up in later chapters.

Proper rehabilitation is vital in the prevention of a recurring injury. It is folly to allow an athlete to go back into action with an injury that is not fully rehabilitated. The trainer and team physician must supervise the program of exercises and other training activity so that maximum benefits result. An athlete who is "partially" ready is not ready. To be less than 100 per cent fit is not enough if the athlete is to perform at his best. The substitute is a better man than the regular under these circumstances.

Treatment of Injuries. The trainer and the team physician, working together, are responsible for the treatment of athletic injuries. Thorough knowledge of the injury, the sport, and the method of treatment help the athlete's return to activity in full physical capacity. Treatments must be prompt, intelligent, and conscientious. Do not put off until tomorrow the treatments that may help the athlete. There are acute injuries for which immediate treatment is mandatory if early recovery is to be made. To send a man home with the "wait and see" attitude may result in much loss of time on the part of the athlete as well as the training staff. It is better to err on the good side than to be wrong; just a little of "wrong" can mean a whole lot in the case of an injury. Many times an injury has been passed off as a minor casualty only to return the next day with much swelling, pain, loss of motion, and a thoroughly disillusioned athlete. When an injury is reported it must be treated. In the acute stage there is no such thing as a minor injury. Never treat an injury halfway; go all out and the response will be gratifying.

The treatments discussed in this manual indicate the specific responsibilities of the trainer and those of the physician. Discussion of the physician's procedures are intended solely to give the trainer an idea of the extent of the treatment that is needed for proper handling of the injury. Furthermore the suggested treatments are those used by the team physicians at Yale. They are not to be regarded as instructions for team physicians or as the final word on treatment. Specific conditions not covered in the chapters on injuries are not to be handled by the trainer and have therefore been omitted.

Trainers should not give medication by mouth unless ordered by the team physician of the health department. Aspirin has been the exception, but then only after specific history has been attained. The use of salt tablets and vitamins are ordered by the team physician and are supplied to the athlete when indicated. Medications for "upset stomach" and other such conditions should be dispensed only on the advice of the physician.

Rehabilitation of Injury. To allow an athlete who is not completely rehabilitated to return to activity is the same as asking for an injury. In all injuries a certain amount of atrophy will be found. If the athlete is allowed to participate in this condition, he will not be able to protect himself fully, since he will not have the necessary muscle quality, and he will be back with you again. There is nothing more aggravating to the training staff than a recurring injury. Many times the staff is not at fault, but it may be questionable whether the injury was ready to be tested by a return to play. One trainer in the profession feels that a recurring injury is his responsibility. In other words, the athlete's reinjury is an indication that he was allowed to return to activity too soon. As has been mentioned, there are some injuries that cannot be prevented. If the reinjury is of this type, the trainer may not be just in his self-criticism. In ankle, knee, and shoulder injuries, the degree of atrophy is usually visible. Exercises to eliminate this condition should be started when the team physician feels that the time has arrived. The exercises should be continued until full recovery has been attained. General exercises for the athlete must be incorporated in the recovery plan along with the special exercises for the injury. In the case of a shoulder injury, the athlete may be able to continue with such an activity as running to keep his legs in shape. This program may be varied in the case of an ankle or knee injury, when the athlete will do exercises and drills to keep the remainder of his body in condition.

GENERAL QUALIFICATIONS OF A TRAINER

Intelligence. A trainer must have a sound knowledge of anatomy and physiology, must know how to apply adhesive strapping and bandages, must do physical therapy under direction of the physician, and must be fully capable of conducting conditioning programs and rehabilitation exercises. He must be ever alert to the scientific advancements in his field and must stay abreast of events in the field of athletic training. New methods are being advanced every day, and he must be intelligent enough to analyze these for adaptability to his work. He must be willing to talk over all matters pertaining to his work with the team physician.

Judgment. He must have good judgment and must know his limitations and when to treat and when to refer to the team physician. In some men this is inherent, whereas others must acquire this with experience. A trainer must bear in mind that he is not a physician and that his training is limited. To refer an athlete to the physician is good judgment and not a sign of inability. The trainer must be able to differentiate between the chronic complainer and the athlete who is genuinely in need of care. The best way to acquire good judgment is to anticipate constantly situations that may arise and require his services.

Industriousness. The trainer must be industrious; he must be resourceful, thoughtful, and patient. His work is hard enough and very demanding, and if he is not industrious, he will have a very hard time of making a success of the position. He will have to work hard, long, and efficiently. Many things occur that may seem trivial to others but are very important to the trainer and, depending on how well he handles trivial things, will determine his success in athletics. To ignore a little pimple because of laziness can affect his status with the athlete and those who surround him.

He must be ever mindful that he is handling a person as well as an athlete, dealing with the person as a whole and not only with the injury. Athletes suffer extreme apprehensions over a condition that the trainer may know to be of little consequence. To pass this off is being very unkind. The trainer must try to alleviate the mental as well as the physical suffering. In the case of "prima donnas" the trainer is put on the spot, and the only solution is to try to be patient with this type of athlete. For some reason or other the athletic world delivers athletes of this type to the training room, and year in and year out every trainer always has a few. His ability to "get along" with these personality problem players is very important if his professional standing is not to be affected. A good sense of humor is very effective in solving this problem.

Cleanliness. Cleanliness of body, clothes, and surroundings is very essential to good training. A trainer who is sloppy in his dress and habits does not make a good impression on the charges he has to handle. The training room must be kept clean and neat. Uniforms must be clean. Training is a profession, and as a professional man, the trainer must do all that is necessary to retain respect from his charges.

Calmness. Calmness is very contagious. When an athlete is injured and the trainer shows signs of nervousness, this will be reflected to the athlete, the coaches, and all who are at the scene. Calmness will be enhanced by a thorough knowledge of the field and experience by exposure to conditions that are not considered normal. A distraught leader will lose the faith of all who work with him. He must be confident but not overbearing, and poised but not egotistical.

Fairness. The trainer must at all times be fair. To favor the first stringer will not only handicap the athlete, but the rest of the squad will feel neglected. Justice must prevail in the training room. Remember, these athletes are people as well as athletes, and if this is not considered, no treatment will ever get these injured athletes well again. A kind word to a "scrub" will pay dividends in a short while. Many times the "scrub" of today will be the star of tomorrow.

Ethics. Every man must live by a code of ethics. The trainer must and does. He will work diligently with the team physician and carry out his orders to the letter. He will conduct himself in the best interests of his profession by working only with conditions that he is capable of handling, referring others to the team physician. Second-guessing the coach or doctor is a poor practice and is a breach of ethics. The coach does not want to be the trainer, and therefore the trainer should not be the coach.

Understanding. The athlete who is injured must be considered as a whole person and not just an injured part that is to be repaired. Too often the athlete is made to feel that he is only a piece of machinery that has been sent to the mechanic for repair. The athlete should be treated as a whole person with feelings rather than a machine that needs overhauling. The athlete is entitled to the best that is available, and this includes the intangibles such as understanding. Athletes are pictured as being big and strong. This they are, but injuries have a way of leveling this stature to that of a little boy. Athletes' emotions are often skin deep and are easily affected by a remark or a so-called wise crack. Tempers flare up at odd incidents; the trainer must be alert to pour the oil on the injured feelings. Athletes have many motivations for participating. They wish to do something for recognition by their classmates. They are doing what they are doing because they like it, and some are in sports only to prove their masculinity.

All these incentives must be taken into consideration when decisions are made and handed down to the athlete. By being a part of the athlete's life, the trainer may make or break him by the way he words or explains the extent of the disability. Many times an athlete has been told that he is finished only to have this decision changed by proper and speedy recovery from the injury. Hasty judgments of the condition of the athlete may backfire and if they prove to be wrong may seriously affect the athlete's confidence in the trainer. A successful approach to an athlete's confidence is to assure him that everything possible will be done to keep him in the game. However, this is not a one-man job and must have the athlete's complete support. If, at the end of the treatment period, the response has not been good, the athlete as well as the trainer will know that he cannot continue and he will be satisfied with the results. This approach is generally successful.

A good trainer does not allow personal feelings to influence treatment or postinjury playing qualifications. If he agrees with the athlete only because he likes the boy, he is not doing the athlete a service. The athlete must be told the truth even if it hurts. A recent editorial in the Journal of the American Medical Association said:

Medicine recognizes that a fractured ankle may leave less of a scar than a personality frustrated by reason of parental timidity over participation in contact sports. Medicine does recognize, however, that there are contact sports which have for their main purpose, rather than competition and victory, injury to the opponent. Medicine recognizes also that there are contact sports and degrees of competition which are too severe for the immature. In standing out against the abuse of highly desirable exercise and highly necessary competition, medicine in no way objects to activity, competition, and risk, in its proper place. All life is a risk and without courage life is not worth living.

A "scar" may result from improper handling as well as from an injury; scars will result from injury but to add a psychological scar is only putting fuel on the fire. It is a wise trainer who uses few words and well-chosen words to explain the inability of the prospective athlete. The prospective athlete feels that the most important thing in the world is making good in the sport he has chosen. Remember, he may be hurt badly by the way his inability to participate is explained. He may not be big enough or strong enough or mature enough to accept an adverse decision, but well-chosen words will convince him that he should perhaps try another less rough activity. The trainer's approach will determine the extent of the scar, if any, on his personality.

Chapter 2

Physical Examination and Medical Coverage

PHYSICAL EXAMINATION

To go into detail about the need for a complete physical examination of all athletes would serve no purpose at this time. There is no doubt in the minds of all concerned that a good physical examination should be part of the athletic program. To rely on the athlete to have a physical at home and bring the report to school is a very poor procedure. A physician well-versed in the intricacies and requirements of athletic competition should be the man to give this physical. Too often, when matters are taken for granted, a minor condition can be aggravated and may result in irreparable damage to the student. Examinations given by family physicians may not tell the true story because the physician, in trying to help, may actually overlook something that does not seem important to him but may be serious in the eyes of a team physician who will evaluate the findings differently.

The first consideration is: Will the boy be physically qualified for the sport for which the physical is being taken? By listening to his heart, taking of blood pressure, etc., the boy may be judged physically sound at the moment, but we must also consider the judgment of the examiner. Even though the boy is physically sound, does he have the physical equipment to withstand the rigors of the sport for which he has applied? It has been found that a boy may be physically sound but not fit for football. Who should take the responsibility for this decision? The examiner, if he has the welfare of the boy at heart, should lead the boy's interest into some other sport. Such an applicant should not be discouraged from sports in general but from football as a sport for him. He may protest vigorously, but in the long run a service will have been rendered to athletics and, by no means last, to the boy and his family. Laxity of the requirements for a good physical report may result in a boy being allowed to play a sport in which he is unfit to participate.

A team physician is the ideal man to perform this very important part of the athletic program. Sports physicians are specialized practitioners, have excellent judgment, and are very alert to pick up conditions that may later become problems. Since the team physician is associated with the applicant from the beginning of his career, it will be easier to handle injuries or other physical ailments that may occur during the playing years of the athlete.

Most schools require a physical examination before the student enters school. When this is received by the authorities at the Department of Health, it is reviewed. Anything questionable is noted and followed up on the physical examination. Example: History of recent serious illness or an acute joint condition that may be arrested and considered as well are brought to the attention of the particular examiner, who will pursue the issue to the fullest. This may include laboratory tests, X-rays. In the meantime the prospective athlete will not be allowed to participate until the condition has been cleared up satisfactorily. Along with this preliminary physical, a complete history of the boy will be obtained and recorded. The history will include all illnesses and injuries. Each condition should be checked by the man who specializes in its respective category. The physician who makes the final decision is the team physician.

The complete physical is repeated each year and kept on file in the Department of Health.

Case Histories. A full afternoon is devoted to the physical examination of the football candidates at Yale. (The same physicial examination is given to all students who wish to participate in sports.) There are many stages in this examination, as listed below:

1. History of all previous illnesses and injuries.
2. Eye examination with and without correction.
3. Height and weight.
4. Chest measurements, normal and expanded.
5. Nose and throat examination.
6. Chest examination by medical man, including heart, lungs, etc. (Blood pressure is taken and recorded before applicant is seen by medical man.)
7. Surgeon makes a general examination and makes note of any condition that is questionable. This examination includes physical appearance (posture, correlation between weight and height, quality of physique, etc.) skin, abdomen, hernias, back (curvatures, etc.), genitals, and extremities.
8. Urine specimen is taken at this time.
9. Chest X-ray.

Name_____ Age_____ yrs._____ mos._____ Date of examination_____ Class_____ A.M._____ P.M._____

General development—excellent—average—poor

Weight_____ Height_____ Hgb._____

Skin and scalp_____

Vaccination { Rt. arm—leg — good
mark   { Lt.   — absent—indef.

Epidermophyrosis (feet)_____

Thorax { Exp._____ Thorax { Normal—flat
circum. { Insp._____   { Pigeon—funnel

Ocular movements_____

Pupil   { Rt. light_____ distance_____
reactions { Lt. light_____ distance_____

Color vision (Ishi)_____ Acc._____

Vision { Rt. eye_____ corr. to_____
       { Lt. eye_____ corr. to_____

Last exam._____ How often_____

Care of mouth—good—average—poor

Teeth—good—average—poor
       right   Upper   left

[dental chart diagram with numbered teeth 8 7 6 5 4 3 2 1 | 1 2 3 4 5 6 7 8]

       right·   Lower   left
Occlusion—good—fair—poor   Class A B C
Gums_____

O To be extracted—Un. unerupted—Dev. devital—Temp. temporary
X Has been extracted—Imp. impacted—Df. defec. filling—G. Cr. gold crown

Nasal obstruction_____

Deflected septum_____

Thyroid—normal—enlarged—moderate—slight_____

Hearing { Rt._____
        { Lt._____

Tonsils { present_____ removed_____ regrowth_____
        { hypertrophied_____ chronic inflamm._____

Lymph { cerv._____ axillary_____
nodes { epitroch_____ inguinal_____

Lungs_____ ref. for x-ray_____

Heart   { Left nipple_____
From   { L. B. D. (deep) 5th space   = cm.
Med.   { L. B. D. (deep) 4th space   = cm.
Line   { L. B. D. (deep) 3d space   = cm.
upright { R. B. D. (deep)_____   = cm.
pos.   { Apex impulse—seen—felt   = cm.

Rhythm_____ A₂—P₂_____

Sounds_____

Murmurs_____

YALE UNIVERSITY · DEPARTMENT OF HEALTH

Abdomen_____

Inguinal { Rt._____
rings   { Lt._____

Genitals { Penis—normal—circum.—phimosis—redund.
         { Testes—Rt._____ Lt._____

Varicocele—Rt._____ Lt._____

Hemorrhoids·_____

Varicose veins_____

Reflexes { Knee jerks—Rt._____ Lt._____
         { Others_____

Bones and joints_____

Muscles and ligaments_____

Remarks pertaining to examination:_____

D. U. H. N. 40

Front of physical examination card.

16

Inoculation history reviewed. In recent years all athletes have been given tetanus shots before being allowed to participate. Polio vaccine has been advocated for all students at Yale. After these preliminaries, the athlete's case history is evaluated by the team physician. The physician reviews it with the boy, and any questionable conditions are evaluated at this time. Should the team physician feel that further study is indicated, he advises the follow-up procedures. If further medical work-up is needed, he makes an appointment with a specialist for the candidate. The procedure is also followed in the case of an orthopedic consultation. The men in this field have the final say and their opinions are final.

Disqualifications for Athletics. When and where to draw the line as to whether a boy should or should not play sports, or a particular sport, is a very hard decision to make. Certainly the examining physician will have to make many decisions that he does not particularly care to make. Even though a few disqualifications may result if the physical examination is thorough, it is folly to minimize a condition that may be aggravated by the boy's participating in sports. There are no set rules to govern this examination, and therefore a few conditions that may warrant further study are given here. At present these are disqualifying in varying degrees in the eyes of the examiners at Yale.

1. *Heart.* Not all heart conditions are disqualifying, but every murmur, etc., must be fully diagnosed to establish whether or not the condition would be aggravated and cause further damage to the participant. To eliminate all heart histories without a full diagnosis is not fair to the candidate.

2. *Hypertension.* This condition should be evaluated because it has been found to be secondary to kidney infection.

3. *Handicapped.* A candidate with one of a pair of organs missing should be disqualified from playing contact sports.

4. *Joint injury.* Many athletes have been allowed to continue sports after a serious joint injury. These conditions should be carefully evaluated, and if instability or incomplete recovery, etc., exists, the candidate should be advised of his condition. If possible a regimen of exercises should be prescribed so that a useful limb for future life may be developed. Too many chronic joint injuries in college result from overzealous management on the high school or lower level. Unfortunately, these boys will be turned down in their request to play sports on a college level, owing to this disability.

Not to be written in by examiner

Follow up notes—

Blood Pressure

Date	Before exercise recumbent			After exercise recumbent		
	Rate	Syst.	Diast.	Rate	Syst.	Diast.

Remarks—

To be filled in by examiner

Findings—

_____ M.D.

Symptoms referable to—

Respiratory system:

G. I. system:

G. U. system:

Cardiac:

Others:

Urinalyses

Date	React.	Sp. Gr.	Alb.	Sugar	Microscopical

Back of physical examination card.

5. *Head injuries.* These are perhaps the hardest decisions to make if the full history is not available or if the candidate chooses to keep the information from the examiner. A boy who has a history of "being knocked out several times" is not a good risk to himself, let alone the sports picture. Posttraumatic syndromes, such as psychological trauma and headaches, should be disqualifying conditions.

6. *Infectious diseases.* A history of an infectious disease, with fever still in existence, should be a disqualification. This category includes infectious mononucleosis, virus pneumonia, hepatitis, etc. The first two, for example, should be treated symptomatically and the student may be released when cured. Hepatitis should be cause for permanent disability in contact sports.

7. *Epilepsy.* Satisfactory control of epilepsy may be attained by the use of the new drugs, proper diets, and good discretion on the part of the individual. However, a seizure in a swimming area or a large stadium is not a healthy sight. Also, in contact sports, a slight lapse of control may result in a severe injury to the participant.

8. *Diabetes.* Intelligent management is the prime control in this disease, and if student can be relied upon to limit or eliminate his indiscretions, only then should he be allowed to participate.

9. *Back disease.* Not all back conditions should be a disqualification for sports. Some sports in which the athlete will not be subject to severe trauma are permissible with many back conditions, but the more severe the condition, the more the applicant should be detoured from contact sports. Spondylolisthesis should eliminate him from contact sports, but he may participate in track if condition warrants. All back-condition histories should be carefully evaluated and, if possible, helped with corrective measures.

10. *Physical make-up.* This is the part of the physical where the examining physician should be alert and should use the power of suggestion. A candidate may be physically fit but unfit for certain sports, and he should not be allowed to participate above his level because serious injury may result. By proper guidance many serious injuries can be prevented. A candidate who shows evidence of poor musculature or obesity should be encouraged to prepare himself before he is allowed to report for a rugged sport. Exercises are prescribed for this individual, and he is advised to report back for further evaluation. If at this time he is considered able to participate, he is then given approval on his physical examination.

11. *Intelligence.* This is most certainly a factor in the ability to participate in athletics. Too many times coaches have wasted their time with a candidate who had absolutely no reason for being a candidate on a team of any kind. This condition should be picked up in the physical examination, and the athlete should be ruled as unfit for athletics.

Medical Staff. A large staff is ideal, but very few places are able to have such a program. The basic examination, as outlined, must be performed. Even if sufficient staff is not available, the same procedures should be followed by the examiner if the physical examination is to be considered a complete one. This will present a hardship to the examiner who performs the task by himself. If all factors are not included, then there is little reason for an examination. In small communities, physical examinations can be given over a period of time previous to participation rather than on one appointment day. Several doctors and the school nurse in a small community can band together to give this full examination.

MEDICAL COVERAGE

After a complete physical examination has been performed and placed on file, the problem of complete medical coverage must be considered. Every athlete should have the benefit of complete medical coverage. Many schools employ a team physician or have at their disposal the services of a member of the local medical society. The practice has been to have the doctor at the field for games, although it is not always possible to have a physician in attendance for practice sessions. The team physician can provide immediate care at the time of injury and then refer the athlete to his family physician.

A program for medical coverage at practice sessions must be considered an important part of complete medical coverage. At the time of injury on the practice field, the coach must make a hurried decision as to the disposition of the injured player. To try to coach and to apply medical coverage is too much to expect of the coach; something must be done to help this situation. The employment of the school nurse has been used very successfully in some areas; she is on call at practice sessions to help in case of an emergency. This will eliminate the coach's having to stop his work and take care of the injured player. The nurse will be responsible for the emergency care of the player and also see that proper medical personnel are alerted for the handling of the athlete.

The student trainer program has also been used effectively in some areas, but he must work under the supervision of the team physician. Adequate training may take too much of the doctor's time, and when this occurs, the student training program falters.

Arrangements for emergency calls to the team physician must be planned so that needed medical service can be available at all practice sessions. Telephone numbers of the doctor, the ambulance service, and the hospital should be placed in a conspicuous place so that these numbers can be called in the event of an emergency. The numbers are often placed in the first aid kit that is always on the practice field.

Illnesses are also conditions that require medical attention, whether they are handled by the team physician or the family physician. The athlete should not be allowed to participate until cleared by the physician, preferably in writing.

Although parents are primarily responsible for the health of their children, it is advisable to have an agreement as to where the responsibility of the school begins and ends. This policy should be in writing and should be known to all athletes and their parents.

Athletic injury insurance policies are designed to cover certain expenses for injuries incurred during participation. The amount of coverage depends on the premium charged. Some schools will pay for this policy in full; others will participate, and others must be paid for by the parents. Some states make a plan of this type available to all schools at a very low rate. The same plan of payment is used: either the school pays in full or there is parent participation.

On the college level, where the student pays a fee for health services, all problems are handled at the Department of Health under the guidance of the medical staff. Many colleges assign a doctor to be responsible for the medical problems of the members of the various teams. This doctor is known as the team physician; he works with the athletic association for promoting the good health of all athletes. He is available at all contests and provides emergency treatment for the home team as well as the visitors. Whenever possible, he attends the practice sessions of all contact sports or sees that the sport is covered by an associate when he cannot attend. Noncontact sports are not covered, but doctors are on duty in the Department of Health or the infirmary and are available for immediate service. Transportation of injured athletes is handled by ambulance service or by a station wagon provided for this purpose.

Whenever there is an athletic contest of an intercollegiate nature on the campus, there will be a doctor in attendance. The doctor is a

NAME	Doe, John J.		CLASS	'61	
Date	SURGICAL NOTES			Diagnosis	Treatment
9/5	Injury to right knee in practice scrimmage.			Strain of medial collateral ligament	Sent to Infirmary ice, compression and elevation
9/6	X-ray rept. 22567 Negative	Right knee	Req. of Dr. Dr. Roentgenologist		
9/6	This patient was examined on September 6, 19--, at the Infirmary. He had been injured in varsity football practise on September 5, 19--. He was hit apparently on the lateral aspect of the right knee and believed that he felt something snap. On examination the knee is entirely encased in an adhesive strapping at about 160° of extension. Felt splints are applied with an ace bandage over the top of the adhesive strapping. The knee is well mobilized. He was treated in the Infirmary on bed rest, elevation and ice pack along with the immobilization. On examination the adhesive tape was stripped off. There is no increased fluid in the joint. The knee can be extended to 180° without pain. Flexion is possible to 30° without pain. There is very slight rocking in abduction, adduction. There is slightly increased swelling over the medial aspect of the knee on the tibial insertion on the collateral ligament. There is slight tenderness over this area. The anterior and posterior draw signs are negative. DIAGNOSIS: Strain, medial tibial collateral ligament. TREATMENT: Continuation of splinting with felt splints and partial weight bearing with crutches. Physical therapy was advised. I should expect that the patient would be able to go back to playing football. Dr. Orthopedist				

Result of X-ray and orthopedic consultation.

22

member of the staff of the Department of Health and is equipped to do work of a minor nature at the site, such as suturing lacerations and splinting fractures. He then directs the athlete to the proper area for further study, if necessary; i.e., X-ray or other services. The services of the attending physician are available to the visiting team members as well as our own athletes.

In football and hockey a doctor is in attendance at all practices as well as the games. In the case of an injury seen at practice, the attending physician advises the trainer as to the condition of the athlete and starts immediate treatment. On the next day the athlete is seen by the athletic surgeon, who thereafter assumes full responsibility for the treatments. After the diagnosis has been made, the athletic surgeon advises the head trainer of the status of the athlete. The head trainer sees that the coach and trainer of the particular sport are fully aware of the condition and know the procedures that they are to follow until the athlete has been cleared by the athletic surgeon for resumption of full activity.

At the time of examination the athlete may be put on a full disability or a competitive disability. Full disability means that the athlete cannot participate in his sport in any way, whereas competitive disability means that the athlete may be able to work partially in practice sessions but may not compete until fully cleared. For example, an athlete with a shoulder injury will be allowed to run but not allowed to use his shoulder for blocking or tackling. This helps the athlete retain the fitness of his legs and other parts of his body. A full layoff is not necessary in some minor injuries, since an athlete may be able to do some good work even though he cannot participate fully in all drills.

In basketball an athlete may be able to shoot free throws even though a foot condition keeps him from running. The same routine is carried out in other sports. In swimming, a shoulder injury restricts a participant to practicing his kicking, but this limited activity keeps the athlete from losing as much time as he would if he were placed on full disability. The coach and trainer of the sport are fully responsible for seeing that the orders are carried out.

The medical coverage is as complete as the surgical coverage. Should an athlete suddenly become ill, he would be seen by the attending physician, who would evaluate the condition and advise proper procedures. The next day the medical doctor who was responsible for the medical coverage of the athlete would examine this athlete, and the procedures as outlined for injuries would be followed out. The physician would inform the head trainer of the athlete's condition, and in turn the trainer would see that the coach was advised of the athlete's status. A prediction as to the prognosis of the athlete's recovery would also be part of the report from the medical doctor. The prognosis is very important because it enables coaches to make a replacement if necessary or to make an adjustment of some kind for the full benefit of the athlete and the team.

Notices of the above procedures are posted in all areas and each athlete is familiar with the organization. All means of communication to athletic director, coaches, and trainers are very direct, and there is very little time lost in evaluating the condition of the athlete who has been injured so that his status can be made known to all concerned.

Care of Athletes. Athletes requiring surgical or medical care report daily to the Department of Health at stated hours, except Sundays, regardless of whether initial treatment has been rendered or not. It is at these daily examinations that the status of the disability is established. *Full disability* means that no athletic activity of any kind will be permitted. In the event of a limited disability, the athlete may be permitted to work out to some extent with the team under the careful supervision of the team physician, trainer, and coach; but he is not allowed to participate in contests until his disability is fully cleared.

Visiting Teams. Visiting teams need not bring along their physician, since there is usually a physician in attendance at all intercollegiate contests. The service of the physician in attendance is available to the visitors as well as to the home team. The following is an example of a *notice posted for all visiting team physicians and trainers:*

It is the express purpose of the Yale University Department of Health to provide facilities and assistance to all visiting teams in accordance with this policy.

1. There is a supply of equipment for suture of *minor* lacerations as part of our own team physician kits, to which you are welcome should the need arise.

2. There is home-team medical coverage for all sports available to assist you at all times.

3. *Football:* In addition to our team physician there is an experienced general surgeon, an experienced orthopedic surgeon, and a radiologist *on the field at all times during all Yale Bowl Football Games.* Hence, should the need arise, expert consultation, emergency treatment, and hospitalization are immediately available simply by calling the Yale bench for assistance.

It is our hope that you will avail yourselves of these facilities and personnel without hesitation, and thereby avoid, as has happened in the past, unfortunate delays in the treatment and disposition of injured athletes because of unfamiliarity with local hospitals, ambulance service, X-ray services and the like.

Should the physician feel that overnight observation is necessary, the infirmary of the Department of Health is available, or the hospital may be preferred. The attending physician notifies the parents of the athlete, if necessary, and all others who may be involved.

Athletes requiring treatments while on the campus are examined by the athletic surgeon who prescribes necessary treatments while they are guests. The services of the Physical Therapy Department are available to visiting teams while on the campus.

Procedure. To have proper control of athletic injuries, and also to have a full record of them, a procedure for medical coverage should be spelled out in detail. The following paragraphs and forms illustrate the procedures developed at Yale over the years and are good examples in a well-planned system.

DATE STAMP WITH TIME	NAME Doe, John J.

(form reproduction)

DATE STAMP WITH TIME

NAME........Doe,........John........J.
(Last)   (First)   (Middle)

Class....'61........Dept........

Check service you wish to consult

4th Floor	☐ Director
1st Floor	☐ Employee Health ☐ Insurance Office
2d Floor	☐ Ear, Nose, Throat ☐ Eye ☐ Nurse ☐ Physician ☐ Surgeon
3d Floor	☐ Dental Hygienist ☐ Laboratory ☐ Mental Hygiene
Basement	☐ Allergist ☒ Athletic Surgeon ☐ Inoculation ☐ Orthopedist ☐ Physical Therapy

Check Sport Below

	Inter-College	Varsity	Freshman	None
	☐	☒	☐	☐

Sport....FOOTBALL

For Office Use Only:

Code No.

Diagnosis *Strain of Rt. Knee*

Disability: ⟨Yes⟩ No

On entering the Department of Health, the athlete fills out the above form.

When a student reports to the Department of Health, he fills out a slip for the service which he needs. In case of an athletic injury he checks off "Athletic Surgeon." Upon being directed to the surgeon he presents the case history, which is then recorded on a blue card kept in his file. The card describes the injury, the doctor's diagnosis, and the treatment. If X-ray is indicated, the athlete is given a form filled out by the surgeon, and is sent to the X-ray room.

If physiotherapy is ordered, the physician fills out the form and sends the athlete to the Physical Therapy Department. All treatments are then listed on his card and are also on file in his folder. The athlete is checked every day by the team physician and progress is noted on his card.

In case of a minor injury the athlete may not be placed on a disability list. There are two types of disability; one is a full disability, which places the athlete out of action until released; the second disability is known as a competitive disability, which permits the athlete to participate partially in his drills and practices but forbids his full competition until release by athletic surgeon is made.

In the case of an illness, the athlete is directed to the medical doctor assigned to the athletes. A record of his complaint, the doctor's diagnosis, and treatment is recorded on a white card that is kept as part of his permanent health record while at Yale.

Disabilities for illnesses are essentially the same as for injuries—full disability or competitive disability. The athlete cannot return to full duty until released by the medical doctor. As with injuries, the athlete who is ill is checked daily until his return to full activity.

Should the athlete require care of a nature that he cannot perform for himself, he is admitted to the infirmary on the campus. The

DEPARTMENT OF UNIVERSITY HEALTH

Physical Therapy and Rehabilitation

Name:.. DOE, JOHN J.... ..Class:.. '61 ....Dept.:.........Date:.. 9/8/..

Diagnosis:.. *Strain of Med. Coll. Lig. Rt. Knee* ....

℞ Treatment desired must be specified and requisition signed by a doctor.
"Personal Charge" must be signed by the patient.

☒ Baking	☐ Sedative Massage	☐ Conditioning Exercises
☐ Infra-red Heat	☐ Stimulating Massage	☐ Corrective Exercises
☐ Short-wave Diathermy	☐ Steam Bath	☐ Postural Exercises
☐ Whirlpool Bath	☐ Adhesive Strapping	☐ Active—Exercises—Passive
☐ Ultra-violet Light	☐ Bandage—2″—3″	☐ Relaxed Motion
☐ Hot—Fomentation—Cold	☒ Splints—Felt—Wood—Metal	☐ Muscle Training
☐ Paraffin Dip	☐ Sling	☐ Bicycle—Pulley—Rowing
☐ Scotch Douche	☒ Crutches—Cane	☐ Passive Stretching
☐ Analgesic Pack	☐ Progressive Resistance	☐ Head Traction

Charge:
   ☐ Personal: Non-athletic or Intercollege   ☒ Accident
   ☐ Personal: Non-athletic or Intercollege (self-supporting: B. of A. partial remission)
   ☐ Department
       (Phys. Th. $1.00 a visit)   Sign...........................M.D.
       (Ultra-violet $1.00 a visit)

Patient's Signature...

D.U.H. No. 34

The request for physical therapy is filled out by the athletic surgeon and sent to Physical Therapy Department.

Name	Doe, John J.		Class	'61	
Date	PHYSICAL THERAPY		Date	PHYSICAL THERAPY	
9/8	Treated with Baking + Felt Splints applied.				
9/9	Treated				
9/10	Treated				

Report of Physical Therapy Department.

NAME	Jones, Fred Thomas	CLASS	'60	
Date	MEDICAL NOTES		Diagnosis	Treatment
10/17	Student complains of sore throat, running nose and slight coughing. To return tomorrow. T 99²		ARD	Medication Rest Disability for 2 days

Medical report.

doctor who admitted the athlete checks his daily progress. In case of illness, the medical doctor treats the athlete; and in an injury, the athletic surgeon is responsible.

Orthopedic as well as other services are available. If the physician in charge feels the necessity of this service, he sets up an appointment for the athlete. Specialists are available at the Department of Health on an appointment basis.

Chapter 3

Diet in Athletics

NUTRITION

Nutrition is the science of nourishing the body properly. There are as many theories on nutrition as there are days in the year. When we get to the bottom of the theories, we come up with one factor, and that is food. All are agreed that we need food. The question is, how much and what kind?

Food consists of substances that give energy, build tissues, and regulate body functions. Food is broken down into three groups: fats, proteins, and carbohydrates.

Fats are found in butter, salad oils, and meat fats. Fat is made up of carbon, hydrogen, and oxygen. Fats are used in the body for the production of energy, heat, and for lubricating purposes. Excessive consumption of fats will result in adipose tissue.

Proteins contain carbon, hydrogen, and oxygen but in different proportions than fats. In addition, proteins contain elements of nitrogen and sulphur. Proteins are needed to build and repair our bodies. Proteins are found in eggs, meat, fish, cheese, legumes, nuts, and various grains.

Carbohydrates are divided into sugars and starches. The general belief is that we have only one kind of sugar, the granulated sugar that we find on our tables. However, five sugars are found in our foods. Granulated sugar comes from the sap of the sugar cane. Some of the sugar on the market comes from the juices of the sugar beet. This is called *sucrose*. Glucose and fructose are commonly found (usually together) in the sap of various plants and in the juices of many of our fruits. Two other sugars are found in our foods; one is lactose, which is found in milk, and the other is maltose, which is also found in milk.

The proper proportion of the three foodstuffs in an athlete's diet should be:

Carbohydrates	50%
Fats	40%
Proteins	10%

Energy needs of the average person at rest is about 1,600 calories per day. The athlete's intake should be variable; the more activity of the larger muscles of the body, the more the intake should be. In an athlete who is inclined to use the smaller muscles, the less intake is needed. The football player or lacrosse player will probably need about 4,500 to 5,000 calories a day during the season. If this diet is continued in the "off" season, an obese athlete is the result. Therefore the diet should be regulated to the amount of work to be done at the time.

There is no magic formula for the increased performance of an athlete through nutrition. Nutrition is a long-term process, and effects of individual foods may not be evident at the time of ingestion. A diet that is full of calories is not essentially a good diet; there may be the proper number of calories but not the proper proportion of the nutrients. Proteins and carbohydrates yield about 4 calories per gram, whereas fat yields about 9 calories per gram. For proper nutrition the diet must:

1. Include a supply of energy-yielding nutrients.
2. Help counteract fatigue.
3. Maintain the athlete at proper weight for maximum performance.
4. Furnish essentials for growth, development, and function.

This program cannot be a one-shot deal. To eat super foods only on the day of a game and not during the progressive training period during the preceding week will not make for satisfactory nutritional habits. The athlete must be supplied with a well-rounded diet containing proper nutrients that have a variety and are attractively served. Serving a well-planned meal is only the first step; the next step is to see that the athlete consumes all that is necessary for full energy.

You must eat a balanced diet if you are to get all the vitamins and minerals that your body needs. If you eat a balanced diet, it will not be necessary to take vitamin pills or mineral pills unless they are specifically prescribed.

The best way to get a balanced diet is to eat a variety of foods. The combination of foods will enhance the value of the foods that are placed before you. For example, grain cereals may be lacking in proteins even though they are high in vitamins and minerals, but when they are consumed with milk added, you will get the essential proteins. The ingredients of a balanced diet include:

Proteins	Fats	Vitamins
Carbohydrates	Salts	Water

We have mentioned before the three big items (proteins, fats, and carbohydrates), but we have not mentioned water, salts and vitamins. Salts are very necessary for the production of bone and for the growth of the body. The main sources of salts are milk, cheese, and green vegetables.

Water is a food. Most people do not consider it as such but it is a necessity of life. You can live on water alone for weeks, but you can live for only a few days on solids alone. Water is a source of important minerals such as calcium. Water is necessary to dissolve foods so that they in turn may be changed into tissue. Water is necessary as a regulator for heat; it acts by cooling off our bodies when we get too hot, as evidenced by the perspiration on warm days.

Vitamins are necessary for proper nutrition, but just how they act is still a mystery. Some scientists have supposed that they act as a catalyst in physiological reactions. It is known, however, that if we eat a variety of food, we are practically assured that all the required kinds and quantities of vitamins will be present. Vitamins are present in all natural foods such as fruits, vegetables, grains, and animal and plant fats.

CALORIES

A food calorie is the amount of heat required to raise the temperature of 1 kilogram of water 1 degree centigrade. One kilogram of water is equivalent to 2 pounds or 1 quart, and 1 degree increase in centigrade is from 15 to 16 degrees centigrade. A calorie, then, is the unit for measurement of energy. An athlete who is going to perform in a certain sport will require certain amounts of calories to perform satisfactorily in that area. Scientists have developed a method of measuring the caloric needs of athletes in various sports. The amount of work to be done, plus the time needed, and the amount of energy to be expended are taken into consideration, and the calorie needs can then be established. There are many factors, such as emotions, the amount of energy lost through incomplete digestion and absorption, and the incomplete oxidation of proteins in the tissues, which may make a variance in the caloric intake. However, the average is such that there is an equalization by normal body processes.

Calorie Requirements. A very simple way to tell the amount of calories needed per day is watch your weight. If there is a weight loss, this is an indication that the caloric intake is not sufficient to meet the demands of the body. On the other hand, an increase in weight, persistently even though slowly, is an indication that the fuel value of the food intake is greater than the energy needs of the body. When the weight remains constant, the energy intake just about balances the outgo, the body neither gains nor loses in weight. Variations of a pound or two from day to day may be considered normal because the water content of the body will account for this variance. It is impossible for a person to put on weight unless there is a surplus of energy supplied in the food. Regardless of the type of food, if weight persistently increases, the fuel value is greater than the body needs. Therefore the first law to observe in losing weight is to cut down on the food intake, especially in foods of high caloric value. If you are losing weight unduly, or if underweight, increase the total amount of food, being sure to include the foods that are rich in fuel value.

REGULARITY OF MEALS

The regularity of meals is most important; the digestive system works best when it performs at regular intervals, and to disrupt it may cause a derangement of the digestive system. Breakfast should be on schedule and should consist of a very hearty meal. The need for a good breakfast is apparent because the body uses nutrients for the tasks of the morning. Lunch is also important, as this is the meal that is eaten immediately before the practice session. Lunch should be consumed early enough so that the stomach is empty before strenuous exercises are performed. The evening meal is after practice and should be planned so that it does not come too close to the end of practice. A sufficient amount of time should elapse so that the athlete has "calmed down" from the work-out and proper digestion can take place. Eating too soon after a hard work-out or game may lead to indigestion and a very uncomfortable athlete.

Missing meals in order to reduce is not good nutrition. As mentioned earlier, the digestive system works best when it is regulated. Digestion and nutrition are best served if a light meal is eaten rather than eliminating the meal completely.

Eating between meals taxes the digestive system.

The training meal table at Yale is supervised by the Department of Health, and the meals are carefully planned by dieticians under the supervision of the nutritionists of the medical school. There are no "fads." The diet is essentially "solid" foods and is varied to be more palatable. The meals are planned for maximum energy requirements, not necessarily meal for meal but from day to day.

Therefore it is necessary to eat all the meals and all the foods that are served. The dining area is well located, and the atmosphere is conducive to "good fellowship" and very pleasant and relaxing meals. The recent addition of a Hi Fi set has been a wonderful means of relaxing the athlete so that full enjoyment of the meals is at its maximum.

Quantities of food to be served to an athlete cannot be set; the more active and larger athlete may require more food than the less active athlete. Common sense prevails in the serving of the meals. The steward is in attendance and is constantly observing the appetites of the athletes. His findings are reported to the trainer, who will make suggestions as to necessary changes. If an athlete is genuinely hungry, he may have more food, but he will have to finish all that he has on his plate, and then he will have to eat the vegetables as well as the meat in his second serving. The athlete who will eat this second portion is genuinely hungry, whereas the athlete who would like to have a little more meat is not genuinely hungry.

Foods are prepared very simply and are served in very pleasant surroundings; fads and fancies are not a part of the menu. Care is taken that no fried foods, pork, condiments, mushy foods, heavy gravies, or under- or overripe fruits are served. Iced drinks are not served with the meals; when they are on the menu, the tea or juice is chilled in large vats and served out of pitchers. No ice is allowed in the drinks at any time. Milk is kept refrigerated but not to an extreme. On the other hand, hot foods are controlled so that they are not served hot enough to burn the athlete. Extremely hot foods will irritate the mucosa of the stomach and will not be enjoyable. All meals are served on plates, and all plates are equal in size and amount of food. Therefore every meal is a production by the members of the kitchen staff. The serving of sandwiches, hamburgers, etc., is not a part of the menu for the athlete.

Along with the servings, the table will have honey, melba toast, and rolls, which may be eaten and enjoyed with the meal. In some instances honey is alternated with various flavors of jelly or jam to be used as a spread on the rolls.

FOOD FADS

It is impossible to evaulate the effect of a food supplement in relation to the athlete's performance. Quite often we read of an athlete who has performed above normal. He relates that he did so because of the intake of some "miracle food" previous to the contest. There are many factors involved in the good performance—psychological factors of motivation, the type of work performed, and the progressive training that has taken place on the practice field. Progressive training is designed for the athlete to better himself as he goes along, and therefore to test efficiently the value of a specific food is almost impossible.

Racial and religious backgrounds plus environment contribute to the individual's requirements for nutrition. Various athletes have food idiosyncracies that also must be considered. With this in mind there cannot be a specific diet that is applicable to all athletes in all sports.

There is no magic formula that can be taken the day of a game or practice session to enhance performance. Various fads and fancies have been in evidence since the beginning of time. They will continue to flourish until more scientific data are available. Who is to say that these fads do not work? We have only our good judgment and proper sense of proportions to guide us in our planning of adequate training diets for athletics. Advances have been made and will continue to be made with the increase of interest by members of the professional organizations. The use of "pep pills" has been investigated and the results have been published. Vitamin supplements are now under study by many nutritionists and a conclusion will be available at a later date.

Vitamins are being used and the nutritionists have maintained that the value is only psychological where the athlete has an adequate diet.

It has been stated that it is practically impossible for a normal healthy person living under ordinary circumstances to avoid the inclusion of adequate vitamins in his daily food intake. The need for vitamins should be established by proper medical authorities after specific examinations have been made. Prominent authorities have stated that there is no evidence that muscular activity increases with the taking of supplementary vitamins.

Feeding large amounts of sugar to an athlete has also been a practice in some areas, basically advocated for quick energy. This may backfire, as there is a possibility of an athlete being hypersensitive to sugars; sugars will promote the production of insulin in the body. When this happens, the blood sugar falls below normal. This results in a hypoglycemia; the symptoms are headache, nervousness, anxiety, irritability, an insatiable desire for sweets, and finally tension. All these factors are contraindicated for good athletic performance because they will have a direct influence on coordination and endurance.

Vegetarianism is a form of diet that comes to the front every now and then, especially when an athlete performs in record time or makes some other outstanding performance. A true vegetarian is one who eats the so-called plant foods only; to use milk, eggs, etc., does not fully comply with the true vegetarian's thoughts of the vegetarian's regime. Those athletes who subscribe to the latter (including the vegetables, etc.) are not true vegetarians but are abstainers from meats. Those who have success with this diet are high in its praise; those who read about it are very critical of its value. Who is right?

The fact that certain foods when eaten together will cause gas, heartburn, and other discomforts has been advanced for the purposes of special diets for athletes. The literature today tends to label this an erroneous conclusion, a result of psychic influences rather than the foods themselves. Athletes would be able to eat these foods except for the power of suggestion.

The eating of certain foods to purify the blood and to ward off bacteria and the alkalizing of the body to combat disease is also a plan adopted by some athletes. Normally the blood does not carry toxic substances, as these are removed very efficiently by the kidneys. That there are foods for promoting immunity to bacteria is also a false claim. Adequate diets of vitamins and minerals will aid in preventing infection but cannot promote immunity to disease. Alkalinizing is also exaggerated; again a substantial diet is the best aid to health. That meats will make athletes fierce and mean is a thought that is a part of a well-known athlete; so much so that he believes raw meat to be the answer to great athletic ability. There is little if any evidence that proves that meat, eaten raw or cooked, will affect the disposition of an athlete.

TRAINING TABLE MENUS

The training table menu at Yale (which is varied through a two-week period) is shown. The dormitory system at Yale makes it unnecessary to serve breakfast at the training table, except for the first two weeks of practice in the fall when school is not open. Breakfasts consist of the standard foods and are served at hours convenient for the students to get to class on time. The training table starts with the noon meal on Monday and goes through the week, closing on Saturday after the game. Sunday meals are served at the college dining rooms. The noon meal is the meal preceding the afternoon practice. The meal is served from noon until 1:30 P.M. Practice is held at 4:30 P.M. in the afternoon, so that plenty of time

YALE A.A. TRAINING TABLE

LUNCH	DINNER

Monday

Orange Juice	Cream of Chicken Soup
Chopped Sirloin Steak	Yankee Pot Roast
Buttered Carrots—Parsley Potato	Mashed Potato—Green Beans
Hearts of Lettuce—Russian Dressing	Tossed Salad
Melba Toast	Rolls and Butter
Dessert—Tea	Dessert—Milk

Tuesday

Orange Juice	Cream of Spinach Soup—Croutons
Swiss Steak	Roast Prime Ribs of Beef
Green Peas—Au Gratin Potato	Mashed Potatoes—Corn and Lima Beans
Lettuce and Tomato Salad—Mayonnaise	Pancakes
Melba Toast	Romaine, Chicory Salad—French Dressing
Dessert—Tea	Rolls and Butter
	Dessert—Milk

Wednesday

Orange Juice	Consomme Alphabet
Baked Meat Loaf	Broiled Chicken
Rissole Potatoes—Vichy Carrots	Whipped Potato—Buttered Lima Beans
Lettuce and Tomato	Tossed Green Salad
Melba Toast	Rolls and Butter
Dessert—Tea	Dessert—Milk

Thursday

Orange Juice	Puree of Lentil Soup
London Broil	Roast Leg of Lamb
Boiled Potato—Peas	Delmonico Potatoes—Green Beans
Shredded Lettuce	Chefs' Salad
Melba Toast	Rolls and Butter
Dessert—Tea	Dessert—Milk

Friday

Orange Juice	Beef Bouillon with Rice
Broiled Swordfish	Roast Prime Ribs
Mashed Potatoes—Vichy Carrots	Baked Potato—Spinach
Lettuce and Tomato Salad—French Dressing	Hearts of Lettuce—French Dressing
Melba Toast	Rolls and Butter
Dessert—Tea	Fruit Jello—Milk

Saturday

Sirloin Steak	Consomme Garni
Baked Potato—Spinach	Roast Young Tom Turkey
Melba Toast	Mashed Potatoes—Green Peas
Fruit Compote—Tea	Tossed Green Salad
	Rolls and Butter
	Ice Cream—Milk

YALE A.A. TRAINING TABLE

LUNCH	DINNER

Monday

Orange Juice	Puree of Green Split Peas
Chopped Sirloin Steak	Braised Swiss Steak—Jardiniere
Mashed Potatoes—Peas	Buttered Macaroni
Hearts of Lettuce—Mayonnaise	Lettuce and Tomato Salad—Mayonnaise
Melba Toast	Rolls and Butter
Dessert—Tea	Dessert—Milk

Tuesday

Orange Juice	Chicken Broth with Rice
Pan Broiled Calves Liver	Roast Young Tom Turkey
Boiled Potato—Lima Beans	Sweet Potato—Green Peas
Shredded Lettuce—French Dressing	Tossed Green Salad
Melba Toast	Rolls and Butter
Dessert—Tea	Dessert—Milk

Wednesday

Orange Juice	Puree of Lima Bean Soup
Ragout of Beef—Buttered Egg Noodles	Roast Top Round of Beef
Green Beans	Rissole Potatoes—Spinach
Lettuce and Tomato Salad—Mayonnaise	Lettuce and Tomato Salad
Melba Toast	Rolls and Butter
Dessert—Tea	Dessert—Milk

Thursday

Orange Juice	Consomme Julienne
Chicken Fricassee and Rice	Roast Leg of Lamb
Green Peas	Whipped Potato—Green Beans
Hearts of Lettuce—French Dressing	Chefs' Salad—French Dressing
Melba Toast	Rolls and Butter
Dessert—Tea	Dessert—Milk

Friday

Orange Juice	Consomme
Roast Meat Loaf—Bordelaise Sauce	Sirloin Steak
Whipped Potatoes—Buttered Lima Beans	Baked Potato—Spinach
Chefs' Salad—French Dressing	Shredded Lettuce
Melba Toast	Rolls and Butter
Dessert—Tea	Fruit Jello—Milk

Saturday

See Pregame Meal	Consomme Vermicelli
	Broiled Chicken
	Mashed Potatoes—Green Peas
	Heart of Lettuce—Mayonnaise
	Rolls and Butter
	Ice Cream—Milk

Lunch desserts are usually jello with fruit or puddings. Evening desserts are cake, ice cream, or puddings.

is allowed for proper emptying of the stomach before exercise period is started.

Orange juice is included in all the lunch menus, as is tea. Athletes have shown a preference for cold tea at lunch, so this is on the daily menus.

Pregame Meal. The pregame meal for football is set from 8:30 A.M. until 10:00 A.M. Due to Saturday classes, etc., it is practical to have "one setting," and therefore the athlete may report to the training table when his classes will permit. Buses are necessary to transport the athletes to the field; the first one is scheduled to leave at 11:30 A.M. on game day; the second, at noon. Prior to boarding the bus, the athlete is served a cup of bouillon and melba toast if he desires this; some will feel hungry after eating early that morning; others will feel satisfied and will decline the bouillon.

PREGAME MEAL MENU

Cup of bouillon.
Steak (approximately 10 ounces), cooked medium rare.
Baked potato, one pat of butter.
String beans.
Toast with honey.
Hot tea with lemon and as much sugar as needed to taste.

WEIGHT CONTROL

Gaining Weight. The most effective method of gaining weight is to increase the amount of fat and high-caloric carbohydrate foods in the diet. The increase in the number of meals per day is also an important factor. The use of foods with excessive fats may decrease the appetite, as fats are harder to digest. This type of food should not be included in all meals. An increase in the amount of sleep is very effective; also, afternoon naps are helpful. Relaxation and serenity are important in the weight-gaining program.

Reduction of Weight. Findings in recent studies reveal that the reduction of weight can be accomplished by exercise. Findings also indicate that an increase in strength of muscle groups is considerably enhanced by this form of program.

Combining an exercise program with proper diets over a period of time will result in weight reduction.

To evaluate properly the results of this type of program, body measurements should be taken. Quite often the increased circulation and added muscle weight may not indicate the amount of fat that has been lost. Athletes who have participated in this type of program have often felt that they had lost more weight than the scales showed, using as a guide the fact that their clothes no longer fit them.

The main cause of overweight in normal healthy athletes is their desire for and consumption of too much food or too much food of the wrong kind. To tell an athlete that he must lose weight and then not spell out in detail how to do it is folly. Diets are printed daily in the newspapers and are classified as "crash" diets or called by other special names. How effective a diet is depends on the will power of the individual. Proper physical examination and advice from the doctor must be obtained before any attempt at a drastic diet plan is started. One of the more common and very successful diets is the "Mayo diet."

SMOKING

In a recent bulletin put out by the American Medical Association, called *Tips on Athletic Training*, smoking is the prime topic. It has this to say:

Tobacco smoke is irritating to the mucose membranes of the nose, throat, and other respiratory passages. Smoking is known to constrict the small blood vessels and to increase the heart rate. There is little doubt that smoking can influence athletic performance, particularly in stress situations. Some persons appear to be more resistant to the effects of tobacco than others. Even assuming the effects on a particular athlete to be slight, the difference between winning and losing may often be just as slight.

WATER DRINKING ON FIELD

Many theories are presented for and against the use of water on the field during practice sessions. The example of the laborer is given—when he is thirsty, he drinks. The theories of drinking and not drinking have been used without much evidence to prove either to be correct. Athletes have been allowed to drink water during practices; others have had water withheld; the results of both practices have been exactly the same. When water was allowed, the athletes had no desire for it; when it was eliminated, they felt that they should have it. At one time the athlete was allowed to drink when he wanted to; at other times there was a "break" in the water-drinking routine. After the first few days of practice in the early fall, athletes do not seem to have the desire for water; thereafter the water "breaks" are not generally utilized. One approach is to use water on the field only to rinse the mouth, but a drink is available in the locker room after practice for those who want it. When the weather is warm, a cold, soft drink is very palatable and refreshing. In the colder weather hot bouillon is served as soon as the athletes are off the field. With this practice, the need for excessive water intake has been eliminated after each practice session, which is preferable because water fills the stomach so that players do not have an appetite for the meal served at the training table. Serving the drink after practice obviates the necessity for filling up with water in the shower. Then the athlete arrives at the training table with a full appetite.

Chapter 4

Physical Conditioning

There are as many conditioning programs as there are coaches and trainers. We know that sports basically require physical strength, endurance, and skills. The better the condition of the athlete, the longer he participates; the poorer the condition of the athlete, the quicker he "retires." Those with good physical condition are the athletes who are part of our teams of today; the group lacking of condition falls by the wayside, and these do not participate for more than a short time in athletics.

Physical condition and an adequate warm-up will prevent many an injury. Adequate strength and flexibility will help the athlete avoid injury by being able to "get out of the way" of a collision or by allowing him to get into a position to roll with the impact. Lack of good conditioning will result in the athlete's overtaxing his muscles, which in turn produces the strains and sprains that trainers must treat. By forcing a muscle or ligament to go beyond its normal limitations in either strength or endurance, an injury of variable magnitudes results. The degree of injury will be established by the way in which the injury occurred and the physical condition of the athlete. Athletes who are in good physical condition are seldom injured.

Exercises of low resistance with many repetitions will increase endurance rather than strength. The more resistance, the more strength. For the best results, the muscles should be worked short of fatigue; to force the muscles to go beyond this point will result in soreness and a decrease in strength. Muscles should be worked in "full range" of motion. To do exercises that do not include the full range of motion means that the work load is too much; then it should be lessened to allow for full capacity. In fatigue the muscles stiffen up and there is a considerable loss of reaction time that may lead to an injury. Conditioning programs are designed to work an athlete along steady levels. This results in better physical conditioning, skills, and pacing.

The physical conditioning results from the organs of the body being able to hold their efficiency at higher levels of activity. Skills are developed because the athlete learns to perform the act with a better economy of muscular effort. He is also able to develop a rapid rate of movement. Motor skills are carried out by reflex action so that many times the athlete will not be consciously aware of what he is doing.

Pacing is hard to develop. The athlete must find the level of his maximum rate and maintain it over a long period of time. With work on the conditioning level, his endurance time increases. An inexperienced athlete will fall by the wayside early because he has not learned to adjust the ability of his body to the demands of the exercises or drills he is performing.

STRENGTH

The dictionary defines strength as the quality or state of being strong; bodily or muscular power, whether for exertion or for endurance. The size of the muscle, the number of fibers that are working on command, the ability of groups to work together, general condition of the muscles, and the structure of bones and muscles in relation to leverage are factors involved in strength of muscles. The size of muscles will grow with exercise, but the number of fibers will remain the same. Each fiber must become larger; therefore the muscle becomes larger. The tendon or tendons of the muscle also become stronger. Size of muscle will include the fat that surrounds the muscle. Fat will interfere with all actions of the muscles and will definitely impair strength, speed, skill, and endurance. A muscle will increase in size if it is required to exert force against resistance. The best principle is the overload theory, by which the muscle is asked to perform progressive exertions. Lack of use results in atrophy, which means a decreasing in size of the muscles.

The number of fibers that respond is dependent on the impulse as the result of a nerve stimulus. A fast motion is the result of a short burst of impulses, whereas a slower motion is the result of a more prolonged impulse at a lower frequency. In the latter, of course, fewer motor neurons are called into action. Needless to say, the former cannot be continued so long as the slower action without fatigue setting in very rapidly. This is in proportion to the condition of the muscles involved.

The condition of muscles is determined by the athlete's ability to postpone fatigue. This is also gauged by the temperature of the muscles, the available sources of energy (foodstuffs, etc.), the condition of the muscles at the time, and the ability to recover from activity. Muscles function at their best when the temperature is

slightly higher than normal body temperature because the viscosity
of the muscle is lowered, the circulation is increased, and the chemical reactions in contraction and recovery are expedited. This is
very evident on cold days when the viscosity of muscle is very high,
thus making the muscles stiff and sluggish. The elements of the
chemical structures are essential for muscle action; when these are
used up, the amount of muscle function is diminished. Muscle
strength is increased by exercise, which not only increases the size
of the muscle but also the ability of the muscle to react quickly and
easily. The exercises will also increase the circulation, which improves the feeding of the muscles and also the drainage of waste
products as a result of using the chemicals needed for functioning.
The ability of muscles to recover from activity is dependent on the
proper nutrition and proper drainage. If this is not adequate, the
muscles lose their ability to perform properly; hence they will lose
their energy and fatigue will set in. The well-trained muscle will
have less waste deposits to remove; they are readily removed by
the increased circulation.

To increase strength, the athlete must work with increasing loads,
starting with light work and gradually building up to heavier drills.
In order to become proficient, the athlete must work on a daily basis
and with increased loads that improve physical conditioning and
also maintain a high state of training. The rate of improvement is
in proportion to the work done; layoffs will result in a decrease in
size of the fibers and a fatty infiltration of the muscle tissues. Long
layoffs should be avoided if possible. However, if necessary, the
athlete will have to start his training from the beginning rather
than from where he left off. If on return to activity he forces the
training, exhaustion will occur, which will result in loss of efficiency
in the work that has already been accomplished. Properly planned
work-outs for this type of athlete are important, as are adequate rest
periods for recovery. Daily training rather than intermittent programs is the best for maintaining a high degree of physical conditioning. The more graduated the routine, the better the body will
respond to increased loads and demands.

ENDURANCE

Some of the terms associated with endurance are the following:
the act or power of enduring anything, a lasting quality, to sustain
without impairment, not yielding to hardships, to hold out, to
harden and resist without giving in. In athletics the ability to
endure continued contractions of muscles over a long period of

time is essential. Muscles must be supplied with food and oxygen to carry on this type of activity. In training, it is necessary that the fuel be made available, the food be stored in greater amount, and the oxygen be more abundant. This requires the athlete to have a greater respiratory and circulatory capacity so that oxygen can be supplied when needed and waste products of the process of metabolism can be removed. Training increases the strength of the muscles and also the heart so that the body will be more efficient. As the athlete's endurance increases, he finds that the work from day to day becomes easier. In the beginning, he found himself enduring pain and discomfort and at intervals gasping for air. As the body adjusted by compensating through developing larger vital capacity and increased blood supply, these conditions were lessened.

Large muscles do not necessarily indicate capability. Quite often large muscles act as a handicap instead of a help. Large muscles are very effective in the work they are trained to do, primarily strength situations. For athletic purposes, the large muscle is not necessarily a muscle that demonstrates endurance. The primary element in endurance is the increased capillarization, which is increased by physiological usage. In training for athletics, the hypertrophy, or enlargement, of muscles and increased capillarization occur simultaneously if proper exercises are performed. It is possible that either one or the other may result if the impulses act separately. Large muscles develop if much resistance is applied, whereas endurance develops if sustained bouts are performed with light loads. The increase in endurance is a result of the adequate use of the muscles of the body. Training contributes to the capability for reorganizing the central nervous system, which in turn controls the motor control part of the central nervous system.

Endurance is developed by work, work, and more work with increased loads. This is very easily said, but how is it done? There is no short cut to endurance, although many theories have been advanced as to how this can be accomplished easily. If we would spend the time working that we expend on trying to avoid work and to figure out short cuts, our athletes would be in a better frame of mind to accept the work-outs that have been planned for them. A few methods that are not "new" and that have been used very satisfactorily over the years will be listed.

An athlete will take the path of least resistance unless specific standards are set up for him. Many are happy to perform the chores of the day in a very efficient manner, utilizing an efficient speed which becomes more efficient with work. However, the demands of a grueling contest or event may find the athlete lacking in endurance because he has not taxed himself during his daily work. With this idea in mind, the athlete must run or perform every act at full speed. In practice, every assignment is carried out at "full speed," stressing the fact that "it is not how fast you run but how hard you try that counts." Today, when time is of the essence, much work must be done in a short period, so every drill must be performed at full effort for proper results.

Practice makes perfect, is an old adage, but if the practice is not full speed, a very inefficient athlete is the result.

SKILLS

Skill in athletics is the ability to accomplish a large amount of work with a small amount of effort. Skill can be acquired by persistent application that results in a refinement of coordination. The ability of an athlete to make his job look easy is skill. An athlete lacks skill when his movements are awkward and he seems to expend great effort in accomplishing the work. There are those who will never succeed in acquiring great skill; they are limited by the following factors:

1. Body weight: They are too large or to small, or subject to obesity.
2. Body height: Too short or too tall.
3. Timing: Lack of coordination of the contractions of muscle fibers.
4. Accuracy of movement: The inability to coordinate all parts of the body to work at once. The eye sees before a group of muscles functions. Balance is catalogued in this category; if the athlete is constantly off balance, his skills will be crude and awkward.

If the athlete is overweight, there is a possibility that by correcting this condition, the continuance of practice may result in some skills. However, there are some sports that a "big" man will not be able to do. He should content himself with the many other sports that are available in the curriculum.

A tall athlete has his problems; his center of gravity is such that when motion is necessary, too much muscle activity is needed to perform the task, and therefore he will be a little slow and a bit behind in his responses. On the other hand, the short individual will have problems; he may not be able to outjump a taller man, but he usually has the advantage of being more skillful than the larger, and he will be able to adapt himself faster than the taller athlete. To increase skill, fine coordination must be developed. In some athletes this coordination is not developed because of the slowness of a group of muscles to act in unison. One group may contract or relax before the other, thus throwing the timing off. This is primarily a deficiency of the central nervous system and may never be overcome in some athletes.

The ability to coordinate sight with action is a skill that is very difficult to develop. The ability of the eye and the muscles to work simultaneously involves interrelation of the inner ear, the sense of balance, and the proper position. This skill improves with practice, providing practice is designed to coordinate the eye with action. Developing peripheral vision is a part of this type of program. The athlete may be able to see the ball but not the man; through training, he may be better able to see the man, the ball, and the field.

WEIGHT TRAINING

Weight training consists of performing exercises with weights at a fast rate. They are designed to improve strength, fitness, speed, and endurance. Exercises for the specific sport that the athlete will play should be similar to and directly related to the event. A series of exercises (usually six to eight) is designed for the athlete, and he goes through them in a rapid manner, returning to the starting position after each attempt. As ability increases, the number of repetitions is also increased, but the weight remains the same. Along with the increase in repetitions, the speed of the exercise is also increased, and the rest time between each exercise is shortened.

Weight training has not been established as an integral part of the program for all athletes at Yale. However, a weight training program has been used with some success on specific individuals. The program was instituted to "build up" and "put weight" on a few smaller athletes. The program consisted of a three-times-a-week schedule, using a heavy weight with few repetitions for strength and a lighter weight with many repetitions for endurance. The athlete also participated in handball, basketball, and squash, either immediately after the work-out or on the "off" days. These games were instituted to lessen the drudgery that may be associated with exercise programs during the "off" season. The response by most students was excellent—they put on weight and became larger and stronger.

INTERVAL TRAINING

Interval training is new and a very important part of the training program for the conditioning of athletes. It has led to great improvement in the middle-distance runners during the past ten years. Interval training consists of running a specified distance in a specified time and then resting a specified time after each run. An example of interval training is to run 220 yards in 30 seconds, rest about 2 to 3 minutes, and then repeat again. The rest period usually consists of jogging during the interval period. The number of repetitions may vary from a few to many. One of the features of this type of program is the terrific demand placed on the body. The result of this type of work-out leaves the athlete with difficult or labored breathing at frequent intervals. The athlete, as he progresses, learns to put up with this breathlessness and is able to tolerate this condition as an aid to generally good conditioning.

CIRCUIT TRAINING

This is a form of interval training that is gaining in popularity in this country after many years of great success in England. Circuit training consists of a series of about ten different types of exercises at various stations. The exercises may include a rope climb, ladder walking, and so on. The circuit is performed as fast as possible. When the athlete has mastered the circuit, he is then increased to two or three or more rounds of the circuit. All these rounds are against time. A very low target time is set for the athlete, and he strives to do all the exercises and the number of circuits in this time. When this is accomplished, the degree of fitness desired has been attained.

FARTLEK

Fartlek is a Swedish word meaning speed play and is a method of training that originated with Swedish athletes. This is a type of work-out designed to produce endurance, vitality, and the psychological benefits that result from the athlete never being forced. The work-out can be varied from day to day. Fartlek comes closest to cross-country running because of the need for wide-open spaces and the demand for much oxygen, running in the woods in a relaxed, back-to-nature attitude. This has a very stimulating effect on the athlete and his training.

Fartlek means playing with speed; however, a very common interpretation today is demonstrated in jogging bouts without the speed play. Due to lack of a watch and perpetual supervision, some athletes feel that this type of work-out is a play toy and therefore they will not work at the task ahead. A typical Fartlek work-out provides for a series of exercises like the following:

Jog for about 10 to 15 minutes on an open field. Do general calisthenics and stretching exercises. Jog another 10 minutes at a fairly fast 8-minute-mile clip for about a mile to a mile and a quarter; then walk from 3 to 5 minutes.

Run about 5 minutes full speed. Walk 3 to 5 minutes. Run another 8 minutes; this time take about 5 to 7 50- or 100-yard sprints.

Walk another 3 to 5 minutes. Run a fast 660, full speed all the way. Walk another 3 to 5 minutes.

Jog 10 minutes, as in the beginning, but take ten 5- to 10-yard sprints as fast as possible. Finish with a relaxing 10-minute jog.

The work-out can be varied to include 220's, 440's, and so on, on the running track.

GRASS DRILLS

The coordination and agility exercises of grass drills involve a series of fast moves that will increase reactions and speed of movement in the athlete. All commands are to be executed as fast as possible.

With the athlete standing, the first command is:

Run: (running in place with knees high); then the command,
On your stomach: (the athlete falls on stomach facing coach).
On your back: (roll over as fast as possible with head away from coach).
Stand: (jump to feet and continue running in place).
Forward roll: (full forward somersault, finishing on back).
On your stomach: (roll over on stomach with head to coach).
Stand: (running in place).
On your stomach: (athlete falls on stomach).

These commands are variable, depending on the location of the athlete on the preceding command. By going through the drills slowly until all commands are learned, the speed will depend on the ability of the group to respond to commands.

This is an excellent drill for all athletes and may be used in all sports where there is action of the body in variable positions (football, basketball, soccer, etc.)

PHYSIOLOGY AND CONDITIONING

Oxygen Debt. When the body is forced to use up the normal amount of oxygen in the tissues, particularly during strenuous exercises, the result is an "oxygen debt." In short work-outs, the incidence to this state is not very likely to occur; also, in mild exercises, this condition is eliminated. The symptoms are cyanosis (bluish color) due to the lack of oxygen in the blood, coldness, and "out of breath." The rapid breathing that results is a reflex action due to the tension of carbon dioxide in the blood and also to the lactic acid and carbon dioxide in the blood, which changes the chemical balance. Much of the lactic acid is taken up by the liver and heart, and some of it passes from the system through perspiration and other means of elimination. While it is present, it accounts for some of the uncomfortable feeling of fatigue. In mild cases of "oxygen debt," the recovery period is enhanced by light exercise; after the completion of a hard race, it is better for the athlete to keep moving than it is to rest. In the severe case, the athlete may not be able to continue to exercise. He should be kept warm and quiet until normal respiration rate has been recovered. Time may be from a few minutes to hours. The use of oxygen as a supplement has not shown any specific value to date, inasmuch as the condition results from the failure of the circulation to supply oxygen and not the deficiency of the respiratory system.

Second Wind. The physiological basis for "second wind" is not clear. It seems to be a phenomenon of the athlete. In intensive work the athlete feels that he cannot continue to perform; he may be dizzy, unable to breathe, have a headache and a feeling of much discomfort. By continuing the exercises, the general feeling of discomfort is replaced by much relief. This is called "second wind." The change is usually quite dramatic—all symptoms disappear and the athlete is clear and ready to resume activity as though nothing had happened.

Some of the changes that occur are:

1. Breathing returns to normal.
2. Decrease in oxygen consumption.
3. Heart rate drops to a more regular rhythm.
4. Relief of stiffness in muscles.
5. Temperature in muscles increases and sweating appears.
6. The head is relieved of fogginess and dizziness.

Many theories have been advanced for this phenomenon of second wind. One theory involves the necessity of carbon dioxide to whip the respiratory center in the brain. When carbon dioxide is decreased in the blood, breathing stops. When carbon dioxide accumulates, the respiratory center is again whipped, and "second wind" results. Another theory is that there is a lack of circulation necessary to remove the lactic acid from the blood. The combination of lactic acid and carbon dioxide results in a decrease of the oxygen necessary to perform at best.

Temperature also plays a part in this phenomenon; the warmer the playing area, the less the time necessary to produce second wind, whereas the colder the area, the longer the delay in reaching the stage of second wind. The better the condition of the athlete, the easier it is to obtain second wind.

PHYSICAL CONDITIONING FOR PREVENTION OF INJURY

Conditioning to prevent injuries is a full-time procedure which cannot be turned on and off at will if good results are expected. The program can be divided into two parts, preseason and seasonal. The total time of both groups amounts to a full year. There is generally not too much trouble with the sports that start after the beginning of the school year, such as baseball, basketball, and track. The biggest problem is with football, where one must have the utmost cooperation from the athlete himself over the vacation period.

The preseason schedule for football starts on May 15 or thereabouts. Each candidate is called in and a personal interview is held. All injuries that the athlete may have encountered in the past year or any chronic disability he has sustained are reviewed. At this time a complete program of summer work is outlined for him verbally and then later confirmed in writing. Suggested exercise programs are set up for him at this time, and a routine is planned for maximum results. Records are made of measurements (such as quadriceps muscles in the thigh in post-injury knees), and these are checked during physical examination in the fall.

At this time the height and weight of the athlete is recorded, and if necessary, a suggested weight at which to return is noted. An overweight athlete is always a problem. At Yale this is solved by assigning a weight at which the athlete should return on September 1. Since the athlete who reports back with an extra burden does not help the team, no uniform is issued to the candidate who returns with excessive weight. In order to expedite this, a letter is sent, reminding him of his obligation; six preaddressed postal cards are enclosed. He is instructed to report every two weeks, with his weight and signature recorded on the card. This program starts as soon as vacation begins, and the cards start arriving in New Haven the first week of July. If all is going well, the findings are recorded; if not, a campaign of letters reminds the athlete of what is in store for him if he does not make the weight. The cards provide a completely current story of his condition so that there is no guesswork when anticipating his return in condition. A very helpful factor in the card system is that sudden weight loss is no problem just before the athlete returns to the training site.

Football shoes are issued at this time. There is a twofold purpose here: first, the shoes constantly remind the player that he has work to do; second, toughening feet during the preseason workouts lessen blister problems. Blisters, although they cannot be classified as injuries, may take a loss of the athletes' time equal to that of injuries.

In the rehabilitation program during the year, or as part of the summer program, a valuable program is Dr. De Lorme's *Progressive Resistance Exercises** with minor variations. The use of weight exercises is encouraged also for conditioning of any kind. You will notice that we say *weight exercises* rather than weight lifting. Our opinion on routine weight work is "many repetitions of a moderate weight rather than few efforts with a heavy load." The use of pulleys and medicine balls is also encouraged.

One cannot send a boy home with the advice "Come back in shape." At this point the athlete is at home. The June letter will greet him on his arrival and will tell him of the work prescribed. The letter contains the following:

To ALL VARSITY FOOTBALL CANDIDATES FOR _____:

Football is a contact sport and you will reap the dividends during the football season if you start at this early date to harden yourself to withstand falling, tackling, and blocking.

The enclosed list of exercises will help you condition yourself and prepare for the football season. Start today and avoid hasty training later. What is your weight today?

These are the demands that the football season places upon you:

1. The desire to make the Varsity squad
   a. Proper attitude.
   b. Cooperation with others.
   c. Endurance.
   d. Organic strength.
   e. Toughness: (1) being able to withstand bruises and stiffness; (2) go both ways for 60 minutes without complete fatigue; (3) carry out assignments efficiently when temperature is 90 degrees.
2. To carefully and conscientiously follow the suggested conditioning program three days a week during July and five days a week during August.

* Thomas L. De Lorme and Arthur L. Watkins, *Progressive Resistance Exercises* (New York: Appleton-Century-Crofts, Inc., 1951).   •

3. Report on August 31 to the coaches with the self-satisfied feeling that the July and August football conditioning program has been well done. The pros say that conditioning is just running, running, running.

What is your attitude towards the demands of football? Complete football conditioning cannot be achieved in a matter of days. It is a matter of months.

Exercises available for inclusion in any given program are almost limitless. Limber up the muscles, ligaments, and tendons slowly and carefully before subjecting them to vigorous effort.

Coaches today realize more than ever the importance of squad members reporting in perfect condition for fall sports. After a vacation in June, July, and August, a squad candidate cannot hope to compete in competition with other conditioned boys. He finds it impossible to maintain the grind in the hot and humid days of early practice. There is no easy method to condition yourself at this late date of participation. No vitamins, no massage, no diet, and no possible short cuts in this short time of preparation. Some few disregard this experience and advice and fall by the sidelines of fatigue. Yes, *they fool no one and let their teammates and school down by their indifference and attitude.*

FOOTBALL SQUAD
EXERCISES FOR JULY
Do not do exercises unless you are warmed up.

1. *Running:* Forward, sideways, and backward.
2. *Arm Swinging:* Arms at shoulder level. Make large circles with arms; reverse and circle opposite direction.
3. *Jumping Jack:* Spread legs apart and clap hands over head. Return to regular standing position.
4. *Belly Grinder:* Arms at shoulder level, touch opposite hand to opposite toe. Return to upright position after each count.
5. *Stretching:* Spread legs 24 inches. Bend over on count 1. Stretch on counts 2 and 3. Return to standing position on count 4. Do not bend knees. Do not jerk.
6. "1,"-"2,"-"3,"-"4"–Stand. (1) Squat with hands on ground; (2) thrust feet and legs backward; (3) back to (1); (4) stand. Start slowly and gradually increase speed. This is an agility exercise.
7. *Sit-ups:* Hands clasped behind neck. Sit up and stretch arms beyond toes.
8. *Leg Raising:* Hands clasped behind neck. (1) Lift legs to right angle. Lower legs on (2), (3), and (4). Do not let feet touch ground. Hold and repeat.
9. *Back-Stretcher:* Flat on back. Raise up and touch toes. Return to flat position and raise legs over head with toes touching ground. Roll front to back.
10. *Bicycle Ride:* Shoulder stand and ride bicycle from shoulder stand position.
11. *Bridge:* Balance on top of head. Push belt buckle up in air. Walk to left, balancing on head. Walk to right, balancing on head.

12. *Rock and Roll:* Flat on stomach, arms out to shoulder level. Raise head, chest, and feet. Rock back and forth. Place hands on small of back and hold.
13. *Push-ups:* On finger tips, keeping body in straight line. On occasion raise up and clap hands.
14. *All Fours:* Raise up on hands (as in push-up). Walk on hands, dragging body. Do not use feet to push.

This letter is the "work" letter. Here we stress work that will toughen the athlete's body. In the follow-up letter, we stress the need for speed and the ways in which this can be accomplished. The second letter reads as follows:

To All Football Candidates:

Now is the time to take an inventory of ourselves. We must check back and see if we have worked hard enough for the ultimate of conditioning that we will need in September. Did I do enough chins, push-ups, etc., to be in good physical condition by the 1st of September? If not, I'll have to go a little harder in the remaining time to try to catch up. Unfortunately you cannot make up what has been lost, but it is possible to catch up by working a little harder.

The more intensive the training routine, the more efficient the body will be. We urge you to establish a daily routine rather than exercise in "spurts and spasms." If you do not take the time now to get in condition and stay in condition, the chances of making the team will be lessened. Do not subject yourself to being disabled early in the season by reporting out of shape. The football season is a short one; take advantage of all the time that you can. Believe me, it's a great game when you are in shape to play it. Conversely, it's pretty tough when you are not in condition.

The average length of time that is required to get in good physical condition is from six to eight weeks. This means that you will have to report in good condition on the first of September or you will not be in shape until long after the season starts.

Will you be able to go through two regular practices a day in full equipment when you report to Yale Field in September? Will you be able to run down under punts, go through blocking and tackling drills on this day? Physical condition is never at a standstill; therefore, if you do the planned exercises you will enhance your physical condition.

Condition and spirit will win many a ball game.

In the July letter, the exercises were intended as building up exercises. The August list includes all those, plus a few more exercises designed to increase speed. The greater part of conditioning is running, and then more running. In your running program, it is advisable to change direction suddenly; also change pace. We are all aware that a change of pace and also a sudden change in direction is a fine asset for a football player. Both of these can be attained by working on them.

In the present day football, *speed* is an important factor. Contrary to the opinion of many, *speed* can be developed and increased. The best way to increase *speed* is to force yourself to run a little harder every time you run. If you will bear in mind "that it is not how fast you run but how hard you try," your *speed* will increase.

Exercises designed to increase *speed* are essentially stretching exercises and should be done with this idea in mind. There is to be *no* jerking or forcing but steady traction. A few are listed below and they will suggest others that you can do.

These exercises are not to be done cold; a good warm-up is essential for the full benefits.

1. Standing: spread legs 30 inches apart, *keeping knees stiff;* bend over on the count of one, gradually increasing the bend on two and three, and returning to straight up position on four. The ultimate in this exercise is to be able to touch your elbows to the ground. (You will notice that there is a pull in the lower back and in the backs of your legs. Eventually this pull will leave and the muscles stretched to where maximum length will be reached. This exercise should be done ten times.)

2. Flat on back with arms outstretched at shoulder level: bring opposite leg to opposite arm on one and gradually increase stretch on two and three and back on four. Five times each, alternating each side.

3. Sitting on ground with legs spread 30 inches: stretch both hands to left toe on one, further on two and three, and back on four. Alternate on right, ten times each side.

4. On stomach: reach back and hold each ankle and gradually pull heels to buttocks. Ultimate is to bring heels to buttocks without strain.

5. Hurdlers stance on ground: bend over and touch both hands to toes; change legs and do the same. Ten times each leg. These are sprinters exercises and if conscientiously performed, your muscles will be stretched to where you will be able to increase your speed and lessen the chances of "pulls." A muscle pulls because it is forced to go beyond its limitations. Let's beat them to the punch and have them stretched.

Football is a tough sport and you must be ready. You should report with all your aches and pains behind you. In your work-outs, wear your football shoes so that the problem of blisters will not hit you in New Haven. By wearing your shoes now, your feet will be toughened. Blisters can sideline you just as well as an injury, so do not let early-day blisters delay you from making the starting line-up.

A big bug in our early training is the "groin pull." The only way to beat this is to be doing your pulling out and change of direction exercises now and not wait until the fall. We do not "pull" groin muscles when running straight ahead. The more pulling out we do now, the better off we will be. This should also be done by the backs as well as linemen.

If you are overweight when you report, you will probably be delayed in your conditioning, thus lessening your chances of being in the starting line-up for our first game. You should figure on reporting at no more than 5 pounds

above your best conditioned weight of last season. We cannot wait for you to
get in shape. The games are scheduled and must be played. If you are not
ready, somebody else will be.

An injury in the early part of the season is costly. Not only do you miss
the early games, but you will be so far behind that you will have a hard time
winning back your position. Do not let an easy summer do this to you.

BE READY!

Now is the time to be cutting down on your smoking; also getting into a
good routine of sleeping. At least 8 hours of sleep is necessary for good habits.
Park the car and do a little more walking than usual. Golf and tennis are great
sports for summer conditioning. Check your weight and do not let it get ahead
of you. Watch your diet; good simple food in moderation is essential to build
good bodies.

Games of any type are excellent ways of getting in shape. Organize a
touchball game in your community; play handball or basketball in the local
playgrounds. If you are close enough to a beach, running in the sand is an
excellent way to develop stamina in your legs.

The season offers a wonderful opportunity. Will you be ready? Remember,
September can be an easy month for you if you work now. Let's make it an
easy month and do not let the people down who are counting on you for this
season.

BE READY!

IN-SEASON CONDITIONING

On arrival at the campus, a complete physical examination awaits
the athlete. A complete file is kept in the Department of Health,
and the previous physical examination is available for comparison.
A large staff available for this examination includes medical men,
surgeons, orthopedists, and the various laboratory personnel. After
the examination, and before the athlete leaves the building, his
record is reviewed by the team physician. The facts then are referred to the trainer who will handle the protective strappings,
preventive exercises, etc., as prescribed by the physician.

After the issue of equipment, we are ready for the first practice.
The weather is very hot and we must try to get in two work-outs a
day. Weight loss at this time is extremely important, and in order
to check this, the athletes weigh in and out at every practice. A
manager is posted by the scale and every boy is weighed in his
athletic supporter only before he goes out on the field and in the
same attire when he comes in. The weight is checked after every
work-out, and any unusual loss of weight is reported to the team
physician who in turn follows the case through. The average weight
loss is noted and the work-outs are governed according to the

average weight loss. The loss of weight at this time of the year is not usually made up from practice to practice but from day to day. Salt tablets are available and all athletes are advised to take one or two 15-grain tablets daily.

This marks the start of in-season training. The practices are timed and broken into periods which are divided equally among the linemen and the backfield athletes; a horn designates the change of periods. The first period and last period is handled by the trainer.

After two laps around the field, the men line up for calisthenics. From left to right the position is: ends, tackles, guards, and so on. With the lineup like this, the coach of the respective position can pass among his athletes and keep tab of their performances in the exercises. After the exercises, the men go to their respective coaches for instructions.

Calisthenics. The calisthenics used are:

Work-out starts with two laps around one field; circling the goal posts; finishing up the last 100 yards with a full sprint.

STANDING

Exercise 1: Arm thrust. Extend both arms forward with vigor and then draw back to chest.

This exercise is done while catching breath from the run and also serves to help loosen the shoulders.

Exercise 2: Arms at shoulder level. Rotate arms, first one way and then reverse; big circles are the ultimate to loosen shoulder girdle and upper back.

Exercise 3: Jumping Jack. Start with feet together and hands at sides. The first move is to jump to spread-leg position (approximately 24 inches) and clap hands over head. The second move is to come back to starting position. This exercise is done at a moderately fast count. All leg work should be done on toes. This is a general loosening up exercise.

Exercise 4: Stretching. Spread legs approximately 24 inches; fold arms on chest. First move is to bend over, keeping knees stiff; (2) press folded arms lower to ground; (3) stretch to maximum; (4) back to origin. This exercise stretches hamstring and low back muscles.

Exercise 5: Belly Grinder. Spread legs approximately 24 inches, with arms extended sideways at shoulder level. (1) Bend over and touch right hand to left toe; (2) back to standing position; (3) reach left hand to right toe; (4) back to normal.

This stretches lower back and shoulder-girdle muscles for relaxation.

Exercise 6 (1-2-3-4): First squat and place both hands on ground; (2) with weight on hands, fully extend body; (3) back to squat position; (4) stand upright.

This is an agility exercise, starting with slow count and gradually increasing speed.

On Back

Exercise 7: Flat on back. Arms locked behind neck. (1) Raise both legs up to right angle; (2) lower legs slowly; (3) lower still further; (4) drop legs to parallel position of ground, but do not let legs touch ground. This is for strengthening stomach, back, and neck muscles.

Exercise 8: (1) On back, raise up to sitting position and extend arms beyond toes; (2) roll back with legs flexed over the head, with toes touching ground; continue to roll back and forth.

This loosens and stretches all long muscles in body.

Exercise 9: Neck bridge. Flat on back. Raise up and put all weight on top of head, pushing belt buckle to the sky; hold. This strengthens neck muscles.

Exercise 10: Neck bridge. Flat on back. Raise up and balance on top of head as in Exercise 9. Using head as a pivot, circle around head, moving feet in a wide circle; after complete circle, then reverse.

Exercise 11: On stomach. Arms at shoulder level extended to sides. Raise trunk and legs up off ground, balancing on belt buckle; hold and drop; keep head up looking at sky. This relieves hyperextension of back; a loosening-up exercise.

Exercise 12: Same as preceding position. Roll from head to toe, loosening up as before.

Exercise 13: Push-ups. Body in full extension, not bending at knees or sagging in low-back area; balancing on finger tips. Push up and down; head is to be held up looking to sky.

Exercise 14: In push-up position, that is, with arms extended. Walk 15 yards on hands, dragging feet. This is a shoulder exercise.

The calisthenics mentioned will take about 15 minutes; this includes the two warm-up laps. These calisthenics are varied slightly as the season progresses but not to a great extent. Some of the strain-type exercises and substitute exercises for agility and stretching may be eliminated. These calisthenics are given every day except Friday (the day before a game), which should be a very light day with little practice. These exercises are also used as a pregame warm-up. Every practice starts with a drill; even the two-a-day practices will be started with this series of exercises.

The trainer and team physician attend all practice sessions, and a big part of the job is to watch the amount of work that each group gets during the work-out. The result of this observation will establish the amount of work in conditioning required at the end of practice. On days when there is a great deal of instruction and close work, more sprints will be planned then for a day when the players are doing much wide-open work (i.e., pass defense, running down under punts, etc.). Perhaps the most dreaded part of the practice is the running of sprints after the practice is over when players line up and run the number of sprints that have been decided on for that work-out. Athletes are always told how many sprints and what distance they are to run. The reason for this is that the athlete will have no reason for holding back, and therefore he should run each sprint faster than the preceding one. The sprints are run by position, and thereby the speed should be the same all across the line; if there is a bad start by anyone on the line, the full group will have to run over again; by calling out the name of the offender, the pressure is put on the group rather than the trainer.

Short distance runs, with a little rest in between, stress the fact "that it is not how fast you run but how hard you try," keeps competition going. This type of program seems to get more results and a better conditioned athlete in the end.

The distance covered in sprints never exceeds 25 yards. This distance is worked up by starting with 5 yards and adding 5 more step by step. On a given day the schedule may call for a 5–5–10–5. This is interpreted by the boys to mean five of 5 yards, five of 10 yards, ten of 10 yards, and five of 5 yards. All sprints are started from a regular stance, and the start of the sprint is on the movement of the ball. The purpose here is twofold; there is a definite improvement of starts, and the ability to get off with the snap of the ball is enhanced. On occasion a quarterback calls cadence for the starts.

In present-day football, speed is essential; this is the reason for the number of stretching exercises given, plus the type of sprint used. The time allotted for the sprints varies from 5 minutes to the maximum of 12 minutes. This is a very strenuous period in the work-out and must be watched closely. Naturally, athletes will be tired at this time, and it is important to keep them from reaching the exhaustion stage.

Many years ago it was very common for practices to last 3 or 4 hours and on some occasions much longer. We felt that this was "milking the cow dry," and as a result practices are now limited to 1¾ hours. This time is broken down into periods, and the work for each period is noted and placed on the bulletin board so that the athlete will know exactly what is expected of him for the day.

When an athlete knows how long he must work and the extent of his work, he will be able to go full speed for the full practice; thus we are assured of a reasonably alert athlete. When the athlete "dogs" in favor of some other drill, this is when he is susceptible to injury. Scrimmaging is now of concern to staffs; in the past, it

Tuesday, September 1—Forenoon

9:45—Calisthenics
10:00—QB's—ball handling, cadence, hand-offs
      HB's—stance, charge, ball reception
      BACKS—individual pass defense
      ENDS—blocking stance, knee drive, shoulder charge
      LINEMEN—blocking stance, knee drive, shoulder charge
10:30—BACKS—blocking vs. bags
      BACKS—4 deep pass defense
      LINEMEN—pulling techniques, then signal blocking and bucker
      ENDS—pass courses
10:55—BACKS and ENDS—pass offense vs. 4 deep
      LINEMEN—continue signal blocking and bucker
11:20—BACKS—401 and 402
      BACKS—continue pass defense
      LINEMEN—individual defensive maneuvers
      ENDS—individual defensive maneuvers
      LINEBACKERS—individual defensive maneuvers
11:35—BACKS—tackling drill
      ENDS and LINE—tackling drill
11:45—Finish

Tuesday, September 1—Afternoon

3:15—Calisthenics
3:30—BACKS—defensive drill
     BACKS—pass blocking vs. bags
     LINEMEN—defensive maneuvers
     ENDS—defensive maneuvers
     LINEBACKERS—pass defense
3:50—BACKS—blocking vs. ENDS and WINGS
     BACKS—tackling sled
     LINE—pass blocking technique, then check pass blocking assignments vs.
     all defenses
     ENDS—pass courses vs. 4 deep
4:15—BACKS—continue defense
     BACKS—square (add 447-428)
     LINE—signal blocking (include 401-402, 447-428)
4:40—Lay out scrimmage on above plays and passes
5:00—Finish

Wednesday, November 11—Afternoon

4:30—Calisthenics
4:45—LINE—bucker drills
     ENDS and BACKS—pass patterns
5:00—BACKS—square
     BACKS—pass defense vs. PRINCETON
     LINE—review defensive details
     ENDS—one-on-one, then defensive scrimmage with LINE
5:30—BACKS—continue as above
     LINE and ENDS—offensive review
5:45—Full offensive review vs. PRINCETON
     Full defensive scrimmage vs. PRINCETON
6:10—Field pass offense vs. PRINCETON
     LINE—wind sprints
6:25—Finish

was not uncommon for teams to scrimmage for many hours during the week. Scrimmaging is now regulated to where there is just enough to help the athlete while still leaving him hungry for the game on Saturday. Two scrimmages a week for one-half hour after the season is under way is sufficient to keep the athlete in good physical condition. On a Monday after a game, there is a scrimmage for all those who did not participate in the previous Saturday's game (those who played are given a short limbering-up work-out, and then a meeting is called to go over the next opponent's scouting report). This scrimmage is a short one, just long enough to give these men a chance to catch up in contact work. On Tuesday the scrimmage is a defensive one in which there is a try-out of the defenses to be used against the next opponent. Wednesday, the scrimmage is an offensive drill, reviewing old plays plus new plays instituted for the coming Saturday. Each of these scrimmages is limited to 30 minutes each.

With the regulation of activities, etc., as mentioned above, stress is placed on other elements of fitness and conditioning, such as sleep (at least 8 hours), diet (strict attendance at training table, stressing breakfast and the prepractice meal), and the abstinence from all drugs (in this category are tobaccos and alcoholic beverages along with other medications). These items are mentioned at regular intervals by the trainer in general conversation, by the team physician when possible, and by the coaches at their individual group meetings.

To establish a conditioning program for each individual sport would be repetitious and would take up more space than this manual allows. The preseason and in-season routines that have been used in football may be varied and used for all sports. The calisthenic schedule given here is one that may be used as a standard routine. The exercises listed are of the kind that develop the big muscles of the body. By adding stretching exercises and rapid-motion exercises to this group, a well-rounded program for all sports will result. Variations may include skipping rope (for foot work), medicine-ball drills for arm strength and coordination, pulley exercises for all parts of the body, to increase strength and endurance. Some trainers and coaches may feel that certain exercises are contraindicated in other sports. If so, different exercises may be substituted for them in the program.

Chapter 5

Common Problems in Training

SYNOVITIS

A traumatic synovitis is a very common joint condition found in athletics. It is a reaction of the joint itself to an injury. Fluid in the joint is one of the first signs of synovitis and is manifested by swelling, obliteration of the normal landmarks, and a feeling of fluctuation on palpation. The swelling in the knee will cause the patella to be lifted from its normal position, and by pressing on the patella, the click can be felt as well as heard. To demonstrate the amount of swelling in a joint, compare with same joint on other limb. Symptoms are swelling, pain, limitation of motion, and muscle spasm.

Treatment consists of compression strapping and elevation, if possible. If found immediately, the application of ice packs to the area will help to control the amount of hemorrhage in the joint. If conservative treatment (as above) does not result in a recessing of the fluid, aspiration of the fluid should be attempted. This is usually a sure way of reducing the swelling and of identifying the type of fluid. Aspiration will relieve the pain and swelling. Should the swelling be allowed to remain, the surrounding tissues will become distended and thus retard healing of this tissue if it is injured.

After aspiration, cold packs and compression should be continued. If the condition is in the leg, the use of crutches is definitely indicated; in the arm or hand, the use of a sling should be routine.

To resume activity too soon will increase the swelling and the condition will be prolonged. After the fluid has indicated a tendency to resorb, the use of heat will help the rate of this process.

ATROPHY

There are several types of atrophy. The most common one in athletics is the type caused by disuse. When we have an injury, the immobilization and lack of use of the limb results in a wasting away of the muscle structure. As most of the joints in the body depend on good musculature to enhance the strength of the joint, we must be aware of the condition of the muscles after an injury. Atrophy is very rapid in appearance, but with proper exercises and treatment, the normal strength and tone of the muscle may be regained. Atrophy as a result of a nerve injury is not so common as atrophy from disuse. As a result of complete or partial subluxations, this condition may be evident. The response depends on the ability of the nerve to regenerate.

CONTRACTURES

A contracture is the result of immobilization and is often found around the elbow joint. It is caused by the application of an appliance or cast that is too tight and which therefore cuts off the venous circulation. The blood is pumped into the tissues but cannot return; the swelling causes a pressure that also obstructs the arterial flow of the blood. The treatment consists in correcting the cause. Casts or appliances should be checked regularly for this condition. Symptoms are: swelling, pain, cyanosis (blueness), loss of function, and tingling and numbness. If these symptoms develop, the athlete should report them, and the loosening or removal of the appliance should be performed immediately. If the condition is allowed to go unnoticed, the contracture will become permanent.

PERIOSTITIS

The periosteum is made up of a fibrous membrane consisting of two layers that covers the surface of bones except at the points of tendinous attachments, ligamentous attachments, and on the articular surfaces where cartilage is substituted. The membrane is very essential to the life of the bone because many blood vessels which nourish the bone lie in the periosteum. The very fine nerves and blood vessels may be seen in the periosteum. Should the periosteum be pulled away from the bone, the bone will die; this is called necrosis.

Periostitis is an inflammation of the periosteum. It may be acute or chronic, the latter being the more frequent form. It is caused by trauma or infection. The exudative forms show a serous, fibrinous, leukocytic, or purulent exudate. The proliferative forms are characterized by a local diffuse formation of collagenous fibrous tissue on bone. A characteristic of this type of condition is the "cellulitis" or red area over the site. It will be warm to the touch and painful. This condition should be referred to the team physician immediately.

The more common type of "bone bruise," where there is swelling of the normal surface of the bone, is a result of the periosteum raising from the bone. The space between the two layers of the periosteum will be filled in by bone, thus making a hard, firm surface. This is a common occurrence on the shin bone where many lumps or bumps may be found. These are painful in the early stages, and heat and protection by means of a pad is usually the only treatment needed.

Severe bone bruise should be watched and reported to the team physician. It is not uncommon to see a bone bruise "flare up," i.e., a violent red area over the site of the bruise. There will be heat to the touch, and pain. Often this condition is accompanied by a lymphadenitis (swollen glands under the arm, groin, etc.). This condition may manifest itself from weeks to months after the initial injury. Treatment will be handled by the team physician, who may apply ice or heat to the area and prescribe various medications. Sometimes drainage by incision may be indicated.

REPAIR IN HEALING

Repair of injured tissues begins as soon as inflammation starts. Inflammation is a local reaction of tissues to injury. As a result of trauma, a gap is formed; the gap is filled with plasma and interlacing strands of fibrin. Small capillaries grow in the fibrin, become filled with blood, and form a network between the walls of the gap. Fibroblasts form and grow into and completely replace the framework of the fibrin, which is absorbed. The scar is reddish in color because of the capillaries and fibroblasts; later, the fibroblasts contract, the capillaries are absorbed, and a white glistening scar remains.

Healing may be complicated by the formation of adhesions or the contraction of scars. Adhesions occur when two surfaces are in contact with each other and the healing process knits them together. Contraction of scars may lead to limitation of function and loss of motion. Stretching of scars has helped to eliminate this condition. Muscles regenerate very poorly, and the wounds are healed by the formation of scar tissue. Periosteum and bone regenerate very well.

HEEL BRUISE

This is seen more in track and basketball than most other sports because in these games the athlete lands hard on the heel. This is very painful and sometimes quite disabling. In order to compensate, the athlete walks on his toes, and as a result the calf will "tie up." When this injury occurs, swelling takes place between the bone and the periosteum; the periosteum, not willing to yield, becomes tight and very painful. The best treatment is the prevention of this injury by use of heel cups or sponge-rubber inserts in the heels of the shoes. The process for making a heel cup is outlined in Chapter 16. The injury will be very painful on pressure and will manifest itself by a localized swelling. The immediate treatment consists of ice to stop the hemorrhage, strapping, and a sponge-rubber pad with a hole cut out so as to eliminate direct contact with the shoe. After the first 24 hours of ice applications, heat is very beneficial. Whirlpool baths are very effective in this injury (see Chapter 16). The athlete will be able to continue with workouts if padded properly. This is a slow-responding condition; the length of duration is usually from ten days to three weeks.

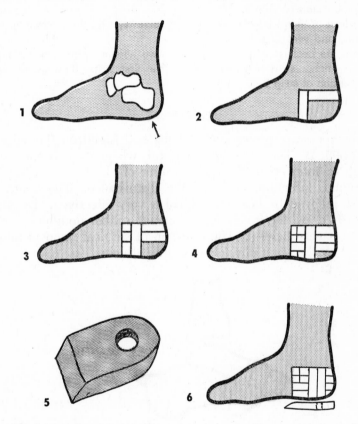

Bruise of heel (stone bruise). (1) Arrow points to area of bruise. (2) Start of taping for compression and protection. (3) Second step in taping. (4) Third step in taping. (5) Sponge rubber cut to fit heel (hole cut out to lessen direct pressure). (6) Completed strapping with sponge rubber protection.

The fiberglass heel cup is frequently used for prevention of heel bruises. Track men who participate in the jumping events use these routinely; the results are, no heel bruises.

HEEL STRAPPING

Strapping is best applied with the athlete on his stomach.

Step 1. Use a piece of 1-inch tape approximately 8 inches long. Place the center of the tape on the heel and apply with pressure toward the toes. Tape should be about 1 inch below the ankle bones and just above the attachment of the tendon Achilles.

Step 2. Use a piece of 1-inch tape 6 inches long. Place the middle of the tape directly on the middle of the foot and apply pressure toward the knee. This piece of tape should end on the ends of strip 1.

Step 3. Overlapping at least halfway, apply this strip parallel to strip 1.

Step 4. Same as step 2.

The heel is completely enclosed in adhesive tape by the alternating of the horizontal and vertical strips.

When the heel is completely encased, two anchor strips may be applied. The first anchor strip is a repetition of the first strip. The second anchor is a repetition of strip 2.

BONE SPURS

Bone spurs are projections of bone and found on the calcaneus (heel bone). They are very painful when they become large enough to interfere with proper fitting of shoes. The cause may be trauma, infection, or metabolic disturbance. The acute pain may be relieved by heat (whirlpool is very effective). To prevent further injuries, the use of felt or sponge-rubber doughnuts around the site is very helpful. The question of surgical removal must be decided by the team physician and the athlete.

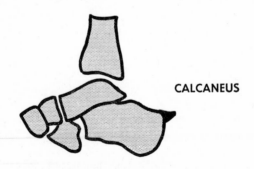

CALCANEUS

CALCANEAL SPUR

Illustration of bone spur.

COLDS AND HEADACHES

Colds. One of the most common conditions seen in the training room is the cold. It is found at all times of the year, and each sport is well represented by athletes who have colds. The literature tells us that colds are caused by a virus infection and that the early symptoms of a cold are the allergic reactions to the infection. The modes of transmission of the germs from one to another are sneezing, coughing, spitting, or transmission of any article that contains saliva. The symptoms are:

Irritation and fullness of nose and throat	Chills
	Fever
Sneezing	Headache
Running nose	Temperature (may or may not be very high)

Complications of a cold may be very serious and hard to handle. Sinus infections, ear infection, tonsils, lungs, pharynx, trachea, and bronchi are sometimes the complications that may set in if proper treatment is not undertaken. For best results see your team physician and follow his advice. He will prescribe rest, light food, liquids, and medication.

The best way to treat a cold is to prevent it. Stay away from those who have colds. Avoid crowded and close quarters. Use your own towel, drinking glass, etc. Proper health habits such as adequate sleep, proper diet, exercise, and recreation will help keep your resistance high. Dress properly for the weather at the moment. Perhaps the old tale that wet feet, cold heads, etc., do cause a cold is not true, but they may lower the resistance of the body to the point where an infection may get a foothold and result in a cold.

The use of disposable tissues is excellent if you have a cold, and you should stay away from people. Cover mouth when coughing or sneezing.

Headache. The Department of Health usually permits only members of the staff to give students medications of any kind. However, in the case of mild headaches not associated with any specific cause, the swallowing of one or two aspirins is allowed. In the case of persistent headaches, the athlete is referred to the team physician for a check-up. Headaches are not necessarily diseases in themselves but symptoms of colds, eye strain, sinusitis, upset stomach, constipation, fatigue, and so on.

EYE CARE

Foreign Body in Eye. This condition is extremely frequent and remarkably disabling. The pain is immediate, and the athlete will not be able to continue to participate. Localizing the foreign body may be difficult; a small cinder in the eye has the feeling of a mountain, and the athlete may not be able to tell where it is. The object should be removed carefully and immediately. Do not remove imbedded cinders, etc. These conditions should be treated by the team physician.

To remove a foreign body, grasp the lash with thumb and forefinger of one hand, pulling gently, and by depressing the cartilage over an applicator stick, evert the lid. The athlete is instructed to move his eye to a position where the full surface may be visible (look up, down, toward nose, etc.). The everted lid will stay in place and permit the trainer to find and remove the object. The lower lid may be moved without resistance to any position so that the lower part of the eye may be investigated. Remove the object gently with a cotton-tipped applicator. Replace upper lid by gentle traction; pull the lid down slowly and it will fall back into place. After the object is removed, there will be a feeling that it has not been removed. This condition will be present because of the irritation that the object set up; it will leave in a few minutes however.

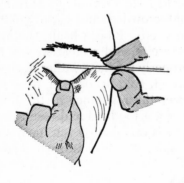

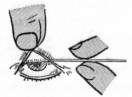

Procedure for the removal of a foreign body from the eye. Place applicator stick in fold of upper lid; grasp lid and pull back over applicator stick.

Stye. A stye is an infection at the root of an eyelash. It manifests itself with much redness at the base of the hair and swells quite profusely. There is a constant aggravation due to the pressure and a continual feeling that something is in the eye.

Treatment consists of applying hot applications to the eye with the aim of bringing infection to a "head." A spontaneous drainage will usually take place with this treatment. Should response be slow, the team physician may remove the hair or nick the top for drainage. To apply hot compresses to the eye, use sterile pads approximately 4 by 4 inches. Soak the pads in hot water and apply to area until cooled; then heat in water and reapply. Soaks of 30 minutes about three times a day is essential for proper treatment.

Conjunctivitis (Pink Eye). This is an inflammation of the eyelids of the eye and affects the conjunctiva, which is the mucous membrane lining on the inside of the eyelids. It is caused by an irritation of some kind and is very uncomfortable. Very often the athlete will complain of his lids being stuck together on arising. The general feeling is that there is sand in the eyes. This condition should be treated by team physician, since it can be very serious if allowed to remain untreated. The application of cold compresses is very comforting.

Purulent conjunctivitis is very contagious, and all precautions should be taken to see that an epidemic does not occur.

Lime in Eye. Wherever lines are laid with lime, the possibility of eye problems is of a certainty. Nowadays, when chalk or marble and many other powders are available, the use of lime should not be tolerated. Lime in the eye is very painful and may cause considerable damage to the athlete's vision. Immediate first aid consists of irrigation with water. This is applied gently with either a dropper or saturated sterile gauze pads squeezed into the eye. Much water should be used and irrigation should be continued until medical help can be summoned. The use of various chemicals may be indicated, but these should not be used without the consent of the team physician.

LIME BURNS

Along with lime burns of the eyes, we must consider that we run into burns of the skin as well. Treatment consists of diluting the lime with water to lessen its caustic effect on the skin. Prevention of infection is essential, and the proper antiseptic procedures must follow the dilution of the lime. A bland-ointment dressing is applied and kept in place with elastic adhesive. This dressing may be left on for a few days at a time. Healing is often disturbed by the continual changing of dressings, which pull the newly formed tissue with them. The use of an antibiotic ointment may be prescribed by the team physician, when and if indicated. Lime burns are slow to heal and quite often will leave a scar. The best treatment is to eliminate lime as a means of marking fields.

UNCONSCIOUSNESS

When an athlete is knocked unconscious on the field, the trainer's first duty is to get on the field as soon as possible. (Unconsciousness is differentiated from an athlete being down on the field by what you see from the bench. If the athlete is very still and not "wiggling," this is a sign that he is unconscious and needs your help.) Do not touch this individual until you have made a complete observation of the athlete. Look for abnormal position of head and neck or any unusual position of any part of his body. Loosen all tight and constricting clothing. Examine mouth, looking for position of tongue. If tongue is swallowed, pull with thumb and index finger to normal position. If you cannot pull the tongue back to normal, direct and upward pressure on the rib cage should disengage the tongue. Look for bleeding about the mouth; if profuse, turn head to side for elimination of blood from mouth.

The use of ammonia may help to hasten recovery. Aromatic spirits of ammonia is a very strong stimulant and should be administered with caution. A strong dose may tend to make the athlete "jerk" his head to get away from it, and you may aggravate his condition by a sharp move. When the athlete comes to, he should be removed from the field on a stretcher, and further examination should be made by the team physician. (Do not hesitate to call your team physician to the field when there is an injury of this type. The officials will give you all the time you need in a game, so do not hesitate to do what you think is right.)

Do not try to administer a drink of any kind to an unconscious person. After the check has been made by the doctor, the boy should be admitted to the infirmary for observation for at least 24 hours. He should not be allowed to play for at least one week after the incident.

MOVING AN INJURED ATHLETE

Do not be in a hurry to move an injured athlete from the field. If you explain to officials that the athlete has a serious injury, they will be very helpful in giving you all the time that is needed. Officials are trained to recognize serious injuries, and they will not require you to do anything that may jeopardize the athlete. Serious injuries (where athlete cannot move an extremity, which may mean a neck or spine injury) should not be moved without medical supervision. Moving an athlete in such a condition may cause further serious damage.

Many institutions require that all joint injuries be removed from the field on a stretcher, and an insert in the program explaining this policy is very consoling to the spectator. If there is any doubt about the degree of injury, the stretcher should be used. The practice of dragging an injured player from the field does not constitute good medical coverage and often will have a bad effect on the spectators. The use of the stretcher is usually fast and does not cause any commotion, and the safeguards provided this type of removal are innumerable.

A stretcher should be available at all athletic contests, and if possible, a stretcher should be made available to both teams to expedite the safe removal of an injured player. The army folding-type stretcher is easily transported and easily stored out of the way but accessible when needed.

Under no condition should you move an athlete who is unable to move an extremity, without first obtaining medical supervision. This is a sign of either a neck or a spinal injury, possibly a fracture. Moving a player with such an injury may cause further damage and may result in permanent disability, even death.

TYPES OF BLEEDING

Capillary oozing is a small flow of blood from a superficial injury. Bleeding is usually from small capillaries or very small veins. The flow will not be rapid and may be controlled by local pressure. Place a sterile compress over the wound and apply gentle pressure; bleeding will stop in a matter of a few minutes. The compress may be held in place with an elastic bandage or roller gauze.

Venous bleeding is evident by steady flowing of blood under low pressure. The blood is usually dark in color, shading toward blue. Elevation and compression is usually sufficient to stop venous bleeding. Placing a compress over the site with an elastic bandage will stop this type of bleeding. The purpose is to apply pressure until a clot forms.

Arterial bleeding is evident by the spurting of blood from the wound. It spurts very rapidly, and the color of the blood is a very bright red. Delay in handling this type of bleeding may lead to

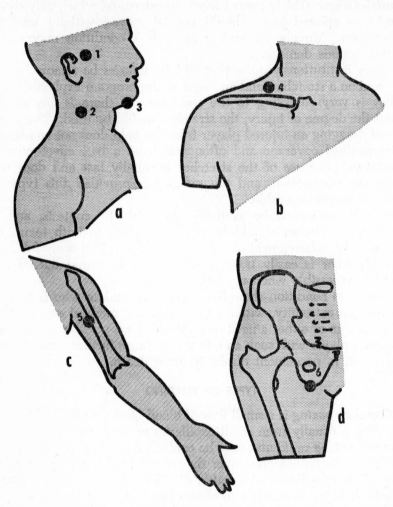

The six major pressure points for the compression of the artery for the control of hemorrhage. (1) Temporal artery (a). (2) Carotid artery (a). (3) Maxillary or facial artery (a). (4) Subclavian artery (b). (5) Brachial artery (c). (6) Femoral artery (d).

serious problems. The use of pressure over arterial sites will stop the bleeding, as will the application of a tourniquet.

Direct pressure over the arterial sites is best applied by compressing the artery over the underlying bone. The six major pressure points are:

1. *Carotid artery.* For neck and wounds of the head, place fingers over the windpipe and feel for pulsations. When found, direct pressure over artery will stop bleeding of carotid artery.
2. *Temporal artery.* In head wounds and lacerations of the scalp, the temporal artery will be located just in front of the ear.
3. *Femoral artery.* For control of bleeding to leg, this artery is easily found in the groin. It should be compressed against the pelvic bone.
4. *Brachial artery.* This is the main artery of the arm and is located in the groove of the biceps muscle. The arm should be turned outward so that direct pressure can be applied over the artery, with direct compression on the bone.
5. *Subclavian artery.* Wounds of the axilla (arm pit) cannot be controlled by the use of a tourniquet. The artery can be felt by placing the fingers in back of the clavicle (collar bone). Compression by fingers will stop this artery from bleeding.
6. *Maxillary or facial artery.* This artery controls bleeding in the face and is located in the back of the mandible (jaw bone). The pulse can be felt at this point and pressure on it will stop bleeding.

Hematoma. A hematoma results from a bruise of the tissues; blood vessels are ruptured and the blood is formed in a "pool." It is an organized mass of blood that is held in a small circumscribed area. The hematoma may be felt as a soft spongy mass that is very slow to absorb. The blood will remain in a liquid state for a few days and then will clot. While in the liquid state, the process of absorption will enhance the drainage; however, if the blood clots, the drainage will be very slow. In the liquid state, aspiration is sometimes used to eliminate the pool of blood. When the clot is formed, an incision may be needed to evacuate it.

Treatment consists of ice, compression, and elevation. Compression may be made effective by using a piece of sponge rubber slightly larger than the hematoma and wrapping it securely over the mass with a firm elastic bandage. This procedure may be carried out for a day or two, depending on the size of the hematoma. After the ice treatment, the use of mild heat to hasten absorption is very effective. Massage above and below the hematoma is helpful; care must be taken so that the massage is not directly over the site of injury.

Occasionally a hematoma will become infected. This infection will manifest itself in a red area that is warm to the touch and also very painful. The nodes of the area will be swollen and tender. When this condition is seen, the team physician should be contacted for treatment under his direction.

Ecchymosis. Ecchymosis, or "black and blue," results from a bruise to subcutaneous tissues. The blood vessels are ruptured (small vessels) and the blood infiltrates into the tissue and is visible to the eye as a black-and-blue area. Treatment consists of ice packs, and after 24 hours, heat in the form of hot soaks will be very beneficial in the removal of the discoloration.

TOURNIQUET

A tourniquet is meant to constrict; it is placed around a limb to stop blood flow. It should be a broad, flat band (this can be an elastic bandage, belt, etc.) applied around the limb very tightly. The use of a series of compresses, or a folded handkerchief under the tourniquet (applied directly over the artery) will produce greater constriction. If a nonelastic strip is used, a place should be left open so that a lever of some kind can be introduced so that the tourniquet can be tightened by twisting the lever. This will result in quick constriction, but caution must be observed to avoid the possibility that the skin may be pinched.

A tourniquet that is too loose is of no value; if too tight, it may cut the skin and severely bruise muscles, nerves, and blood vessels. If a tourniquet is used, *do not cover; make sure that it can be seen. Do not leave the tourniquet on for more than 20 minutes without loosening it for a few minutes. Failure to do so will result in serious damage to the tissues. If, after loosening the tourniquet, the bleeding has stopped, the use of a compression wrap may be all that is needed.*

SHOCK

Shock is a common condition associated with severe injuries. It is a general depression of all the bodily functions. It may be recognized by the following signs:

1. A feeling of weakness.
2. Faintness.
3. Dizziness.
4. Nausea.
5. Breathing shallow and irregular.

The skin becomes very pale and then turns ashen; also, a cold clammy skin is present. The eyes are glassy and present a vacant stare. The pupils are dilated. Also a general depression of the mental condition is evident which, if allowed to progress, will cause the athlete to go into a stupor. Pulse is weak or absent.

Shock is a very serious condition. Fortunately we do not see this very often in athletics. The general feeling that an athlete is big and strong, and therefore will not be subject to shock, is foolishness. In the event of a serious injury, all precautions for the prevention of shock should be instituted. The same principles for the treatment of shock are used for the prevention of shock.

1. Keep athlete warm; the use of blankets, hot water bottles, etc., are recommended.
2. Lower head so that blood may enter upper body. Elevate lower limbs 8 to 10 inches.
3. Hot drinks, coffee, tea or broth, etc. should be administered with caution as the watchword. Do not pour or force liquids down the throat of an unconscious athlete.
4. Relieve pain as much as possible. In the case of a fracture, etc., use splints so that motion, etc., will not cause more pain.

LYMPH NODES

Lymph nodes are placed at strategic places over the body and act as a sieve to prevent invasion of bacteria to other parts of the body. They are found under the arm, groin, chin, behind knee, etc., and when active with bacteria, they become distended and painful. When this condition occurs, it is secondary to inflammation in the local region. An open wound that apparently is of no consequence may be the cause of this condition. A seemingly minor condition on the bottom of the foot may cause the lymph glands in the groin to be swollen and painful. Local examination may not reveal anything, but on investigating the foot (or below the node), the actual site or portal of entry may be found. In the case of a very prominent infection, this condition will also exist.

When the glands become distended or filled, this is called *lymphadenitis*. This condition is usually seen within 12 to 24 hours following the entrance of bacteria to the area. If allowed to go untreated, the nodes become violently inflamed and quite painful. Local redness over the site may also be evident. This condition clears readily if the primary infection is cared for. The lymph node will assume normal size in a matter of a day or two.

Treatment is usually the same as treatment for local infections but should be ordered by the team physician. Rest and the application of hot packs to the primary lesion are part of the treatment. The use of medications as ordered will also be part of the treatment. In the case of an abscess the incision and drainage may be carried out.

Lymphangitis is a result of an acute inflammation and is evident by the red streaks that run up the limb from the portal of entry. It is seen following mild infections or in a serious invasion of the part by potent bacteria. If allowed to continue, fever, chills, etc., may result. It will subside in a short period of time if proper treatment is started. Again, this condition must be shown to the team physician immediately, and he will order the treatment for the condition. Treatment is usually the same as for lymphadenitis.

Lymphangitis has resulted from an infected blister, ingrown toenail, and many minor abrasions that have not been reported until the "redness" appears. Care should be stressed in the athletic set-up, and the immediate reporting of all injuries should be stressed. Little scratches often wind up being more disabling than a joint injury, and for this reason all injuries—no matter how minor—should be treated immediately.

ABSCESS

An abscess is a circumscribed focus of infection. It is composed of pus surrounded by a wall of inflammatory tissue. If the abscess is directly beneath the skin, it enlarges and attempts to "point" through the skin. The drainage takes place through channels sent out by the abscess. If the abscess is deep and cannot drain of its own accord, incision and drainage may be necessary. The cardinal signs of an infection are:

1. Redness.
2. Heat.
3. Pain.
4. Swelling.
5. Loss of function.

Swelling of the inflamed area is due chiefly to the presence of the inflammatory exudate and the increase of blood in the area. Heat is due to the increase of blood to the part and the increased rate of blood flow. Pain is caused by pressure, and the loss of function may be due to pain and interference of the nerve supply. Limitation of muscle action is also brought on by the exudate and the destruction of tissue.

CELLULITIS

Inflammation is the body's response to invasion by foreign matter, and in the case of cellulitis, it is more severe and more pronounced. The findings will be redness, swelling, pain, and localized heat. The redness is called *hyperemia*, which is due to the increased blood supply to the area; the increased blood supply will also have the effect of swelling. The pain is due to pressure of the swelling, and the local heat is produced by the rapid flow of blood. The acute inflammation is soft and less painful, whereas the longer the condition persists, the tighter and harder the area will become. The redness will be more intense over the site, diminishing away from the infection. In cellulitis the red streak may be visible, as well as the distension of the lymph nodes.

Treatment should be handled exclusively by the team physician, who will order the athlete to bed and will prescribe medications and proper treatments. Treatments mentioned for other infections may also be used for this condition.

Athletics are contraindicated in cellulitis, and the decision to return to activity must be made by the attending physician.

BOILS AND CARBUNCLES

A *boil* (furuncle) is a type of infection of the skin and is always caused by a staphylococcus. It is caused by a mechanical irritation of hair follicle, such as friction or ingrown hair, and by the separation of the skin in a minor wound. The infection is walled off under the skin and a very red area is visible (cellulitis). This is painful and, depending on location, may be disabling. The infection is localized and forms a core that has to be extruded before condition clears.

Treatment. Simple or small boils may be treated by hot soaks and the application of an antibiotic ointment to the area. The soaks should be of 30-minute duration at least three times a day. The "core" will come out of its own accord when it is ready. Cleanliness of the surrounding tissues must be practiced; boils have a tendency to spread, and by keeping the area clean, the chance of a series may be prevented.

Large boils must be treated with rest, to minimize pain and also to lessen the extension of the infection. Hot compresses as described above and the use of antibiotics are also indicated. The process of bringing the boil to a head and then draining may be hastened by the use of an incision. The treatment along the lines mentioned must be given by the team physician. The discussion here is given so that the trainer will have a working knowledge and will understand that boils are often serious and should not be taken lightly.

Carbuncles are deeper infections than boils. They manifest themselves with many little abscesses that drain through innumerable openings in the skin. A carbuncle may start as a very small boil, gradually breaking out into many channels. There may be an accompanying fever, pain, and loss of function to the area.

Treatment is designed to enhance proper and adequate drainage of the lesion. Incision may be indicated, along with antibiotics. Various treatments are available, and the decision as to what to use in each case should be decided by the team physician.

The participation in athletics of a player with boils and carbuncles may lead to further complications and should not be permitted. The decision as to when the athlete will be able to return is wholly the responsibility of the attending physician.

WOUNDS

The most common condition and the most frequently seen in the training room is the wound. They manifest themselves in the form of abrasions, lacerations, puncture wounds, and burns. There is no such thing as a minor wound; all are serious in that the possibility of infection is constant. The immediate treatment of a wound is to be sure that it is clean. There will always be a certain amount of germs that will reach the tissues, but every effort must be made to keep the increasing numbers away from the site. Overlooking a very small wound can result in a serious infection. Inasmuch as the degree of infection cannot be estimated in advance, all wounds should be treated as potential infectious areas.

Dressings. Applications of dressings are a daily procedure, and the best way to apply these is to tape across the muscle. This will cause less friction and irritation from motion and clothes. If a dry dressing is indicated, a strip of tape across the top and bottom of the dressing should suffice (Step 2). If an ointment dressing is applied, the dressing should be enclosed on all four sides (Step 1). Stick bands (Step 3) should also be applied across muscles. Stick bands may be cut in such a fashion as to fit over joints (Step 4) so that they will adhere better.

Butterflies (Step 5). This is a very effective means of pulling tissue together. It is done by nicking the edges of the adhesive

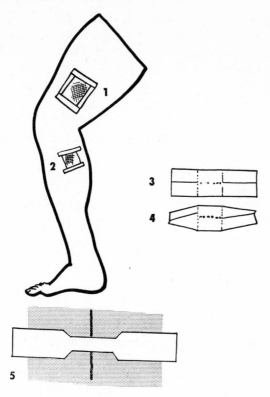

Small and superficial wounds may be approximated by the use of a butterfly dressing. The edges may be pulled together, eliminating the necessity of suture.

tape and turning back the tape to a butterfly shape. To sterilize this tape, you must hold it over the flame of a match, lighter, etc. Do not scorch. Apply by anchoring one side of the butterfly and then pulling the wound together and fixing the remaining end of the butterfly.

Treatment of Abrasions. An abrasion is the tearing off of the upper layer or layers of the skin. Some may bleed; others will just weep. The wound should be thoroughly cleaned with soap and water. Holding the area under the shower and allowing the water to irrigate is a very effective means of cleansing the wound. After cleaning, an approved antiseptic should be applied. In the case of the weeping wound, a dressing with a bland ointment should be applied. The necessity of a dressing on an abrasion depends on the condition of the wound and the location. If the wound oozes, it should be covered. An abrasion over a joint area will heal faster if an ointment dressing is applied daily. All others will progress better if allowed to scab and heal naturally. Scabs that form at a joint are subject to motion, and this causes the wound to break open, become painful, and take longer to heal.

Cinder Burns. Wounds sustained by falling on a cinder track, which results in cinders being imbedded in the scratches of the wound, are very difficult to clean. As much of the debris as possible should be cleaned out of the wound. The best procedure is to irrigate with much soap and water. The use of a small bristle brush may also be advantageous. The wound will bleed with the brushing, and this should help drain the area of the cinders, dirt, etc. An antiseptic is then used, and the wound is dressed with an ointment to help loosen the cinders.

Puncture Wounds. Puncture wounds are usually not much to look at on the surface. The extent of the damage to the tissues under the skin should be the immediate concern of the trainer. A decision by the team physician as to the amount of injury is necessary. Keep the wound open until it has been examined by the team physician. This is done by irrigations and a bland ointment dressing.

Lacerations. A tear of the skin that leaves a gaping wound is a laceration. Any wound that has any degree of separation of the tissues should be sutured. The suturing of the wound will hasten recovery and lessen the size of the scar. Decisions for suturing must be made by the team physician, who will also do the suturing. Immediate first aid consists of cleaning the wound and controlling the bleeding. A sterile dressing is applied, transportation arranged, and an appointment made for the athlete to be seen by the team physician. The use of a butterfly may act as a substitute for the sutures, but this decision should be made by the team physician.

The most common site for this type of laceration is over the eyes where the skin is very thin and the bony prominence very sharp. A blow in this area splits the skin, resulting in a laceration.

Collodion dressings applied over lacerations will protect the wound when the athlete engages in further competition. Collodion dressings may be made by cutting gauze in the size desired, saturating in collodion, and applying to wound. It will dry hard and will protect from water as well as the possibility of reinjuring the wound.

Injections of Tetanus Toxoid. The routine tetanus inoculation of all athletes is part of the medical coverage at Yale. All students are required to have the tetanus toxoid series before admission to school. These series are reviewed by the Department of Health,

YALE UNIVERSITY DEPARTMENT OF HEALTH

----

has completed the initial series of
TETANUS TOXOID injections

Date................   ....M.D.
                          (over)

1. Carry this card at all times.
2. If hurt—no matter when or where—show this card to the
   doctor.
3. Keep immune—return annually for one dose.

Boosters Dates

Wallet-sized cards show status of tetanus toxoid series.

and if necessary, a booster injection is ordered. At the completion
of a series, a wallet-sized card is given to the student, and this is
carried at all times. When a laceration, etc., is acquired, the card
is reviewed and the status of the series reviewed, and if necessary,
another booster shot is ordered.

Ulcers. An ulcer is an open wound with retarded healing. It is
rare in athletes because of the age grouping, but sometimes it is seen
as the result of improper treatment, continuous irritation, etc. Ulcers
as a result of circulatory defects will not be discussed. Quite often
an athlete will have a "sore" that will not heal. In reviewing the
condition, it may be found that the irritation that caused the wound
is still present (i.e., rubbing shoes, etc.). Remove the cause and perhaps good results will follow. The application of innumerable ointments or "wonder antiseptics" may also be a contributing factor.
Cleanse the area with soap and water and then apply a dry dressing;
change daily and observe for healing. The use of infrared heat to
the area may also enhance healing of an ulcer. Ultraviolet rays are
also helpful in clearing up an ulcer.

SKIN CONDITIONS

Blisters. Blisters are caused by friction which results in the separating of the outer layer of the skin (epidermis) from the inner

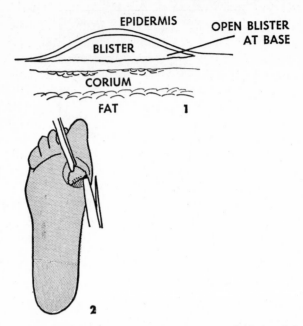

Formation of blister (1). Method of removing dead skin (2).

layer (dermis), and a liquid is welled in this space. The liquid may be pus, blood, or serum. (See Chapter 16 for further discussion.)

A blister that has pus in it is a very serious problem. The area around the blister will be painful, swollen, and quite red. Immediately at the edge of the blister will be a red line encircling the area. Blisters with these symptoms should not be opened by trainer, but the team physician should examine and prescribe proper treatment.

To open all blisters routinely is folly. The skin that surrounds the blister will be a better protection from infection than any medication applied after opening. When the blister is "ready," it will open of its own accord. To prevent further friction to the area, cut a hole just a shade larger than the blister in a piece of 1/16-inch adhesive felt and apply it around the blister. Two thicknesses may be necessary in some places. The adhesive felt may also be worn in dress shoes to prevent further irritation.

In the case of a very painful and disabling blister, it is wise to open and drain. This should be done with the best possible asepsis and is done preferably by the team physician. Only equipment that has been thoroughly sterilized should be used. Dipping a pair of bandage scissors in some alcohol and then using them to open the blister is just inviting trouble. Cleanse the area with soap and water, after which the skin is again cleaned with alcohol. Using sterile scissors, needle, etc., puncture the base of the blister. Drain the contents but do not cut away the "dead skin." (This will act as protection to the tender skin underneath.) Apply an antiseptic and a bland ointment. Ointment will keep dressing from adhering to the blister. Cover with dressing to prevent further friction and also to keep the wound clean. The team physician should be consulted if use of the new antibiotic ointments appears to be advisable.

After two or three days, the skin of the blister may be removed if the underlying skin is ready for exposure. Using a powder dressing for a few days will help to toughen the new skin.

The prevention of blisters is a lot easier than the treatment. This condition, although it cannot be classified as an injury, may keep an athlete out of action for a few days. The daily use of powder in shoes and socks is very effective. Wearing two pairs of socks, a light pair next to the skin and a heavier second pair over the first pair is good practice. Friction takes place between the two pairs of socks rather than the sock and skin. The application of adhesive tape in the early part of the season on known pressure points is also helpful.

In basketball a piece of adhesive felt $\frac{1}{16}$-inch thick and cut 3 inches by 4 inches, with corners rounded, is applied to the ball of the foot to prevent blisters in that area. The skin should be dry, and a medication for the promotion of adherence of the felt should be applied. This felt pad may or may not be left on for days at a time.

The above procedures will also apply to a blood blister.

Callus. Thickening of the horny layer of the skin is caused by friction and irritation from one cause or another, improper fitting shoes, foreign body in shoe (tacks or lumps), or pressure from a fallen metatarsal arch (which shows up as calluses in a small circumscribed area). Too much callus on the hands (such as oarsmen) or on the feet (such as basketball players) may be harmful. With continued activity, the callus pulls away from the skin and a very painful condition presents itself. On the foot, too, much callus has the same effect as a pebble in the shoe. The constant pressure results in a bone bruise, which is worse than the original condition. Calluses should be filed rather than pared. Filing of the callus regularly will prevent it from becoming too large and pulling away from the underlying skin. To prevent the accumulation of callus, the file is used daily; with a few strokes of the file, the callus from the day before is erased and the condition remains "normal." Paring with a knife or razor blade may lead to further trouble in the hands of the "do-it-yourself" athlete; therefore the use of inexpensive callus files will eliminate the excess callus and the danger of an infection due to lacerating the skin while paring the callus.

In painful calluses the use of chiropodists' felt, applied directly to the foot, will relieve the tenderness. In small circumscribed areas, the same felt has a hole cut of the size of the area, to lessen the pressure and friction and keep from further bruising the area.

Toe Nail Care. Toe nails should be trimmed so they do not protrude over the end of the toe. This is done by cutting or filing the toe nail straight across and not with the contour of the toe. If the nail is allowed to protrude over the end of the toe, quick movements of the foot may cause the nail to hit the shoe, and a separation of the nail from its bed will result. The nail will turn blue and become very painful. Relief of this condition may be accomplished by drilling a hole in the nail and releasing the blood that is under pressure. This must be done with caution so that infection will not result. Heating a paper clip and introducing it into the nail is also a very effective procedure. In due time, the nail will come off.

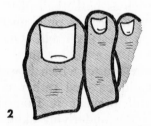

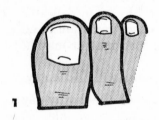

Toe nail care. (1) Improper cutting of nails. (2) Proper method of cutting nails.

This is best accomplished by leaving the nail alone, strapping it down so that it will not be disturbed when the socks are put on or removed. The nail will take about six weeks to come off.

Proper hygiene of the feet is necessary for the good grooming of the nails. Keep feet clean and dry at all times. When the new nail comes in, it may have a tendency to imbed itself at the sides of the nail bed. By soaking, to soften, pledgets of cotton may be inserted between the nail and the bed to force straight nail growth. The time for regrowth of a nail is figured in months and is therefore a slow process.

Ingrown nails are best treated by prevention, cutting nails straight across so that the ends will not become imbedded in the soft tissue of the toe. When the nail becomes imbedded in the surrounding tissues, pain, inflammation, and redness will result. Soaking in hot water, and the use of cotton under the nail at the border, will relieve the condition. If this fails, surgical intervention may be indicated.

Folliculitis. Folliculitis is an irritation to the skin that results in an inflammation of the hair follicles. Friction over a hairy area will result in little pus pockets or very inflamed pimples at the base of each hair. This condition is very annoying and quite painful. The most common site is the thigh and the condition usually develops in early football practice. The thigh pad moves with the action of the leg, and with the thigh-pad pocket wet and coarse, the hairs become irritated and inflamed. Massaging without sufficient lubrication also produces this condition. Avoid massage until condition clears.

Treatment consists of hot compresses applied to the area for about 20 minutes three times a day, the application of an antiseptic, and the use of petroleum jelly extensively over the area to lubricate while practicing.

Warts. These are localized little masses that occur on the skin. They are flat in shape and, looking at them from the top, they resemble a cauliflower. They are cone-shaped and have little black dots through the surface. They often become painful and very tender. Infection is also a condition quite prevalent in a wart.

Treatment. If infected, treatment to control and eliminate the infection must be started. This is limited generally to hot soaks, etc.; otherwise there is no treatment except to remove the warts surgically. Warts are caused by a virus, and they will disappear of their own volition. However, the use of drugs or cautery is employed for the removal of warts. Warts of the hands should be protected by adhesive strapping so that they will not be torn off in competition.

Fungi Treatment. Fungi are everywhere. Some athletes are more susceptible than others. A fungus on the feet resembles a round, scaly, itchy patch on the skin. The type of fungus that affects the feet (called *athlete's foot*) likes the dark moist places of the feet, preferably between the toes. This type of fungus may affect other parts of the body; namely, groin, ears, or scalp.

Improper drying between the toes causes the skin to crack. The dark and damp climate plus the open area caused by the dessication of the skin acts as a wonderful host for the fungus.

The most common type of fungus manifests itself in little blisters. The blisters break and the fluid crusts. Itching is quite prevalent. Scratching the area and then rubbing the ear, etc., may cause the fungus to spread to other parts of the body. If allowed to progress, these little blisters may become infected.

The best treatment is in the prevention of the condition. Proper cleaning of shower rooms, locker rooms, and good foot hygiene will lessen the possibility of exposure. The use of foot baths as the prophylaxis has been frowned upon in recent years, but the use of foot-powder baths has produced excellent results. The reason for failure of foot baths was not the medication used but the inability to keep the solution up to proper proportions. The drippings from the shower, etc., after each use, had a tendency to reduce the efficacy of the drug, thus rendering it ineffective after successive uses. The use of strong disinfectants to clean the shower and locker rooms has no substitute, and along with proper airing, etc., and if used constantly, the rooms will be reasonably clear of the germs that cause the infection. The use of wooden clogs or similar foot gear should be recommended in the locker room.

The proper drying of the feet after the shower, plus the use of a foot powder, will prevent this condition. The changing of underwear, supporters, and socks must be a daily ritual. Fungus, as we have already stated, likes dampness as its host, and wet or damp socks and supporters will enhance the growth of this germ. To wear this equipment when damp, etc., is asking for trouble.

Treatment consists of keeping the area as dry and clean as possible. The use of clean, white socks daily heads the list on our steps of treatment.

Routinely we use a 5 per cent solution of salicylic acid in alcohol, applied daily to the area, and then dusted with a foot powder. The application of powder is also recommended before bedtime. The

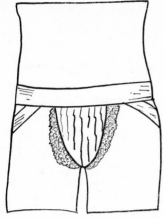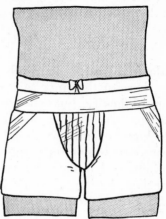

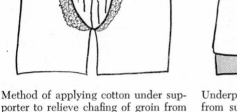

Method of applying cotton under sup-   Underpants worn to prevent friction
porter to relieve chafing of groin from   from supporter.
friction of supporter.

use of Whitfield's ointment or other similar product is also recommended for the moderate to severe condition. The ointment is
rubbed into the area before bedtime and allowed to work overnight.
This ointment burns and is quite uncomfortable for a very short
time. The more severe condition may be treated by a solution of
potassium permanganate. This is a purple solution and will turn
the skin a very dark brown. Directions are given on the bottle label
(usually 5 grams to a quart of warm water). For many years we
have allowed the solution to dry on the feet, rather than dry feet
with a towel. For some reason or other this method has given
excellent results. Many have reported excellent results from the
use of ultraviolet rays for this condition.

Fungus of the toe nails is a very unsightly condition and very
difficult to handle. Scraping the nails and applying 5 per cent sali-
cyclic acid in alcohol has been very effective. However, the treatment is of very long duration, sometimes many months.

There is a very definite tendency for fungus to recur, and good
hygiene must be practiced to keep this at a minimum.

Dermatitis in Groin. Irritation due to the athletic supporter manifests itself in a rash and is very common, being very prevalent in the
early days of practice. There will be itching and redness. Pain is
not severe but resembles a "burn" irritation. Treatment consists of
the application of a bland ointment overnight and the use of cotton

under the supporter to lessen the friction while practicing. The use of cotton underpants is very effective in preventing this condition.

CYSTS

Pilonidal Cyst. As a result of a congenital malformation located at the base of the spine, a cyst is formed. There may or may not be any difficulty, but when it becomes inflamed, the area is very sensitive. The cyst is observed by spreading the cheeks of the buttock and examining directly over the coccyx. There will appear one or more dimples over the mid-line that will give rise to possible draining at a late date. There are sinuses that open and drain, and when they close up, the pain in the area will be intense. Even with good drainage, etc., the condition never heals. Many attacks of discomfort, drainage, etc., should be considered as a disabling factor for qualification in athletic participation. Surgical repair should be considered for the cyst that drains constantly.

Sebaceous Cysts. This is a very common cyst found prominently on the neck, ears, back and scalp. It is a cylindrical mass elevated under the skin. When felt, it may be very soft and very loose. Cysts do not usually present a problem, but they occasionally become infected. Infection should be treated by routine methods. Incision and drainage may be indicated. The removal of a cyst is a decision to be made by the athlete and team physician. Cysts that are a source of constant trouble may well be removed. Those on the back of the neck where the helmet rubs and irritates are cysts that can affect the ability of the athlete to perform.

SUN EXPOSURE

Heat Stroke. Heat stroke or sunstroke usually happens during the hot months of the year when the temperatures are in the high 90's and 100's. The athlete may be unconscious when seen, have a very rapid pulse, hot flushed skin, and a very high fever, due to a disturbance in the heat-regulating mechanism.

Treatment should be immediate and consists of lowering the temperature of the body. The use of cold packs, cold baths, etc., is very effective. Care must be taken so that the lowering of the temperature is not too rapid.

Heat Exhaustion. Heat exhaustion is usually due to severe dehydration and loss of salt in the body. When excessive perspiration takes place and the replacing of fluids is not observed, the condition of heat exhaustion is present. There will be fatigue, cramps of muscles, abdominal pain, nausea, and finally prostration. The skin is moist and pale; there may or may not be an increase in temperature; the pulse will be normal.

Treatment consists of replenishing the liquid content of the body and supplementing salt with this intake. The use of salt tablets is very effective in restoring salt at this time. When nausea is present, the drinking of salt water is not too palatable, and the tablets of concentrated salt are very comfortable and effective. To eliminate this condition, the routine use of salt tablets should be required of all athletes in the warm or hot weather. Salt tablets, will be discussed under separate heading at the end of this chapter.

SURGICAL CONDITIONS

Varicose Veins. There are not many cases of varicose veins in the age group that participates in athletics. Varicose veins are caused by the failure of the valves of the veins: The valves deteriorate and drainage is not complete. Results are a very distended blood vessel that may be seen and felt.

Symptoms are the bulging of the blood vessels, fatigue of the legs, and pain. The pain may be mild but constant and aggravating. The feeling that the legs are constantly "heavy" is also a symptom.

Treatment consists of compression by means of an elastic bandage, or rubber stockings, and elevation. The use of heat and massage may prove effective in some cases.

The team physician may choose to inject the veins with a medication that will alleviate the varicosity. This procedure has been used for a long time and many are happy as a result. This is a decision for the physician and must be performed by him.

Hemorrhoids. Hemorrhoids, or *piles* affect the anal area of the body. Blood vessels are damaged, and if visible, these are known as external hemorrhoids. Those that occur inside the anus are called internal and are not readily seen. The external hemorrhoids are visible, and a very boggy mass of tissue is seen protruding from around the anus. There will be pain, itching, and sensitivity in the area. If bleeding is present, it may be mild or profuse.

Treatment consists of eliminating the cause; straining at stool, constipation, and irritation may be the cause of this condition. The use of mineral oil as an internal lubricant and the use of an ointment (petroleum jelly, etc.) to lubricate the external area will relieve itching and soreness. After a bowel movement, the hemorrhoid will

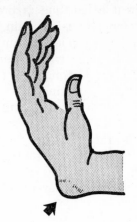

Shape and area of ganglion.

protrude. This should be replaced gently back inside the anus. Using wet toilet paper will ease the pain in wiping. Sitz baths are very effective for the absorption of the blood in the tissue. If conservative treatment is not effective, the team physician may advise injection, drainage, or operative procedures.

Disability depends on the discomfort of the athlete. It is usually not a condition that will keep an athlete from activity.

Ganglion. Ganglion is a condition that occurs as a result of a herniation of the tendon sheath. It is seen most commonly over the back of the wrist. It is usually about ½ inch in diameter (may be larger) and resembles a grape cut in half and placed under the skin. It is very evident on flexion of the wrist and is very soft to the touch. Treatment, to be effective, should consist of complete excision of the mass. Conservative treatment, such as the application of a pressure strapping, is sometimes effective. This involves placing a piece of felt about 1½ inches in diameter and ½ inch thick directly over the mass and strapping it in place snugly. Repeated strappings over a period of time may effect a cure. Aspiration and the injection of a sclerosing solution is used; the results are sometimes effective.

Appendicitis. This is a condition that sometimes presents itself in the training room and must be recognized so that definitive treatment can be started. The athlete will complain of pain in the abdomen, starting at the umbilicus (belly button) and gradually progressing to the lower right quadrant. In addition to the pain, there will be tenderness over the area. Nausea may or may not be present. Temperature may be normal or slightly elevated. Do not give food, cathartics, or medication for "upset stomach." Send immediately to the team physician.

Injury to Spleen. The spleen is a very important part of the body but not indispensable. It has as its functions the manufacture of lymphocytes and also serves as a reservoir for blood. The spleen is well protected by the ribs in the front and the spine in the rear, but it may be subject to a laceration. When lacerated, blood is spilled into the tissues and surgical procedures are necessary. Very seldom is the laceration sutured, but the spleen is removed intact. The removal of the spleen is not detrimental to normal body functions.

The injury may occur as a direct blow to the area, usually severe and very painful; often confused with "wind being knocked out" in an athlete. Owing to the severity of the injury, shock will be present. If the symptoms of shock are not eliminated in a reasonable time, it is wise to assume that the spleen has been injured. In

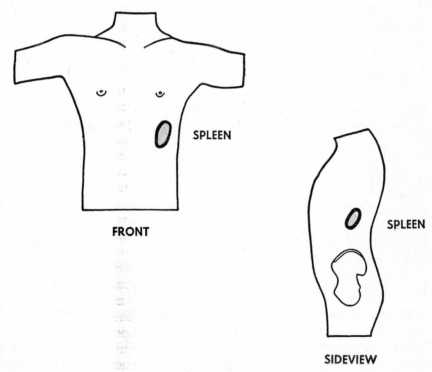

Spleen as seen from the front and from the side.

severe contusions of the abdomen, the athlete should be checked by the team physician before further competition is permitted.

The removal of the spleen is not a condition that will disqualify the athlete from continuing his career in athletics. It is not advisable that the athlete participate in the current season, but he should wait until the next year and then resume activities.

Hernia. A hernia is an abnormal protrusion through an opening of the wall of the body. It occurs in the abdomen more frequently than in any other part of the body and is the result of a weakness in the wall, which cannot tolerate straining. The athlete will recite a very definite story as to the motions that caused the condition. There will be pain and the protruding of a mass. The mass is soft and usually not very tender.

Treatment consists of sending the athlete to the team physician for examination and evaluation. Participation in athletics is usually not contraindicated. However, an athlete with a hernia cannot be too effective, and surgical repair should be considered. If the hernia is acquired in one season, the athlete will be required to undergo surgical repair before the next season so that participation may be allowed.

AIDS IN TRAINING

Additional Oxygen. Oxygen cannot be stored in the body, and any benefit derived from the inhaling of oxygen before or during a contest is purely psychological. If the oxygen could be supplied continuously it might have beneficial results. This cannot be done because of the necessity of heavy and cumbersome equipment, etc. Also, this would reflect on the sportsmanship which we all recognize in athletics. The use of oxygen after exertion may be beneficial and may help recuperation. Although the processes of repair cannot be hurried, the resorbing of lactic acid will take the same amount of time with or without the use of oxygen; therefore the recuperation period cannot be hurried, owing to the many factors involved. The comfort may be enhanced in this period but that is all that can be done; so, the use of supplemental oxygen is slowly becoming obsolescent on the scene of sporting contests.

Sleep. An adage handed down through the ages is that an hour's sleep before midnight is worth two hours after the witching hour. Where the basis for this comes from, or its truth, is not known. However, the indication for going to bed before twelve o'clock usually accounts for more hours of sleep for the athlete. There will always be a disagreement on the necessary hours of sleep needed to keep the athlete at top efficiency. Some say 10 hours; some will go as low as 6 hours. The amount of sleep needed will depend on the individual. Some athletes will sleep "all day" and do a magnificent job; others will have just a few hours sleep and also perform excellently. Where to draw the line is not known, but the magic number is now 8 hours sleep a day. This should be a variable number; in the early season practices, the athlete cannot get enough sleep, but as he rounds into condition, he finds that he does not need as much as he did in the beginning. Good rest and proper sleeping habits are essential, and the number of hours of actual sleep can be leveled off. The athlete will be able to gauge himself accordingly and he will come up with the proper number.

Weight Charts. The daily use of weight charts is very helpful to the coach and trainer. If the chart is used properly, it will tell a story about the condition of the squad. The chart should be arranged so that the outgoing weight as well as the incoming weight can be recorded. The difference between the two weights is very important. The athlete must be weighed in the same attire before and after practice. We specify the wearing of a supporter and no other equipment; any other apparel changes the picture that the weight chart will tell. If at all possible, a manager should be stationed by the chart to see that all players weigh in and out and that all are attired in the same manner.

The average weight loss per practice will be from 3 to 7 pounds, with the average around 5 pounds. This is all water weight and

NAME	Monday		Tuesday		Wednesday		Thursday		Friday		Saturday		Average	
	Out	In	Out	In	Out	In	Out	In	Out	In	Out	In	Out	In

The weight chart.

will be picked up overnight. The fat boys will continue to lose from day to day, but the average athletes will level off very rapidly. As the season progresses, the weights will be very constant. However, if at any time, such as a game, a large weight loss is noted, the indication is that the team or athletes are not in shape.

Many conditions may be picked up by the use of the weight chart. An athlete may steadily lose weight from day to day even though he is in good condition and the weight loss slight. This indicates that something is wrong and he should be examined by the team physician. "Goldbricking" on the part of a few may show up; if other members of a group are losing more than an individual player, the chances are that he is "dogging or loafing." On "hot days" a large over-all weight loss may indicate to the coach that the work-out was too much, and then this can be remedied on the next day. The weight chart may also be used as an attendance record. In the present type of coaching, where there are individual groups working, one group may have more of a weight loss than others. This indicates that one group is working too hard or the others not hard enough.

False accounting must be watched. If the athlete is aware of the findings of the chart, he may falsify his weight with the idea of fooling the coach. For this reason a manager should be in attendance.

Weight charts are kept on a weekly basis rather than monthly. The larger monthly charts present a problem of wrong entries on the chart because the space is far from the name column. A weekly chart with the names separated by a large heavy line at every fifth space is preferable. This eliminates the possibility of an error by writing in the wrong space. The charts are examined daily and changed at the end of the week. The charts are kept on file and weights are examined to establish the returning weight of the athlete in the fall.

Chewing Gum. Chewing gum, and the act of chewing, is a very controversial subject in athletics. There are those who believe that the athlete will swallow the wad of gum during the heat of a contest, thus choking himself. We have never seen this happen nor have we heard of any specific incident that would serve as an example. By and large, the athlete will chew gum before a contest, and when the game commences, throw it away. Most athletes will chew gum until the taste leaves and then discard it. Chewing gum before a contest relieves dryness of the throat and helps to control nervousness. For these reasons athletes may chew gum if they so wish.

Swimming as Conditioning. A daily plunge in the swimming pool between double sessions of football practice in the early season has a very stimulating and energizing effect on football players. For years we have permitted our players to go to the gymnasium and swim between practices. At one time a plunge before the evening meal was well received by the players. As of late they have only used the pool in the midday. We cannot see any deleterious effects from this activity and we now encourage this noon dip. The allotted time for the use of the pool is 30 minutes, but the average time in the water is about 15 minutes per man. The players "bathe" more than swim, but we encourage activity in the water to "loosen" them up after a hard practice. The swim has a very relaxing effect and has been very helpful to those who are sore and have multiple contusions.

Staleness. Staleness is a condition that is often hard to "sell" to coaches and others connected with the athletic picture. An athlete would not play the sport if he did not like it, and therefore how can you become tired or bored with something that you like? As in anything else, too much of anything is boring and tiring. A routine such as reporting to the practice field at the same time every day of the week and doing the same thing has a tendency to weary an athlete. The psychological effect is often carried over to the physical side; namely, loss of weight, loss of appetite, etc. On the other hand, the athlete may be so bored that he indulges in compulsive eating. This in turn leads to laziness and irritability. Loss of sleep is often included in the list of symptoms. On physical examination, results will be negative. The findings are strictly academic.

To combat the element of staleness, change in routines and work-outs proves very effective. A day off at strategic times will also be a very helpful factor.

Symptoms of this condition are readily observed by the trainer who is close to the squad: loafing and stalling in the dressing room, much concern over minor injuries, injuries that are slow in responding, and being "touchy" over slight remarks of team mates. These are the symptoms. They may occur in the squad as a whole, but invariably they are found especially in individuals. By being alert to such possibilities, the trainer can avert them by guidance and by proper handling of schedules. An unexpected day off, a change in practice schedule, or a special dinner of some kind may be arranged.

A work-out in sweat suits, for example, may be all that is needed to stall this condition in football; other sports have similar devices.

Long, drawn-out practices plus a losing season contribute to this condition. Shortened and regulated practices and wins are wonderful solutions.

Injections. Infiltration of an injured area with novocain (procaine, etc.) so that the athlete may resume play has no justification whatever. The use of these drugs as effective means of treatment is recognized by all and may be used by team physicians when indicated. It has not been routine practice at Yale, and the decision for their use in treatment rests solely with the Department of Health. If used for the purpose of disguising pain so that the athlete may play, the dangers of damage to other tissues in the area may result, and a simple injury may then become a chronic and disabling condition. The athlete should not be allowed to return to play unless he is without disability of any kind—*and not before.* The slightest impairment may be the cause of a more serious injury as a result of "favoring" the recent injury that is "not quite ready."

The Use of Amphetamines (Pep Pills). Dr. Allan J. Ryan, chairman of the committee to investigate the use of amphetamines for the American Medical Association reports:

. . . that since it has been demonstrated that amphetamines can artificially improve performance beyond the ordinary capabilities of the athlete, their use for this purpose is in violation of the word and ethical principles of sportsmanship. This principle has already been recognized by the United States Olympic Association, the Amateur Athletic Union, and the International Amateur Athletic Federation, all of whom will disqualify from their competitions anyone found to be using any drug as an aid to improving performance. In view of the fact that the use of amphetamines to improve athletic performances is inconsistent with the practice and ideals of sportsmanship, and since their repeated use may be associated with harmful effect, the committee strongly condemns the prescription of these drugs for this purpose by physicians or the administration or use in athletics by coaches, trainers, or participants.

Relaxation at Half Time. A very controversial subject is what to do at half time to replenish or revive the athlete. The use of many fads and fancies is in existence today, and all have been tried. The most effective routine is:

1. Make the athlete comfortable by having him stretch out so that he can relax.
2. Wipe off face, etc., with cool towel in warm weather and a dry towel in cold weather.

3. Quartered oranges in warm weather are very effective, as is broth, hot tea, etc., in cold weather.
4. Let the athlete rest quietly. Unnecessary movements are very distracting. In other words, the less done for him, the more he will be pleased.

The use of soft drinks and fancy concoctions has not proved to be very effective, and so these have been eliminated. The less you put in the stomach during the heat of competition, the less apt the athlete is to be in discomfort. A small cup of water may quench thirst, but care should be taken to see that the athlete does not fill himself, thus becoming bloated and nauseated.

Cramps. A cramp is a spasm of the muscle and is due to the incoordination of muscle action or to exposure to cold or heat. Cramps may also be caused by fatigue, dietary deficiencies, lack of salt, and vitamin deficiencies.

Considering the type of athlete that we see today, it is reasonable to assume that we are dealing with a normal healthy boy. Therefore we can deduce that the cause of his cramps is due to fatigue or lack of salt. When a cramp is first seen, the treatment is to stretch the cramp to relieve the contraction. In the cramp of the calf, the foot will be pointed downward because of the contracture of the muscles of the calf. By forcing (gently) the toes upward and flexing the foot, the muscles of the calf will stretch and relax. Hold for a few minutes to be sure that the cramp is gone. After the cramp has subsided, there will be residual soreness that may be eliminated by heat and massage. In the leg, calf, or thigh, it is advisable to apply a hot pack to the area to add to the comfort of the athlete.

A hot pack is applied by covering the skin with a balm that is hot in nature (a counterirritant); cover with cotton and wrap snugly with an elastic bandage. The athlete will be able to continue playing with this type of wrap and the tendency to cramps will be eliminated.

Investigate the cause of the cramps, and if it is found that they are due to dehydration, the use of salt tablets should be suggested to the athlete. Salt tablets are easily swallowed without any side effects and will lessen the tendency to cramps.

Salt Tablets. The most common and perhaps the most unpleasant result of heat is the feeling of exhaustion and the inability to carry on the expected work program that has been outlined for the day. There is also profuse sweating, the feeling of faintness, nausea, blurred vision, and near-temporary unconsciousness. There is a body loss of fluids and salts from sweating. In due time this adjusts and the athlete will become accustomed to the heat. The loss of salt lessens and the body becomes conditioned to heat.

To overcome this condition, the use of salt in the diet will help, although often it cannot be tolerated. By using salt tablets, the vital salts are replenished. The use of water alone is not the answer; by filling up with water, the athlete becomes logy and listless and is unable to eat his regular meals. However, the use of salt tablets with a glass of water will be very effective. Some athletes are sensitive to the salt tablets, but the use of the enteric-coated tablet has eliminated almost all the side effects of the salt tablet. The enteric-coated tablet is a salt preparation covered by a thin layer that is not dissolved until it reaches the small intestine. This eliminates the nausea and diarrhea that may result from taking plain salt or the salt tablet. The average daily dose is about 30 grains a day. This may be increased if excessive perspiration is encountered. If the enteric-coated tablet is used, the salt may be taken any time. On the other hand, if plain salt is used, it should be taken after the athlete has "cooled down," so that gastric disturbances do not result.

Cramps or muscle spasm are a common condition that results from the excessive loss of body fluids. Salt tablets will relieve this disturbance, and the cramps and muscle spasms will disappear.

Warm-up. Warming up improves performance and prevents injury in athletics. The essential process that takes place is the saturating of the muscles with blood. By the increased supply of blood, the muscles are softened and more pliable. To attempt sudden, rapid, or vigorous work with stiff muscles may bring on muscle damage. The athlete would not be able to perform at his best and his skills would not be satisfactory for good performance. The incidence to injury would be increased by the lack of pliability of the tissues.

Warm-ups must be organized and complete. To do a few arm swings and jumping jacks is not enough. The amount of warm-up varies with the individual; some men will warm up for 20 minutes, while others will take an hour.

The best warm-up is in the rehearsal of the skill that the athlete is to perform. A pitcher will warm up by throwing easily, gradually increasing his pace. The track man will also warm up by running and, in turn, gradually increasing his pace. The use of stretching exercises also comes under the heading of a warm-up. To have muscles stretched will also improve performance and help prevent injury.

The benefit of a warm-up may be lost if it is performed too early before a contest. In football we do not return to the dressing room after our warm-up. We feel that the time lost will greatly affect the performance of the athlete. We leave the dressing room in time to get a sufficient warm-up; we take more time on a cold day than on a warm day. All the game plans, etc., are discussed, and last minute arrangements are taken care of. Only then do we take to the field, where we stay until the half time. The usual procedure of going out on the field and then returning to the room takes away too much of the advantage of the warm-up.

The use of steam baths, massage, etc., has questionable value over the actual participation of the athlete in active play. Men who have used the above-mentioned procedures have divided opinions on the ultimate advantage of this type of warm-up.

Failure to warm up properly may lead to injuries that may have been prevented by sufficient work prior to the participation. A track man who pulls a muscle because of insufficient warm-up will be very unhappy because of the amount of time lost because of injury. By having the muscles stretched and loose, the incidence of injury is greatly reduced.

Stiffness and Soreness. In the early part of the season, stiffness of muscles is usually the most common complaint. It is caused by the deposits of fatigue in the muscles and the inability of the circulation to remove them as fast as they are produced.

Soreness of muscles is attributed to the tearing of fibers in the muscles as a result of strain put on them. The tears are microscopic. However, even though they are small, they are still painful.

Treatment. Both conditions go hand in hand in the early season. The best treatment is to continue to do the work that has caused this accumulation of waste products. Resting will only delay the process, and the athlete will be affected for a longer period of time. The use of a hot shower, hot baths, etc., will help to eliminate the deposits and relieve the soreness. A light massage is also helpful. As mentioned elsewhere in this chapter, we advocate the use of swimming after early football practices, to help eliminate the conditions of soreness and stiffness.

Stitch in Side. A stitch in the side is a very painful condition and resembles a cramp on onset. The pain is usually over the lower rib margins and is usually severe enough to make the athlete stop running. He will apply pressure to the side affected, in an attempt to relieve the pain. The cause is not readily known and many theories have been advanced. It is due to intestinal gases, excessive demands put on the diaphragm, and lack of condition of athlete; indigestion and constipation also are contributing factors. Most "stitches" occur on the left side; this has been attributed to the distention of the spleen. In others that occur on the right side, the liver is believed to be distended.

Treatment. If the digestive system has caused the condition, the meals of the athlete should be examined, especially the one preceding the contest. If conditioning enters into the picture, this should be taken care of by the work schedule of the athlete.

To relieve the immediate pain, raise the arm of the affected side above the head; this will stretch the side and relax the spasm. Light massage over the area will also help. This is a condition that recurs, usually to the same athlete, and it should be noted that, although painful, the condition is never serious.

Contusion of Scrotum. A blow or kick to the scrotum produces a very painful injury. It produces a very sickening pain and is very disabling. The rich supply of blood vessels and nerves results in a very sensitive and easily injured area. The pain will diminish very readily when the athlete is put on his back with his knees bent. The application of cold packs is also very effective in the handling of this injury. When the pain subsides, examine scrotum; occasionally a testicle may be driven into the abdominal cavity. If the absence of one testicle is evident, the team physician will take over.

The pain will leave momentarily, but should it continue, the athlete should be moved to the training room and the continued use of cold packs applied. If the scrotum swells, the team physician should be called to handle the case.

Wind Knocked Out. The abdominal muscles are a very powerful group; when the athlete is tensed, the muscles are very effective in protecting the abdomen. However, if the athlete is taken by surprise and a blow to the abdomen is delivered, the muscles are forced back into the very complex nerve supply and produce a momentary paralysis of the solar plexus. The solar plexus involves the breathing mechanism: stomach, heart, and lungs. On receiving the blow, the athlete will feel very faint, nauseous, and weak, and will be unable to breathe.

Treatment. The athlete will be in much pain, more from the inability to breathe than the actual blow. He will feel weak and dizzy and possibly nauseous. When examined, the athlete will have labored breathing and will tell you in gasps just what has happened. Loosen clothing from around his neck and abdomen and instruct the athlete to breathe in through his nose and blow out of his mouth as in a whistle. By slowing down his breathing, the athlete will be able to relax, and the spasm of the solar plexus will subside. The use of ammonia inhalant will help at this time. (Do not allow athlete to take a full whiff of the newly broken inhalant.) Holding it under his nose will stimulate the breathing centers.

This injury responds very readily, but if symptoms linger on, beware of damage to the abdominal organs and make sure that the team physician is called to check before allowing the athlete to re-enter the game. To pump the body up and down is not recommended as "good treatment" of this injury.

ADHESIVE TAPING

By the principle of bridging, adhesive tape is applied to the athlete for the purpose of support. Adhesive tape is applied in the case of sprains, strains, etc., for full or partial immobilization, to alleviate discomfort, and to permit more rapid healing.

In athletics, a very important use of adhesive taping is for protection and the support of a previously injured or weakened area for the prevention of a reoccurring injury.

Adhesive tape, if properly applied, will give immediate relief of discomfort and will decrease much of the pain. A thorough knowledge of the anatomic structures is very important so that the application of the tape will be of value. Along with the knowledge of anatomy, the mechanics of the injury to be taped must be fully understood. The purpose of the tape is to pull the injured parts to closer approximation and promote repair. If the injury is pulled apart, not only will the tape be improperly applied, but the injury will be delayed in healing. When the tape is applied in an improper manner, pain and discomfort will be very evident, and if not corrected, healing will be retarded.

The simpler the strapping, the better; if you can get the required support with one piece of adhesive do not apply more. The principle subscribed to in taping is *bridging*. Start from a "good" area, bridge over the "bad" area, and then anchor on another "good" area. Use the proper width of tape for all strappings. Manufacturers have made adhesive tape available in all widths, and there is one to suit the need of every strapping. Use wide tape on large areas and, conversely, use narrower tape on irregular surfaces.

The application of adhesive tape is an art, and in the hands of the inexperienced it may be very difficult. Practice is essential to good taping. Neatness is the trade mark of a good taper. Be neat and the respect of the athlete will be earned. Wrinkles in taping are not only a sign of poor taping but are also constant sources of irritation to the skin. Wrinkles will cause minor blisters or abrasions that are very painful and uncomfortable. To restrap over an irritated area is aggravating to the athlete, and often this condition causes him more concern than the original injury. Adhesive tape will stick to almost anything, and the beginner finds that the tape will stick to everything except the area required. The beginner should start slowly; his application of tape should be very deliberate and neat. After much practice, speed and efficiency will be the result.

Learn the fundamentals of taping. After the fundamentals have been learned, applications to suit the individual needs may be improvised. Do not get in a rut and use a particular type of strapping for everything. All injuries are different, and so must be the application of the adhesive tape. Many types of strappings will be found in this manual. These have been developed over a period of years, but they need not be considered as final. Many are applied with variations when needed.

All strappings should be applied snugly but never tightly. Constriction is always a possibility and must be avoided. When we apply tape to the skin, we cannot fully immobilize tendons, ligaments, or underlying tissues, by tightness. We are relying on skin traction. Skin will move because of its elasticity, and therefore there will be a considerable loss of the immobilization. To fully immobilize these tissues, it will be necessary to immobilize the joint on each side of the tissue involved.

Purposes of Adhesive Strapping

1. Hold dressings in place.
2. Support.
3. Prevention of injuries.
4. Treatment of injury.
5. Protection of injury.
6. Limitation of motion.
7. Increase stability.
8. Compression.

Preparations for Taping

1. Clean the area to be taped; soap and water are excellent for this. Tape will not stick to an oily skin. The skin must also be dry.
2. Shave the hair in the area. Short stubble of hair will actually enhance adhesive strapping, but it is uncomfortable when tape is removed. Also, with the daily application of adhesive over a hairy area, the hair follicles will become inflamed and a very aggravating dermatitis may be the result.
3. If at all possible, tape over gauze or some other material, stockinette, elastic bandage, etc. This will lessen the irritation to the skin, and if daily strappings are necessary, this procedure will be a must.
4. Paint the area with an astringent. Tincture of benzoin or any similar product is excellent for this. By painting with this preparation, many tape rashes are prevented and the tape will remain intact when applied. The use of an astringent also enhances the removal of the tape.

Sensitivity to Adhesive Tape. Some athletes may be sensitive to adhesive tape. This will show up rather readily after the tape has been applied. The athlete will complain of burning, itching, and much discomfort. If this complaint is lodged, remove the tape and cleanse the area with alcohol; then apply a powder or calamine lotion.

Some athletes may not be sensitive to the tape but to the astringent. This will result in the same complaint as before. Remove the tape and thoroughly cleanse the skin with soap and water; in some instances tape remover will be needed to remove the astringent. Apply alcohol and cover the area with powder or calamine lotion.

In such cases it will be necessary to tape over gauze or some other form of padding; stockinette or elastic wraps do very well.

Removing Adhesive Tape. To remove adhesive tape, use a chemical to dissolve the rubber base of the mass. Gasoline, benzene, or similar products should not be used because of the possibility of an irritation to the skin and primarily because of their highly flammable nature. Many rubber solvents are available that will not burn. Use these, and the possibility of irritation and fire will be eliminated.

Strip the tape off about $\frac{1}{2}$ inch; then saturate the area with the solvent. As the solvent works, the tape may be pulled gently from the skin. Remember, always pull parallel to the skin. The pull should be quite fast, instead of the slow torturous type. This is a slow process because the tape is removed in short distances at a time.

If the remover is not used, the tape must be pulled gently and firmly, holding the skin from where it is to be pulled away. Again the pull must be parallel to the skin, to avoid the possibility of tearing it.

After the tape has been removed, check the skin for rash or open lesions. Paint skin with an antiseptic and apply a dressing if the wound is "oozing." When irritations result, repeated taping must be applied over padding of some type.

EQUIPMENT

All those concerned with the welfare of the athlete are very positive in their beliefs that the best protective equipment must be issued to the athlete. The manufacturers have been very progessive in this field and the results are gratifying. These people are sincerely dedicated to the maximum protection of the athlete. The improvement in all fields of protection, ski bindings, wrestling mats, boxers helmets, etc., has been excellent, and the protection afforded the athlete is better than it ever was.

Detail on protective equipment would fill the pages of this book, and it is not the intention to discuss equipment in this manual other than to point out a few necessary items.

Protection of the head in contact sports is vital; to this end the manufacturers have pledged themselves to continual research. Helmets should be fitted carefully for maximum protection. In football, the use of the face guard and the mouthpiece also offers protection to the head.

Other parts of the body should be equally well protected. Many injuries occur as a result of poor protective equipment and from the improper fit of what is otherwise excellent equipment. Care in fitting is extremely important, for the best equipment that money can buy is not effective if the fit is wrong. Cheap equipment is false economy. Buy the best—it will last longer and afford the best protection.

Poorly fitting shoes may result in conditions of the feet that can not be categorized as injuries but may disable an athlete as much as an injury. Proper fit not only enhances the athlete's activity but will eliminate many of the problems of the feet, such as corns, blisters, and painful calluses.

The trainer and team physician are responsible for the welfare of the athlete; they should play a vital role in the buying and fitting of all equipment.

Contact Lenses. There are many advantages to the wearing of contact lenses in athletics. Efficiency of contact lenses for the most part has been very satisfactory. Jolting and jarring, etc., which most athletes are exposed to, do not present a problem to the individual who may under ordinary circumstances wear glasses. The problem of fog, steaming, etc., is also eliminated by the use of contact lenses. A very important factor is the mental attitude of the individual who must wear glasses in order to compete. By the use of contact lenses, we do not have the problem of the glasses being knocked off and broken, etc., thus relieving much of the mental anguish. Recent articles available to the public have proved that the peripheral vision has been found to be larger when contact lenses are worn in lieu of glasses. The lens will rotate with the eye and the frames are eliminated; thus no limit of field. Many of the contact lenses today are worn in swimming, when glasses cannot be worn.

Many athletes may not be able to wear this lens; some may be affected by the foreign body in the eye. However, the newer types of lens almost eliminate this completely. A few disadvantages must also be noted: The cost is high, time is needed for the fittings, and there will be a period of time, which varies with the individual, for the adaptation of the lenses.

Mouthpieces. The use of mouthpieces has been on the advance in the past few years, and rightly so because of the protection afforded the athlete. Not only is there protection of the teeth but also of the jaw, lips, and the head proper. The mouthpiece acts as a shock absorber in the mouth, taking the blows that are directed upward from a force directed to the chin. A mouthpiece, in order to be effective, must fit properly and allow for good breathing, and comfort. Finally it must stay in place and allow the athlete to talk. There are many on the market today that fill these requirements. We recommend the appliance that can be moulded to the teeth and is made to the individual mouth. The process takes only a few minutes and is well worth the time. The use of this appliance is strongly urged on our athletes and the reception is very gratifying.

Chapter 6

Types of Athletic Injuries

DIAGNOSTIC STEPS

When an injury occurs, there are three important steps that must be followed in order to handle the situation properly: They are history, inspection, and palpation. Each step is important and must be carried out to the fullest extent. These steps are listed so that the limitations of the examiner will be clear. Do not overstep your limitations.

History. History of a case is a very important step in the handling of athletic injuries. Many injuries can be diagnosed on a complete and careful history. Establish the mechanics of the injury: Was there a blow? Did he fall? Was there a twist involved? Also establish what the athlete may have heard: Was there a click, pop or a crack? What type of pain is the athlete experiencing? Is there a dull pain, sharp pain, or a constant pain? Does the pain remain in one place or does it travel?

The athlete should spell out in detail all that he is experiencing. Do not ask leading questions until the athlete has told his story as completely as he can. Watch the way in which he points to the injury: placing his full hand over the area suggests a large area of injury, whereas a point with a finger greatly localizes the injury.

Inspection. There is no pain or discomfort from this examination. It can be made while the athlete is telling the history of the injury. Look for an obvious deformity, either from a bone injury or severe swelling. Compare with the other member to note any difference. Also look for wounds or discolored areas. Watch the manner in which the athlete points to the injury, using the finger or hand as a guide. It is also advisable to look in the athlete's eyes. He may try to disguise the injury by minimizing it. This may be picked up by watching the eye reflexes as you examine the injury.

Palpation. *Gently* feel the injured part. Do not jerk or pull the injured area at any time. Be careful to avoid any unnecessary movements. An athlete will resist any efforts to help him if you are rough and overzealous.

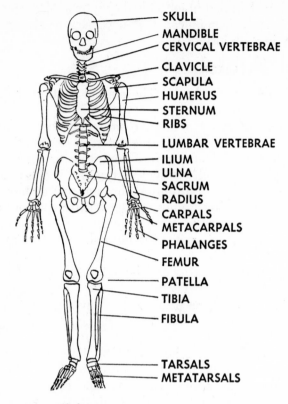

SKULL
MANDIBLE
CERVICAL VERTEBRAE
CLAVICLE
SCAPULA
HUMERUS
STERNUM
RIBS
LUMBAR VERTEBRAE
ILIUM
ULNA
SACRUM
RADIUS
CARPALS
METACARPALS
PHALANGES
FEMUR
PATELLA
TIBIA
FIBULA
TARSALS
METATARSALS

Skeleton.

Avoidance of pain is very necessary, but the examination is designed to locate the tender area, so be very careful in your approach to the injury site. If you feel that the examination will produce pain, tell him so that he will cooperate with you. If, in the examination, pain is found, do not go any further, for you have found the seat of the injury. The tenderness is very important in the diagnosis of injury.

Feel the area for swelling, deformity, tenderness, and temperature. Crepitus is a cardinal sign of a fracture; if found, *STOP*. Do not go any further. Functional tests are included in this category. If motion aggravates the injury, *do not proceed* to the next step.

Do not make a hasty diagnosis. When there is any doubt, send for the team physician or make arrangements for the transportation of the athlete to the team physician or hospital.

Specific injuries will be handled in individual chapters. However, whatever the nature of injury or illness, it is necessary to observe the precautions above in each instance.

FRACTURES

A fracture is the breaking of a bone. The normal continuity of the bone is discontinued.

Fractures are caused by direct action or indirect forces. The direct type of fracture is the one most frequently seen in athletics. These are caused by direct violence, severe contusion or impact, such as a blow to the nose. An indirect type of fracture is one that may be caused by a force being transmitted through one or more bones; i.e., fracture of clavicle by falling on the outstretched arm or elbow.

Another cause of a fracture is powerful muscular contraction. By powerful muscular contraction, bone may be fractured; for example, an injury to the patella, caused by the action of the quadriceps group of muscles reacting violently. Another type is the sprain fracture. The soft tissue, when sprained (forced to go beyond normal limits), will pull a piece of bone with it, i.e., internal or external malleoli of the ankle.

No fracture is a "minor" fracture, but to differentiate, we shall use the term. A minor fracture occurs quite often with the athlete not being too conscious of the injury until after the contest. Or sometimes if the injury occurred early in the contest, the stiffness and soreness that accompanies a fracture will manifest itself later. The excitement of a contest may disguise the feelings of the athlete so that he is unaware of the pain until later. It is not unusual to have a boy report after a contest with a fracture, with which he played much of the game. Even though it may be a serious fracture, we call this type a minor fracture because of the way in which it comes to light. A minor fracture should be handled with the utmost of efficiency even though the athlete may feel that it is not bad. A simple fracture of the index finger is a very serious injury to a passer, or a simple fracture of a toe can play havoc with a runner. As with the major fractures, these should be splinted and sent to the team physician.

The most common fractures seen in athletics are (1) fingers, (2) hand, (3) collarbone, (4) radius (forearm), and (5) fibula.

One type of fracture seen in athletics has a classification all its own. It is known as the March fracture. These occur in the second, third, or fourth metatarsal, and usually there will not be any specific history to indicate trauma. It is found very often in track athletes, more so from running on the board tracks than on the cinder track. This injury will be discussed in detail in Chapter 16.

Handling of Fractures. In athletics, major fractures are usually obvious. These are fractures of the extremities that manifest themselves with a very obvious deformity. These fractures should and must be splinted before they are moved. Fractures should be splinted before they are transported because the motion may cause the fragments to move, and when they do, pain and further damage to tissue will result. An increase of hemorrhage and shock may also result if splinting is not performed. In the case of serious injury, the officials will give you all the time that you need, so there is no reason to hurry and possibly cause further damage. In a major fracture a physician should supervise the moving of the injured athlete.

Whether the athlete should be transported in an ambulance or other means of transportation should also be the decision of the attending physician. If a doctor is not available, you will have to make the decision. Remember—you cannot make a mistake on the side of caution; therefore every detail should be taken care of. All well-equipped athletic set-ups should have available splints for the handling of fractures. The Thomas leg and arm splints should be available where all contact sports are played. A stretcher should also be available for the transportation of the injured. If splints, as mentioned, are not available, the use of boards with padding will aid in the splinting of the injury to help transport the athlete to the hospital without further aggravation to the injury. If there is an open wound associated with the fracture, this should be dressed with a sterile dressing; do not attempt to clean the wound. The cleansing of the wound must be done with hospital facilities and cannot be accomplished on the field or in the training room. If profuse bleeding is present, the use of a tourniquet is indicated. The athlete with a major fracture should also be treated for the prevention of shock. Warm coverings are necessary and should be applied immediately to the injured athlete.

Excessive and unnecessary movements of the injured part may produce or increase shock. If fracture is suspected, treat the condition as such. The injury should be handled as little as possible, but if necessary to handle, be very gentle. When the bone is fractured, the supporting structure is broken, and this must be replaced by adequate support. Splints will hold the injury and supply the necessary support needed. Splints may be made of any unyielding material—wood, metal, etc. If a rigid splint is not available, a "pillow splint" or a bundle of towels will act as a good substitute. A "pillow splint" is the application of a pillow wrapped snugly around the suspected fracture site. When using hard splints, padding is necessary for comfort, and caution should be observed in the applying of the splint. The purpose of the splint is for immobilization. It should be applied firmly and snugly but never too tight. Remember, you are replacing the normal support with artificial props.

All efforts are for the sole purpose of making the athlete comfortable. Pain and discomfort should be relieved as much as possible. Proper handling and assurance will do much to help the athlete overcome some of the discomfort. Proceed with caution; do only the procedures that are necessary; avoid too much handling of the injured part. Expedite the process of transporting the athlete to the team physician or to the hospital.

In splinting, we must immobilize the joint on either side of the fracture so that there will not be motion of any kind in the area. In the case of legs, or any part thereof, crutches are a must. With the arm, or any part thereof, a sling is also indicated.

Reduction of a fracture (put back to normal) must not be attempted by anyone other than a doctor. Splint them as they are. If there is very obvious deformity, do not attempt to correct; apply the splint as best you can and where the athlete is. The handling of this injury should be kept to minimum, and its disposition should be prompt.

Fractures may occur at any time during the course of athletic endeavors. It is not the trainer's duty to treat these injuries, but he should be able to recognize the symptoms so that they can be handled properly. His responsibility is in the proper, immediate treatment and possibly later in the after-care.

If there is any doubt about whether there is a fracture or not, splint the injury at the scene but do not attempt other aid until the diagnosis is made.

The means of treatment concerns the medical profession. Many texts are available for further information if desired.

Types of Fractures

1. *Compound fracture.* Recognized by the fragment of the bone breaking the skin and exposed.
2. *Simple fracture.* The bone is broken but does not pierce the skin.
3. *Comminuted fracture.* When there are more than two pieces of bone involved at the fracture site; there may be many free pieces of bone in the area.

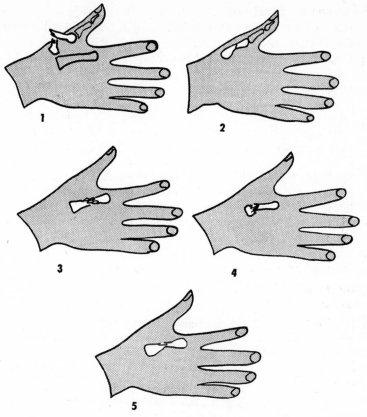

Types of fractures. (1) Compound (bone pierces skin). (2) Simple. (3) Comminuted. (4) Impacted. (5) Greenstick (one side bends; the other breaks).

4. *Impacted fracture.* Results when the broken ends of the bones are jammed together, one against the other.
5. *Greenstick fracture.* Where one side bends and the other breaks, as in breaking a green twig.

Treatment of Fractures. Treatment on the level of the trainer should be designed for immediate first aid and nothing beyond this level. The old adage, "Splint them where they are," is to be observed at all times. *DO NOT* attempt to reduce a fracture! To straighten out an arm or leg may lead to further damage of the surrounding tissues; i.e., muscles, tendons, arteries, or nerves, etc., may be injured with the fracture and unnecessary movements may aggravate the already abnormal condition. Splint the fracture at the scene of the injury, on the field, court, etc., and then make ready for transportation.

Symptoms of Fractures

1. *Pain and tenderness.* There will be a dull ache which becomes very sharp with motion.
2. *Crepitus.* The fragments of the bone when rubbing together will cause a grating effect.
3. *Disability.* Usually a disability will result. However, this is not a cardinal sign. It is very possible to have a fracture and not have disability. (In a fracture of wrist, full motion may be evidenced; on the other hand, a fracture of the leg will result in loss of function.)
4. *Deformity.* Compare with other member. Look for difference in shape or length.
5. *Swelling.* There will be some degree of swelling in a fracture. Swelling may disguise deformity and must be checked thoroughly if fracture is suspected.
6. *False joint.* Evidence of a joint where there should not be one is a symptom of fracture.
7. *Ecchymosis,* a black-and-blue condition, may not show up immediately but must be considered if in the injured area.

Splinting of Fractures

Fracture of spine. Severe straining of muscles, landing on feet quite hard, or being hit or wrenched may result in a fracture of the

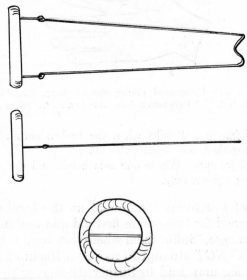

Thomas splint: (top) front view; (center) side view; (bottom) end view. The Thomas splint is made of iron and the ring is on a hinge to allow adaptation to limb. The ring is covered with padding and enclosed in a durable cover. It is a very effective splint where traction is required. The services of an assistant are needed to apply to limb. One holds the limb while the other places the limb through the circle of the splint. This splint is usually used on the leg.

spine. The individual vertebrae have many parts, all of which are potential fracture sites. Injuries to the spine must be handled carefully, as further damage may result. In reviewing the anatomy of the vertebrae, the spinal cord is enclosed in the opening of the

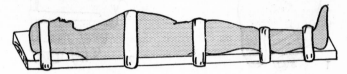

Splint for fracture of spine and neck.

vertebrae, and if injured, there may be pressure on the cord or it may be severed. If the cord is damaged, there will be a resulting partial or complete paralysis. Fortunately we do not see many such cases in athletics. Most spine injuries in athletics do not result in partial or complete paralysis.

If injury is serious enough to suspect a fracture to the spine, treat it as such. It is better to err on the side of caution than to risk permanent damage. Splint the whole body as it lies. This is accomplished by using a hard and firm stretcher. The athlete should be transported face down, if possible, to eliminate the "jack-knifing" of the spine and the possibility of damaging the spinal cord. If this position cannot be attained, the placing of a pillow, etc., under the small of the back will help. Lifting from the ground to stretcher must be carefully planned. Make sure there is enough help to lift the athlete on a level plane. *DO NOT FLEX THE SPINE.*

Injuries to the neck area must be handled very carefully. The head must not be moved in any direction. The athlete should be carefully placed on a firm stretcher and the head held firm at all times. If possible, light traction during the moving will be very helpful. By placing hands on each side of the head with fingers extended below the ears, a steady pull in opposite direction from the feet is applied. This will keep the affected area quiet and the discomfort lessened. The use of sand bags, pillows, etc., should be utilized to keep the head from moving. The head should not be placed on a pillow but on the stretcher itself. Transportation must be by ambulance.

Fractures of foot and toes. Very often the use of a splint is not necessary for the emergency treatment of fractures of the foot or toes. The application of a routine ankle strapping or a compression wrap with an elastic bandage will suffice if the athlete is being

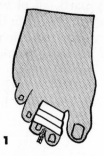 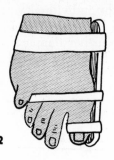

Splint for toes. (1) Strapping toes together with pad between is a very effective method of strapping toes. (2) Tongue blade covered with padding is used to splint the great toe.

transported to the office of the team physician. A compression wrap is made by using sheet wadding or cotton in abundance, over which the elastic bandage is applied snugly. The use of crutches is indicated in foot and toe fractures. The use of a tongue blade (padded) applied to the great toe will immobilize it sufficiently for transportation. Toes that are fractured may be strapped to their neighbors for adequate splinting and the use of crutches is essential to eliminate the undue pressure of weight bearing.

Leg fractures (Lower Leg). There are two bones of the lower leg, the tibia (larger of the two) and the fibula (thinner of the two). The tibia, the weight-bearing bone of the lower leg, is immediately below the skin, and fractures may be felt by looking for symptoms of fracture. The fibula acts as an attachment for muscles in the lower leg; the lower end is the lateral (outside) ankle bone. A fractured tibia is completely disabling, whereas a fractured fibula may not be. The tibia must be splinted with firm splints on each side of the leg. A Thomas splint is very effective, but if it is not available, the use of a pillow reinforced with wooden splints can serve.

Fractures of the fibula, which are in the ankle area, may be managed by the use of an ankle strapping or an elastic compression bandage. The tibia will act as a splint for the fibula, and the crutches may be all that is necessary to support the athlete.

If both bones are broken, there will be an obvious deformity, and other signs of a fracture will also be in evidence. Splinting for this injury should include the thigh as well as the lower leg. The larger muscles of the thigh attach to the tibia, and any motion of the knee will cause irritation to the fracture. By the same token, the ankle should also be splinted with the lower leg because of the possibility of irritation to the fracture by motion of the ankle. The Thomas splint is by far the best splint for this type of fracture. However, if not available, long boards (the length of the leg) may be placed on each side of the leg and wrapped firmly. If nothing is available, the strapping of the two legs together will provide immobilization for transportation. Transportation should be by ambulance.

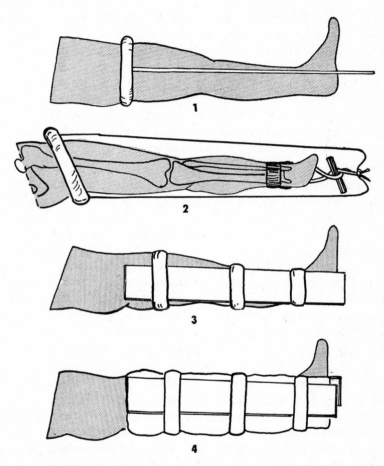

Splints for leg fracture. (1) Side view of the Thomas splint. (2) Side view of the Thomas splint with traction applied to leg. (3) Plain board splint. (4) Combination board and pillow splint.

Fractures of the thigh. This is not a common fracture in athletics but is seen on occasion. This bone is completely buried in muscle

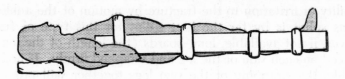

Splint for fracture of femur (thigh).

except for the lower end around the knee joint. Fractures of any part of this bone—head, neck or shaft—should be splinted with a firm splint, to eliminate rotation of the hip. The foot must be in an upright position, to eliminate rotation. The Thomas splint is excellent, but if not available, the use of a long board (padded) should be applied from under the arm to the foot, and wrapped securely. Avoid placing straps over the fracture site. If the board is not available, the two legs may be tied together for transportation. Transportation should be by ambulance.

Fractures of the patella. The patella is located in the tendon of the thigh muscles, and when fractured, the leg cannot be straightened. Fractures of the patella may or may not be obvious by a depression or deformity. If fracture is suspected, a splint should be applied directly to the back of the leg from mid-thigh to the foot. Complete extension is necessary for proper splinting. This may be accomplished by letting the leg rest on the splint until it extends; do not forcibly try to extend the leg. If full extension cannot be accomplished, apply a wedge under the knee, using a towel, etc. Transportation may be by car if space is available for full leg extension without bending the knee.

Fracture of arm (Humerus, Upper Arm). The upper arm has only one bone, the humerus. Like the thigh, it is buried in muscle, except for the lower end near the elbow joint. Fractures are not too common, but it has happened on occasion. If fracture symptoms are evident, treat as a fracture. The whole arm should be splinted in full extension, using a splint the length of the arm. The elbow must be included in the immobilization, as movement of the elbow joint will cause the fracture to result in much pain and increase the possibility of shock. Fractures of the arm may be transported in a car, etc., if properly splinted.

Radius and/or ulna (Lower Arm). The lower arm (forearm) has two bones: the radius, on the thumb side; and the ulna, on the "little finger" side. Both bones are covered with muscles except at the lower end (wrist). Many parts of the bones may be felt, and any question of interrupted continuity should be respected and treated as a fracture. Fracture of the forearm may occur at any location on the bones. The wrist area presents many problems in athletics. The most common fracture of the forearm at the wrist is the colles fracture. The colles fracture is found at the base of the radius and usually results in a deformity. Splinting consists of applying a hard object—wood, metal, etc.—from the elbow to the end of the fingers and wrapping it in place. The use of a sling is also indicated.

This procedure is also used for fractures other than the colles fracture; i.e., fractures of the ulna, either at the wrist or in the shaft or shaft fractures of the radius. A fracture of both bones should be splinted with two firm splints, one on each side of the

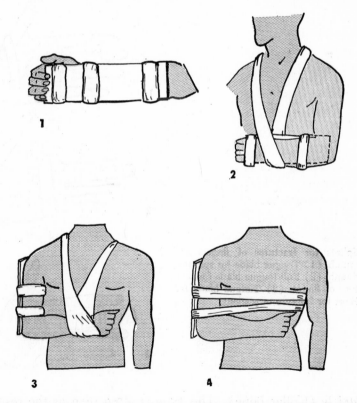

Arm splints. (1) Splint for fracture of forearm. (2) Forearm splint with sling applied. (3) Splint for fracture of humerus, using sling. (4) Alternate method of splinting humerus, using body and board as splints.

forearm. A fracture of both bones may result in a deformity, which should not be disturbed by the splint. Splint and apply a sling. Transportation may be by automobile, etc.

Fractures of fingers. Each finger has three bones, with the exception of the thumb, which has two. There are many parts to each bone and any part may be fractured. Sometimes the fractures are obvious, but most times it is difficult to diagnose a fracture. In a moderate to severe injury of the finger the application of a splint should be routine until diagnosis is made. The use of a tongue blade, trimmed and padded, is a very effective means of immobilizing a finger. The use of a sling may be indicated if, by the arm hanging at the side, symptoms are persistent, i.e., pain, swelling, etc. Transportation may be by car, etc.

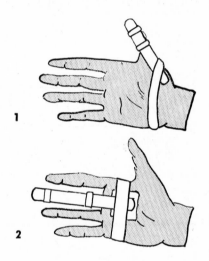

Splints for fractures of fingers and thumb. (1) Tongue blade for splinting thumb. (2) Full tongue blade for fracture of finger. (3) Tongue blade cut short for fracture of phalanx.

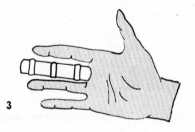

Clavicle (Collar bone). This type is often seen as the result of falling on the outstretched hand or elbow or by a direct blow to the clavicle. Obvious deformity may or may not be present, but if fracture symptoms are evident, apply a sling to the arm of the affected side and transport for further diagnosis. Transportation may be by automobile.

Pelvis. Pelvic fractures are not a common injury in athletics, but if seen, the athlete should be transported on a firm stretcher by ambulance. The knees may be flexed for comfort, and this is accomplished by placing pillows, etc., under the fold of the knee. Quite often a fracture of the pelvis is accompanied by injury to the internal organs, and caution and gentleness is necessary in injuries in this area.

Compound fractures. A sterile dressing must be applied as soon as possible. This will help to stop the bleeding as well as prevent further contamination. If the athlete is bleeding, this must be stopped. If simple bleeding from the wound is all that is in evidence, the application of the sterile dressing with pressure will suffice. Serious bleeding, such as spurting (which indicates arterial bleeding) must be stopped by the means of a tourniquet. In a compound fracture, time is a very serious factor; the sooner the athlete is sent to the hospital, the better the chance of preventing infection. Splinting must be applied, and if a tourniquet is used, this must be exposed.

Epiphyseal separations. An epiphyseal separation is a fracture in which the fracture line is partially or completely through the epiphysis. The epiphysis (cartilage that permits the full growth of the bone) may be wholly or partly separated from the shaft of the bone. This type of fracture occurs in early youth and is not seen so frequently on the college level as it is in the prehigh school or high school age groups. The epiphysis usually unites at age twenty, and this accounts for the lack of these injuries.

Symptoms are exactly like those of a fracture and must be handled as such. Any injury around a joint in a young athlete must be suspected as an epiphyseal separation until ruled out by the team physician. Very often the only way to diagnose this injury is by X-ray.

DISLOCATIONS

Dislocations occur in athletics but do not occur as often as fractures. A dislocation is the separating of the articulating surfaces of the joint. They are invariably caused by a counter joint motion. The more common dislocations occur to the fingers and shoulders. This injury is very painful while "out," and the relief is quite dramatic on reduction.

Every joint is enclosed in a capsule. This capsule is lined with a membrane that gives off a fluid known as synovia, which lubricates the joint. The joint is also held in place by ligaments. Many muscles are closely associated with the joint for motion. In a dislocation all these tissues are affected; first, a tear of the capsule results, a stretching or tearing of the ligaments, and also damage to the surrounding muscles must be suspected.

The degree of damage to each of the above will depend on the force of the injury. Knowing all this makes the handling of a dislocation a serious problem. Many team physicians will reduce a dislocation on the field if at all possible. The reason is that the longer the condition exists, the more spasm (tightness) develops and the more pain will result. The possibility of an associated fracture cannot be eliminated. Some team physicians will permit their trainers to reduce dislocations immediately, splint them, and send them for further treatment. However, for the new man who does not have the experience, it is advisable to splint and send to the physician for further treatment.

Dislocations may be classified in the same manner as fractures. We have two classifications for dislocations: the simple type where the skin is not broken, and the compound where the bone end will be visible through an opening in the skin. The simple dislocation is the more common. The compound dislocation is treated in exactly the same way as a compound fracture. A sterile dressing is applied to the wound, the dislocation is splinted, and the athlete is moved to the hospital for further treatment.

A dislocation as a rule is a very serious injury, not so much for the injury but for the length of disability ensued in the course of the athlete's season. A shoulder dislocation can mean a minimum four-week disability, or longer. After a dislocation has been reduced, apply ice, compression, and elevation. In this instance try to lessen the degree of swelling that will result from the injury to the soft tissue surrounding the joint.

Factors in Diagnosing a Dislocation

Loss of function. With the injury there will be a loss of function due to the lack in continuity of the structure.

Deformity. With the loss of continuity there will be a space where the displaced bone originated and also a corresponding change where the bone manifests itself.

Swelling. Due to the type of the injury, damage to soft tissue and rupture of blood vessels are inevitable, and the area will be infiltrated with blood. Due to trauma of the joint an overproduction of joint fluid will also result, thus swelling the area.

Pain and tenderness. Both are quite acute in a dislocation.

X-rays. These are most important and a requirement in all joint injuries.

Nerve damage. Complications that may arise from the injury are in the form of nerve damage and also circulatory deficiency. In nerve damage a paralysis results from injury to the motor nerve, together with a loss of sensation due to injury of the sensory nerve. The damage to the sensory nerve may result in a numbness or a tingling sensation.

A circulatory disturbance exhibits blanching of the skin, cyanosis (which is blueness of the skin), or coldness of the skin. When any of these conditions result, the athlete should be referred immediately to the team physician.

Details of the management of specific dislocations will be taken up in later chapters.

Simple Dislocations. A simple dislocation (one that is not compound) is one in which a bone is pulled away from another in a joint. There may be a complete dislocation or a partial dislocation. A partial dislocation is commonly called a *subluxation.* Complications of a dislocation are an associated fracture, injury to the blood vessels, and injury to nerves. Injury to blood vessels will result in the blanching of the skin, cyanosis, and coldness of skin below the dislocation area. Injury to the nerves will result in paralysis, numbness, and tingling. These symptoms should be looked for in the immediate treatment of a dislocation.

A dislocation should be reduced as rapidly as possible, so all efforts should be made to see that the athlete is seen by the team physician as soon as possible. No attempt should be made to reduce the dislocation until the possibility of fracture is ruled out. Improper handling or unskilled reduction of the injury may result in further damage to the surrounding soft tissues.

A dislocation will result in much damage to soft tissues. There will be a tear in the capsule, the ligaments will be stretched or torn, and the muscles also will be damaged by stretching or tearing.

When a dislocation occurs, there will be immediate splinting of the area by nature. Muscle spasm sets in to contract the surrounding tissues, resulting in a very tight and spastic condition. Very often this is all the splinting that is necessary to require immediate medical attention. After the shoulder, elbow, or wrist has been placed in a sling, the injured man is transported by car to the physician's office.

Dislocations of the leg, hip, knee, or ankle, should be splinted in the same manner as a fracture before transportation. These injuries should be transported by ambulance.

Dislocations of the spine should be treated as fractures of the spine and should be handled with caution. These are rare but should be suspected. Full emergency precautions should be taken. Place athlete on a hard stretcher, as in a fracture, and move by ambulance.

Compound Dislocations. A compound dislocation takes place when the bone has ripped through the overlying soft tissue and is exposed to the air. This condition should be treated like a compound fracture, dressed with a sterile dressing, and properly splinted to prevent further damage. Compound dislocations are extremely serious, since infection of the joint is very possible, and if it should occur, the recovery is very difficult and prolonged.

Treatment for the prevention of shock, control of bleeding, and splinting are necessary. Transportation to a hospital is very necessary and should be expedited. Surgical reduction must be accomplished as soon as possible.

SPRAINS, STRAINS, AND CONTUSIONS

Sprains. The most frequent injury seen in the training room is a sprain. All athletes are subject to this injury, and oftentimes it is not the participation in athletics that causes it. A sprain results from any manner of activity such as stepping on a rock, which results in a thrust of the ankle or knee; or lifting something heavy, which results in the sprain of the wrist, elbow, or shoulder. A sprain is the partial or complete tearing of one or more ligaments that surround a joint.

Ligaments for the most part are accessory strengthening bands which surround a joint. These ligaments may be separate or may be part of the capsule of the joint. Under ordinary circumstances, ligaments are nonelastic but are very flexible and pliable. They permit variable degrees of motion and allow freedom of movement in a joint. Ligaments serve a prime function, namely, to hold bones together; in some joints, they are more tense than in others. In the knee, for example, ligaments check extreme motions.

Ligaments are composed mainly of bundles of white fibrous tissue. These bundles are placed parallel to or interlaced with one another. They present white shiny appearance. White fibrous tissue is composed of closely packed collagenous fibers with rows of flattened fibroblasts among them.

In addition to the ligaments, there is an articular capsule completely surrounding each joint. The capsule has two layers: the outer, which is composed of white fibrous tissue; and the inner, which is a secreting layer. The inner layer is known as the *synovial membrane*. The synovial membrane gives off a liquid known as *synovia* which lubricates the joint. Synovia is thick and resembles the white of an egg.

When we talk of a sprain of a joint, we must consider that other tissues are also involved, namely, the capsule, the tendons, and muscles. Nerve involvements as a result of a severe sprain may also be present.

A sprain presents manifold problems:

1. The ligaments are injured.
2. The capsule is damaged.
3. The tendons, etc., are also affected.
4. There is possibility of nerve involvements.

Treatment must be designed to limit the degree of further damage to all the mentioned conditions. When a sprain of a joint is seen or reported, the cessation of further activity should be carried out. A mild injury may be the predisposing factor to a more severe injury, and further participation will not enhance the recovery of the condition. Swelling must be controlled; if allowed to swell, the tissues will be in a state of distention, thus putting more strain on the injured tissues. Hemorrhage may be controlled by the immediate application of cold. It is a known fact that the injury cannot be treated until the swelling is eliminated. The more swelling, the longer time for absorption; therefore, to hasten the healing process, the control of the hemorrhage is first and foremost. To enhance the control of hemorrhage, the use of a compression strapping and also elevation are recommended.

The earlier this procedure is started, the faster the recovery. Since the seasons are short in athletics, every possible means must be used to enhance further participation of athletes. Nature does the healing; we are the helpers; and by the control of hemorrhage, we can help nature speed the repair.

The use of crutches or a sling in a limb sprain is heartily recommended for the first few days. The absence of activity and weight bearing will give nature the needed time and the injuries the needed rest to help speed repair.

Our aim in early treatment is the control of hemorrhage. The length of time that the cold should be applied meets with many varying opinions. Some say 30 minutes, since we all know that bleeding stops in a matter of minutes. Others say 24 hours. Others will use the cold treatment for as long as 72 hours, depending on the severity of the sprain. Early and too vigorous treatment may start the hemorrhage over again and all will be lost. The so-called prolonged treatment with cold is used quite extensively. Many experiences of recurring hemorrhages have taught a hard lesson. Many now prefer to err on the side of the cold pack rather than risk the early application of heat.

In the pathology of repair, the area becomes stimulated immediately after the injury. To apply a stimulation, such as heat, to an already stimulated area results in more stimulation and a painful irritation. Early application of heat and massage has increased the swelling in the area and has caused athletes to suffer severely from the resulting pain. The swelling causes pressure and pressure in turn will cause pain. By the prolonged application of cold, we are letting nature get organized and get to work on the injury. The slowing of metabolism is perhaps the physiological condition that results, but the results have been very gratifying.

In the treatment of a sprain to the lower leg, elevation is advisable and heartily recommended. Elevation will have gravity as its ally. Gravity will help to hasten absorption of the hemorrhage present. With this in mind, treat all these injuries by elevation and continue to take advantage of gravity. If moist heat is indicated, hot towels are applied in elevation rather than completely immersing the foot or leg in a tub.

Swelling may be increased in an injury by the early application of heat. Circulation is increased to the area by the arterial flow of blood, but due to the injury, the venous circulation may be impaired and the drainage of this blood from the area may be slow. When this condition is present, swelling will result.

Treatment of all sprains as well as other injuries should be started as soon as the athlete reports the condition. The athlete is referred to the team physician for diagnosis and treatment, and this is done immediately. Allowing an injured athlete to go home and see what the morrow brings is not the proper method of caring for athletic injuries. All injuries reported are treated routinely with compression and ice. If possible, elevation is prescribed. Treatment started this early will enhance the athlete's quick return to activity.

Treatment for specific sprains will be handled in later chapters.

Details and specific injuries will be handled along with the immediate treatment recommended.

It has been said that "once a sprain, always a sprain." Perhaps this is true when sprains have been neglected. However, with an adequate approach to the treatment of the sprain and proper rehabilitation of the ligament, repair will be successful and the adage will prove to be in error.

STRAINS, OR "PULLED MUSCLES"

Before we can talk about "pulled muscles," we should first review the muscles in detail. Muscles are the motor organs of the body and compose 40 per cent of the body weight. Voluntary muscles are composed of bundles of fibers bound together by a connective tissue sheath; this sheath covers the entire muscle. A fiber is approximately 1½ inches long (this will vary with the length of the muscle) and is as thick as a human hair. (Under microscope it shows transverse stripings which are not present in involuntary muscles.) Each fiber is enclosed in an elastic sheath and is attached to other fibers to form longitudinal strands that are arranged in parallel bundles. The belly of the muscle is composed of an enormous number of these bundles.

Each muscle is abundantly supplied with blood, which serves to ensure sufficient nutrition to the muscle as well as to provide proper drainage of wastes. During exercise, when waste products are being formed and more oxygen and nourishment is in demand, there is an increased flow of blood to the area. The increase in blood flow through the muscle is due largely to the contraction of the muscle, which has the same action as a subsidiary pump and which mechanically squeezes the blood outward through the veins. Our demand in athletics for more blood to the muscles is greatly dependent on the fact that we have contraction of the muscle to help the venous circulation in bringing the blood back to the heart. Arteries break up into capillaries, which bring a rich supply to each muscle fiber. Each muscle is equipped with a nerve that contains both the motor and sensory fibers. The main trunk of the nerve breaks up into a number of branches. These branches enter the muscle, usually along with the blood supply, and break up into little filaments that are distributed to each individual muscle fiber.

So much for the structure. To fully understand the injury, a discussion of mechanics will help. Muscles are attached to bones, cartilages, ligaments, skin, or by inelastic white fibrous tissue which is elongated into tendons. The fixed attachment of the muscle is the origin, and the movable one is the insertion. The insertion, by and large, moves toward the origin. Most muscles work as units, but some parts of the muscle have an entirely different function, depending on the nerve stimulus affecting the particular part. The use of one muscle alone is almost impossible. To carry out a movement, a definite combination of muscles is called into play. One or more muscles of the combination is the leading force. All muscles are in a state of contraction. There is no slack in the muscle to be taken up when the command is given to function.

The fleshy part of the muscle is called the *belly*. The origin is usually by fleshy attachment, while the insertion is almost invariably by means of a tendon. However, both attachments may be by tendon.

The term *pulled muscle* has been the expression used in the athletic field to describe a sprain or strain. True terminology of the injury designates either a sprain or a strain, depending on the severity of the injury. A mild "pull" is technically a strain, whereas a more severe injury would be a sprain. This condition is brought about by forcing the muscle to go beyond its expansion limitation. The "pull" usually occurs in the muscles and not too often in the tendon. However, a rupture (complete tear) may occur at the insertion of the tendon on the bone or the origin, and many times at the attachment of the tendon to the muscle. A sprain fracture may happen, which is the pulling away of the bony attachment of the muscle.

Nature's method of warning against a "pull" is tightness (muscle spasm). If this is ignored, the result is a tear of the muscle fibers. This can mean tearing just a few fibers or the rupturing of many. If we tear just a few fibers, then we have a mild pull. If the tear affects many, then we have a moderate-to-severe pull.

As we have stated, the blood supply is very intense in the muscles. With the tear, we have bleeding from the torn blood vessels in the muscle. Our first step in the treatment of this pull is to stop the bleeding. This is done by the use of a compression bandage (usually an elastic bandage made of rubberized cloth, or in some cases, adhesive tape applied snugly to the area; the use of adhesive tape depends on the location of the muscle involved) and the immediate application of ice caps. We try to do this on the field and then send the athlete to the training room for further treatment. Along with the compression, elevation is used if at all possible. (Naturally a leg may be elevated without too much trouble, but other muscles do not lend themselves to elevation.)

Keep the ice and compression applied for at least 30 minutes before allowing the individual to shower. When showering, the athlete must be reminded to avoid heat near the injured area. Hence he showers in cold or tepid water, or takes a sponge bath, whichever is indicated. After the shower, a compression wrap is applied along with the ice cap, and the athlete keeps ice applied to the injury overnight. The elevation is also continued if at all feasible.

The application of the compression, ice, and elevation is intended to lessen the amount of blood in the area. The more bleeding, the more space will be needed in the muscle to store this blood; and this in turn will keep the torn fibers farther apart. The larger the separation between torn ends of fibers, the more scar tissue will be needed to unite the avulsed ends. Muscle tissue will not regenerate, and therefore the healing of the tear will be with scar tissue. This tissue is not elastic, and the more scar tissue in the muscle, the more contraction in the healed muscle. Maximum protection with the minimum of scar tissue is the objective.

CONTUSIONS

Contusion is the medical term for bruise. This injury in athletics is commonly called a "Charlie horse." Sometimes it is referred to as a "frog," and by many other terms too numerous to mention. The origin of these terms is immaterial, but they all describe the injury very well. A bruise is very common in athletics. All sports are possible contributors to this category; none is exempt. The athlete may receive the bruise from a blow or contact of some kind with his opponent, or he may acquire a bruise from a fall. All parts of the anatomy are affected: the skin, soft tissues, and bones.

A bruise will manifest itself in many ways. Some are very painful, some very disabling, and some will not impair activity at all. When the athlete receives a blow forceful enough to cause a bruise, the common result is primarily ruptured blood vessels and torn muscle fibers. This, many times, will result in a very pronounced hematoma (organized mass of blood). This is alarming to the athlete, although in many instances he would not know that he had such a condition if he had not looked at it.

Bruises are quite dramatic. Some are complicated with much pain; others hardly pain at all. The principal procedure is to stop further bleeding and to keep the swelling soft so that it can be readily absorbed. Contusions to the eye, bone, and muscles will be taken up in the respective order of the injuries.

Chapter 7

Physical Therapy

Physical therapy is the employment of physical or other properties of electricity, massage, exercises, heat, light, cold water, and mechanical devices for the treatment of diseases and injuries.

There are many ways of mechanically applying these therapeutics to the field of athletics. Because injuries are variable, the modality used should be fully understood before applying it. All physical therapy should be prescribed by the team physician. He specifies the modality to be used, the length of time it is to be used, and how often treatments should be given. Much of the equipment is very safe; the manufacturers have been successful in eliminating the hazards that were at one time present in this type of equipment. However, a simple application of heat, if improperly administered, may result in a severe burn that will be more disabling than the injury initially treated.

There are many makes and styles of equipment, and to describe all would more than fill this book. A few of the modalities will be discussed from the standpoint of experience and not from literature on the subject.

PHYSICAL METHODS

Cold Applications. The application of ice to acute injuries is a very controversial subject. To use ice for 30 minutes or to use it longer is a topic discussed at all meetings of athletic trainers. The authors' program of immediate treatment in all acute injuries is the immediate application of ice, compression, and elevation (if possible). The length of time the ice is applied varies. However, the ice pack remains at least overnight in all acute injuries. After the first 24 hours, the decision as to whether to continue or not is made. In the case of most joint injuries, the ice pack is applied for another 24 hours. This application is continued with compression and elevation.

Most of the injuries seen in athletics are usually accompanied by a pathologic disturbance which is known as swelling. Swelling, if allowed to continue, will impede the return of the good blood supply so necessary for healing. To lessen the degree of swelling, the lowering of the temperature in the area or the use of compression is required. Naturally the use of both these procedures will be better. Compression may be accomplished by strapping with adhesive or by the application of an elastic wrap. The local temperature is lowered by ice packs on the site. To be successful, the treatment must be started early and continued until the extravasation of fluid ceases. During the time that this procedure is going on, the injured area should be at complete rest and also in elevation if possible.

Swelling will be removed by the elevated position of the part of the body, the application of heat, massage, and exercise. However the early application of heat and massage has caused no end of grief in the past years because it induces an increase in swelling at that stage. Due to the early application of these methods, the prolonged use of the cold treatment is preferred, since it has produced much more satisfactory results.

The increase in swelling at the time of the injury is caused by the rise in local temperature, which in turn creates an increase in tissue fluids brought about by the passage of fluid from the capillaries into the tissue spaces. This prolongs the swelling and retards the rate of repair of the injury. By keeping the local temperature at a lower rate, the process of repair is carried on in an orderly manner. When an injury occurs, there is stimulation of the tissues; to stimulate the tissues further by the early application of heat retards the recovery.

Treatment by cold applications has been used to eliminate pain and congestion for many years, but lately an increase in the length of application time has been advocated by many. Cold, when applied in ice bags (rubber lining and a cloth cover), is very safe. The possibility of injury due to the lengthy application has been eliminated by the use of ice bags. This treatment is very mild in comparison to the full-immersion cold treatment which involves placing ice in a bucket of water and then immersing the limb for a period of time. This is not only barbaric but is not conducive to good treatment, since frost bite may result and the discomfort of the athlete will be great. The throb and ache that accompanies this treatment is usually worse than the original injury. Moreover, the bucket treatment contradicts the theory that elevation is important in early management of injuries. By immersing the limb in a bucket, the limb is placed in a dependent position, thus enhancing the organization of swelling.

Heat Lamps. Heat lamps are a form of convective heat. The depth of penetration of heat applied to the body by means of an outside source depends on the type of lamp used. Infrared lamps have a core that gets hot and the heat of the core is thrown onto the body by means of a reflector. The radiant heat lamp has a tungsten filament bulb which is heat producing and is also enclosed in a reflector. These two types of lamps are those most commonly used for heat applications to the body for producing increased blood flow. The radiant heat lamp is preferred because of the increase of depth in the penetration. Infrared lamps will not penetrate as deep as the radiant heat lamp. Information will reveal that the infrared lamp oftentimes will only heat the skin, whereas the radiant heat lamp will penetrate $\frac{1}{4}$ to $\frac{3}{8}$ inch. Radiant heat energy is rapidly dissipated by the blood capillaries and is more effective in stimulating vasodilation.

Infrared lamps (core type) are quite hard to focus on the area because the rays are invisible, whereas the radiant heat can be seen and can be almost pinpointed on the local area. When using either lamp, it must be noted that mild heat for a longer period of time is more effective than intense heat for a short period of time.

Treatments should be of 30 minutes duration for maximum vasodilation, with the lamp at a distance safe enough to protect the skin from burning. Try the lamp on yourself so that the distance can be accurate. The part immediately under the lamp should be the area observed for this test (at right angles to the source the reflected heat is hotter than at the fringe area). Covering the area with a towel to lessen the amount of heat is very effective if the distance of the lamp cannot be regulated. The application of oil to the skin will also enhance the treatment as well as prevent burns.

These lamps are very inexpensive and are quite often used in home treatments by athletes. Their adaptability is excellent, since they can be plugged into any light socket and used very effectively.

These lamps are the most common and perhaps the most useful forms of heat in the training room. They will do much more than many other modalities now being used and can be used safely in all athletic injuries that are close to the surface. Although they provide a very superficial type of application, they are very effective when used before massage and exercises. Lamps may be used for the application of moist heat by placing a wet towel on the body and focusing the lamp accordingly.

Ultraviolet Lamp. Ultraviolet rays are not used to a very great extent in athletics. We have used this modality on our swimmers with some degree of success for the prevention of colds. The use of ultraviolet irradiation for ringworm, acne, and other skin conditions has been tried, and the results are not too conclusive, since there has been no careful control of this program.

The danger in the use of ultraviolet rays has been the amount of burn received when the modality has been used without proper supervision. Very often the student will buy a lamp and treat himself; usually, when the athletes are ready to go south on their spring vacation, they try to "brown up" before exposure to the sun's rays. This will result in the athlete's falling asleep under the lamp so that proper timing is neglected and a severe "sunburn" results. The use of this equipment should be controlled either by an associate or the use of an alarm clock.

The time of exposure should be controlled. A simple means of establishing the erythema (redness of skin) dose is to apply a piece of paper on the inside of the forearm. A series of holes about ¾ inch in diameter are made in this paper. All holes are covered except the first one; with the lamp turned on, the skin is exposed for 30 seconds, and after that, each hole in succession is exposed to the ultraviolet lamp. This is done over the range of approximately ten holes until the last hole has received about 5 minutes of irradiation. After six hours the skin will be examined and the degree of burn established. The starting time for the first treatment or exposure will be where the redness is at its minimal. From this point each exposure may be increased as indicated for the degree of erythema dose needed. When further treatments are given, care should be taken to see that the lamp is the same distance from the body as when the tests were made.

When applying ultraviolet rays to the face, the eyes should be covered with wet compresses or by sun goggles. The chief complaint is that a white area will result under the area covered. This may be eliminated by removing the pads or goggles about 1 minute before the completion of the treatment.

The maximum treatment recommended is about 15 minutes. When this period has been reached, it is recommended that the athlete discontinue the use of this modality for about three weeks and then start again.

Various types of lamps are available for this type of ray, and care should be taken to see that the proper lamp has been purchased. Some lamps do not give off a sufficient amount of ultraviolet radiation to be practicable. There are lamps on the market for home use that have been very well recommended. However, before purchasing, check to see that the proper amount of ultraviolet rays are irradiated.

Quartz, mercury, carbon arcs, and cold quartz are some of the types of lamp units that are used for this ray. Check each thoroughly to establish the particular lamp adapted to your needs.

Diathermy. Diathermy is a conversive form of heat available in either long-wave or short-wave diathermy machines. The long-wave diathermy machine is no longer used to a large extent in athletics. There is considerable danger involved unless the trainer is proficient in the use of this machine. The machine is a high-frequency apparatus, usually controlled by a spark gap. Its big advantage is the depth of the heat, but the control of this heat is very complicated and very hard to manage unless much time is spent in the application of the electrodes (conductors of the heat). The electrodes must be coated with a solution to make perfect contact, and must be curved and bent to fit the contours of the body. If they do not fit snugly, a hot spot results, and hence a burn. The electrodes must be strapped or wrapped so that they will not move; otherwise, a burn will result.

The heat produced by the short-wave diathermy machine is very evenly distributed and as equally effective. Therefore it has more or less replaced the conventional high-frequency type of apparatus. Short-wave diathermy is of short radiation wavelength and is produced by machines with oscillating tubes. There is no question of the value of this type of machine for the production of heat. It is well to remember that other means of heat can be as effective, and even simpler to apply, when treating a large area of injury or multiple injuries in several joints.

The electrodes vary, depending on the age and type of machine. Pads are applied to the body over toweling for air space, and drums are focused on the injury site, or the air-spaced electrodes may be applied directly to the skin. The "coil," or induction cable, with air spacing has been a useful electrode but has given way to the drum or the air-spaced electrode on an arm extending from the machine.

The application of short-wave diathermy should be prescribed by the team physician, and he should also stipulate the length of treatment. He may prescribe this modality for 20 minutes once or twice a day, either with massage or active or passive exercises. Care should be taken to see that the electrode is not applied over metal on the skin (such as an identification tag), since a severe burn will result.

Instructions for using this machine must be followed closely. All machines are clearly marked and are almost foolproof. Do not operate a machine without full knowledge of the instructions which accompany each diathermy apparatus on delivery.

Diathermy is indicated for deep injuries that may not be reached by heat from either whirlpool or other heat lamps. It is capable of deep penetration and is very effective in sprains of the back. Physiatrists are not in favor of applying diathermy over an acute joint injury. The reason is that there is usually not enough soft tissue to utilize the heat.

Microwave Diathermy. This is a fairly new modality of high frequency, with great value in localizing heat to a small area. By means of directors, the heat can be concentrated on a very small area without affecting all the surrounding tissues that will ordinarily absorb some of the heat from other more dispersed heat radiation lamps. The sizes of the directors are variable, from a small circular type to the oval and also to the longer director for larger areas. The machine may be used in conjunction with other modalities of treatments.

Microwave treatments have become very popular. Microwave therapy will reach peak temperatures faster than other modality and will show a rapid rise in temperature of deep tissues; the ratio of increase of temperature in the deep tissues will be greater than the skin temperature. It is a very effective form of heat for deep injuries, and the indications for use of this modality are deep sprains, strains and contusions.

Heat Pads. Heat pads produce a form of conductive heat which is applied to the body by means of continuity; i.e., the object is hot, and when applied to the body, the local temperature of that area of application is increased. Heat pads may be of a chemical nature (a chemical combines with water to produce heat and is enclosed in a covered pad to prevent burns) or contain electrically heated devices. They are indicated where long periods of heat are to be used, such as the low back area, when athlete is confined to bed, or in other similar conditions. When heat is used for a long period of time, the mild heat is very comfortable and relaxing. A heat pad with controls for low, medium, and high temperatures is superior to the single-switch type of only one heat. The use of the heat pad on low temperature for an extended time is most effective, and there is less chance of a burn resulting. Heat pads should be enclosed in a towel when used where perspiration is excessive.

Heat pads are very effective for home treatments, to supplement daily treatments in the training room. They are easily purchased and may be loaned out by the trainer or coach for home treatment.

Ultrasonic Vibration. Ultrasonics is a fairly new form of treatment and has become extremely popular in the treatment of athletic injuries. Ultrasonic energy is produced by a mechanical vibration identical to that of the sound of a human voice, various noises, and musical notes. Sound ordinarily vibrates at 20,000 cycles per second or less, but ultrasonic vibrations may be 100,000 or more cycles of vibration per second. The latest equipment has been designed for medical use at one million cycles per second.

Directions for the use of this piece of equipment are supplied with the purchase of the unit. Read them carefully, and if necessary, have a trained technician explain all the details. Ultrasonics is contraindicated in many regions of the body and the operator should be well acquainted with these areas.

The ultrasonic equipment should not be used indiscriminately, since this agent has a very specific effect upon body systems and therefore must be wisely applied if benefit of treatment is to be derived. The team physician should prescribe the treatment, amount of energy, method of treatment, and the amount of time for each treatment for each athlete.

In the treatment of injuries with ultrasonic waves, low intensities will be sedative, medium intensities will be very stimulative, and very high intensities may be destructive. When applied properly, pain will be reduced, and if applied with too high an intensity, pain will be provoked.

Ultrasonic energy will not pass through air, and the use of an agent to couple the energy and the tissues must be used. In direct application, mineral oil, glycerin, etc., is applied to the skin and then the sound head or transducer is pressed firmly into the tissue to eliminate an air space. If the sound head should not be in direct contact with the oil, etc., and should make contact with the dry skin, a slight shock may result.

The indirect treatment is used when the area is very sensitive and direct contact cannot be tolerated. This indirect treatment consists of underwater application. The injured part is immersed in water and the transducer or sound head is then submerged and placed directly at the site of injury. The sound head is held about 1 inch away from the injured surface, and the water will very effectively transmit the energy, permitting the same treatment that resulted with the use of oil, etc., on the skin.

Ultrasonics may be used in conjunction with other treatments such as whirlpool, short wave, or other physical measures.

The sound waves may be applied directly to an acute injury, even while the application of ice packs is being used. After the acute stage, the uses are the same as for diathermy treatments. Ultrasonic waves will aid in the absorption of calcium deposits.

Galvanism. A galvanic machine delivers a low-frequency current that is used to stimulate muscles. It is used more for the testing of muscle function than it is for actual treatment in athletics. The specific conditions for which galvanism may be indicated are injuries to nerves or muscles that are fibrosed. To restore power and function in muscles, active motions are the best. However, the use of galvanic currents may help this condition because the contractions are not voluntary but are forced by the stimulus of an interrupted electric current. This is a type of treatment that is not frequently seen in the training rooms today.

Faradic and Sinusoidal Currents. These are currents that are interrupted and are used similarly to the galvanic current. The same comments may be made for this equipment as for the galvanic machine.

The faradic current is produced by an induction coil and causes sharp stinging sensations when applied to the body. It is not used as a form of treatment as much as for testing of muscles.

Sinusoidal current is produced by passing the current through a rhythmically varying resistance which periodically reverses the direction of flow of the current. The rhythmic waves may be varied in intensity and length. It is a current that is not stinging in nature, but it is effective for soothing sore muscles.

Vibrators. A vibrator is a very useful type of equipment. It is usually portable and very handy for a soothing massage. Its benefits for the treatment of injuries may be questioned, but it does have a soothing effect when incorporated with a local massage. It is a very inexpensive piece of equipment and many uses are found for this in the training room.

Whirlpool Bath. Because of its effectiveness, the whirlpool bath is very common, being seen in most training rooms. It combines moisture with heat and is therefore a very effective modality. Water at a temperature above body temperature is agitated in a tub and this motion of the water gives a mild massage that produces a hyperemia (redness) and stimulates blood flow. The usual temperature prescribed is between 106 and 110 degrees. The duration of the bath is usually 20 minutes.

The agitation of the water by means of aeration or by a motor-driven turbine will cause a vigorous action of the water which is very effective for the loosening of stiff joints, softening of scars, promotion of healing, and the loosening of tissues. A particular advantage of the whirlpool bath is that the athlete is able to exercise the limb while being immersed in the water.

We are inclined to use the whirlpool as the only modality available because of its ease in operation. All that is necessary is to put the limb in the tank and turn on a switch. It becomes a lazy man's necessity. The early application of the whirlpool may promote hemorrhage because of the necessity of lowering the limb into the tub for the treatment. In our early treatment of an acute injury, we stress elevation, but by recommending the use of the whirlpool, we contradict ourselves. We do not use the whirlpool until a considerable time has elapsed from the onset of the injury. We have seen too many "normal in size" limbs immersed in the whirlpool come out with a considerable amount of swelling, thus causing aching and much discomfort. The production of swelling will retard the healing time, and of course this is a very important factor. Where moist heat is indicated, we use hot towels, applied in elevation, or infrared lamps directed over moist towels also applied in elevation.

In the case of an ankle sprain, we will not use the whirlpool until the athlete has been weight bearing for a few days. The same is true with a knee or other limbs.

Whirlpool treatments are indicated in all sprains, strains, and contusions which can benefit from a modality of moist heat application. They may be used prior to massage and various types of rehabilitation exercises but are not recommended in the acute stage of a sprain.

Whirlpool has the ability to remain at a known temperature throughout the treatment and is known for its ease of application.

Hydrocollator. This provides moist heat to an area by use of a chemical pack (salicylate gel) which has been previously heated in a controlled steam cabinet. The packs are kept in water and are constantly heated. By wrapping the pack in a towel, it may be applied to the area and left in place for the length of time prescribed (usually 20 to 30 minutes, and sometimes longer). This is a very safe application of moist heat to an area, provided insulation (either towels or a special cover) is used. The packs are effective for fairly deep, moist heat, are easily applied, and may be used over and over again.

This piece of equipment is of low cost and provides excellent heat. By having several packs, more than one athlete can be treated at a time.

The hydrocollator is very effective for moist heat treatments for a period of about 30 minutes. It is indicated in all sprains, strains, and contusions and can be used very effectively before massage and exercises. Hydrocollator applications are very relaxing by producing enough heat that will be superficial in nature.

Contrast Baths. The contrast bath is a very simple method of producing a hyperemia (redness of skin) and consists of applying alternating hot and cold applications to the injured area. The first and the last applications are always with hot water. The time for each type of application is variable, from a 10 to 1 (10 minutes hot to 1 minute cold) to the more common figures of 4 to 1 (4 minutes hot to 1 minute cold). The length of time for the treatment is usually 20 minutes. This type of treatment is very popular because there is no need for equipment and therefore it may be used very effectively in the home. Immersion in buckets, etc., is not so effective as the actual use of a hose attached to the faucet, spraying first with the hot water, then changing to the cold water at the intervals prescribed. Application of towels, either hot or cold, is also a very effective means of applying the contrast bath.

Except for the use on the limbs, this is a very difficult treatment for an athlete to apply to his back. However, the use of the shower may be made to substitute for the hose or towels.

Temperatures of the water should be: hot water about 102 degrees Fahrenheit, and the cold application between 40 to 50 degrees Fahrenheit.

Hot Baths. Hot or warm baths are a very effective means of eliminating general soreness of the body after a game. Water will eliminate the loss of heat from the body, and heat is readily conducted from the water to the tissues. Hot water is by far the best method of raising body temperature and therefore it may be dangerous. Hot baths should be limited to not more than 30 minutes, and the athlete should be supplied with salt tablets and water to drink to prevent exhaustion that may result from the loss of fluids from the long exposure to the heat.

The baths should be started at about 98 degrees, gradually increasing the temperature of the water to about 105 degrees. If the athlete steps into the tub with the temperature at the maximum, unusual side effects may result.

Too long an exposure to hot baths has a tendency to exhaust the athlete, to make him listless and logy, and also produces excessive perspiration. The use of long, hot baths is usually not indicated in athletics, but when indicated, an interruption by taking a cold bath will help to invigorate the tissues.

Steam Baths or Cabinet Baths. This is a very effective method of relieving the aches and pains of multiple contusions on Sunday after a very rough game on Saturday. In the use of this procedure, the athlete does not have to remain in the "hot area" for more than 15 minutes. After the treatment, the use of a hot shower followed by a cold shower is very effective. In winter months the athlete should be thoroughly cooled down before he enters the elements. This is accomplished by taking a nap for about an hour after the bath.

Paraffin Baths. Another means of applying local heat to a small area is by means of a paraffin bath. Paraffin melted over a double boiler in mineral oil (mixed about ten to one, ten parts paraffin to one part mineral oil) is heated to about 120 degrees, allowed to cool, and then the limb is immersed quickly into the paraffin and immediately withdrawn. Paraffin will adhere to the skin and repeated dips will thicken the paraffin coating. Remove when paraffin is about ⅛ inch thick, cover with a towel, and retain this condition for about 30 minutes. If the area is particularly hairy, mineral oil applied to the skin will prevent the paraffin from adhering to the hairs. After the treatment, the paraffin can be peeled off and then reheated.

This treatment must be well supervised because the possibility of a burn is quite prevalent. Paraffin baths are used for fingers, hands, feet, and the lower leg. Paraffin baths will produce the maximal amount of conductive heat to the parts, but we fail to see its advantages over the whirlpool bath or just plain hot soaks.

Hot Packs. This is a form of treatment that owes its origin to athletic trainers. It is used universally for the treatment of injuries in athletics and has many advantages:

1. It is easy to apply.
2. No expensive machines, etc., are necessary.
3. Heat is local and may be varied from intense to mild.
4. The athlete is able to perform while action of treatment is working.
5. It allows for the longer application of heat to an injured part.

The "hot pack" is made by applying a counterirritant to the skin, covering this with cotton, and then applying a snug elastic bandage. The counterirritant produces the heat, the cotton holds the heat in, and the elastic bandage will, because of its elasticity, present a local massaging action each time the area is moved.

A counterirritant or hot ointment is made of a petrolatum or similar ingredient as a base and then the addition of oil of wintergreen, capsicum, or any other irritant. The mixture must be in proportion to prevent the possibility of a burn. Many on the market are very effective and reasonably priced, so it is just as economical to buy a ready-made preparation as to try to make it yourself. The manufactured products have been thoroughly tested, whereas the "home made" may have a few flaws that may produce a burn or irritation to the skin.

MASSAGE AND EXERCISE

Massage. A very ancient method of treatment, which seems to come and go with the years, is massage. Today it has taken a back seat to the physical methods more recently developed. However, massage is indicated in most injuries. The application immediately over the site of injury may be delayed until tolerable, but the use of massage above and below the site is necessary for proper treatment. In recent years the method has been neglected, but fortunately for many athletes, it is now making a comeback. Hippocrates realized the value of massage many years ago when he advocated the rubbing of the injury with soft hands in a gentle motion, combining this with mild exercise, without producing pain.

Massage is the scientific and systematic manipulation of the tissues for therapeutic purposes. Massage will increase circulation, thus bringing better nutrition and drainage to the injured area. Massage may be stimulating or sedative. The sedative type is used mostly in the treatment of athletic injuries.

Three types of movements are used in medical massage. They are: stroking, kneading, and friction. *Stroking* is technically known as *effleurage*. It is a stroking movement, with the palm of the hand applied directly to the skin with a firm and even motion. Stroking may be light or deep and consists of long sweeping movements following the contours of the body. The more pressure, the deeper the massage. The direction of the stroke is toward the heart; the return motion of the hands should be very light but should remain in contact with the skin.

Kneading, technically known as *petrissage,* consists of wringing the tissues by compression methods. Tissues may be lifted, rolled, or squeezed, with variable intensities of pressure. Kneading may be deep or superficial, depending on the area being treated.

Friction massage consists of deep, circular rolling movements with the tips of the fingers, palms of the hands or thumbs. It is used for the breaking down of scars or chronic conditions around joints and helps to loosen stiff and sore muscles by hastening absorption of fatigue products. The use of a lubricant is unnecessary. Again, the type of friction may be deep or superficial, depending on the condition to be treated. Even though friction massage has been prescribed, the treatment is always preceded and concluded by stroking.

When massaging, use a lubricant of some kind (unless friction massage is ordered). The more hair on the skin, the more lubricant will be needed. Mineral oil, cocoa butter, olive oil, petroleum jelly, or talcum powder may be used. In the case of a massage with a counterirritant (hot liniment, usually made by adding wintergreen, etc., to the oil), be careful that this does not burn or get into vital areas, such as the eyes.

Massage should be started from the distant part of the limb and directed toward the heart. After several stroking movements, kneading may be applied. After sufficient kneading is performed, finish the massage with several stroking movements.

Exercise. Exercise is a very important part of the physical therapy treatment. To rely on physical therapy alone without exercises will not produce the results needed for active recovery. Exercises have many physiological effects:

1. They increase circulation.
2. They increase muscular strength.
3. They prevent atrophy.
4. They assist normal range of motion.
5. They help re-establish motion.

Passive exercises. Passive exercises are performed primarily by the trainer. He puts the injured part of the athlete through the full range of motion of the exercises indicated. The athlete will not participate in the movement. Passive exercises are rarely used in athletics. The primary form of exercise indicated is active rather than passive. Passive exercises are used in the event of paralysis or other nerve involvements. Passive exercises should not produce pain or muscle spasm; if they do, they are no longer passive exercises. Stretching is considered a part of passive exercise. Stretching should be regulated and handled carefully.

Active assistive exercises. The athlete attempts to do the exercise, with the trainer assisting him. This type of exercise is used primarily in stiff joints and is prescribed in post-fracture work where there has been immobilization and a loss of function in the area because of lack of use. This type of treatment requires considerable judgment on the part of the trainer in determining the amount of forcing indicated. Pain will result, but if it disappears readily, the force has not been too great. Pain over a period of hours after the treatment is evidence of too much forcing and should be avoided.

Active exercises. Active exercises are those which the athlete performs by himself. They are the most preferable type of exercise in the athletic program. Active exercises promote full range of motion, prevent atrophy, stimulate circulation, strengthen muscles, and condition athletes. Active exercises are given in tolerance, and the number of repetitions is regulated according to the ability of the athlete.

Active resistive exercises. The athlete performs certain exercises with resistance, i.e., quadriceps exercises performed with weights attached to foot. Weight training, pulleys, medicine balls, etc., are considered active exercises with resistance. This type of program plays a very large part in athletics and is used quite frequently for the rehabilitation of an injury.

GENERAL COMMENTS

Dr. Ernst Jokl stated in his book, *The Clinical Physiology of Physical Fitness and Rehabilitation,** that "the use of exercise in clinical practice is the most neglected sector of medical therapy." There is a tendency to apply physical means of therapy to the athlete and then dismiss him. All treatments should be followed by a form of exercise, either passive or active. Physical methods (machines, etc.) will not completely rehabilitate the athlete. Therapeutic exercises are more important than some of the physical agents used for some conditions. In an ankle injury, for example, if the normal gait is not established as soon as possible, the athlete will be delayed in his return to activity. The same holds true with all other joints in the body.

* Ernst Jokl, M.D., *The Clinical Physiology of Physical Fitness and Rehabilitation* (Springfield, Illinois: Charles C Thomas, Publishers, 1958).

Do not be in a hurry to apply heat to a new injury. The early and vigorous treatment of an acute injury may cause further hemorrhage, thus resulting in delayed recovery. The physical methods are for assistance to the injury; they do not represent a cure-all. The body will "work" on the injury and proper help will enhance the recovery. The trainer or technician does not effect a "cure"; he only assists. Dr. Bilik states that "heat in itself has no curative powers that we are aware of, but by producing an active hyperemia, profoundly influences the physiology of the body, locally or generally, as desired, with beneficial effects."

Part II

Injuries of Body Areas

Chapter 8

Head and Neck

FRACTURES

Skull. In a serious skull injury the presence of a fracture is incidental to injury to the brain itself. Some fractures of the skull (namely, the linear fractures) may present no symptoms of fracture at all. There also may not be any symptoms of concussion in this injury. Fractures of the skull may be of all types, simple, compound, etc. There is a common type of fracture of the skull, namely, depressed fracture, that is not listed in types of fractures and is associated with the head: injury caused by a sharp blow to the head, knee on head, or head-on collision.

The athlete may not be conscious, so that a history from him will be lacking. Coaches will be able to give a complete story that will help. Symptoms are:

Conscious or unconscious.
Pulse may be very slow.
Respiration may be labored.
Vomiting (indicates cranial pressure).
Bleeding from openings, ears, nose, or mouth.
Pupils of the eyes may be unequal, large, or pinpointed.
Twitching, localized pressure.
Bleeding from ears (fracture at base of skull).

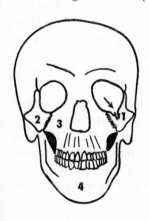

The skull, front view. (1) Fracture of the zygoma. (2) Zygomatic bone. (3) Maxilla. (4) Mandible.

Treatment. The athlete should be moved from the area only on a stretcher. Keep him absolutely quiet, with ice packs to head and blankets to remainder of body to prevent shock. Summon the team physician immediately.

Do not attempt to give liquids; do not allow athlete to sit up.

The use of an ammonia inhalant may be indicated, but the athlete should be cautioned as to strength of inhalant so as not to cause a twitching of the head as a result of the sting.

Bed rest and complete quiet are indicated for a long period of time and disability varies with the injury. Many team physicians will not allow the athlete to participate in contact sports as a result of this injury.

Fractures of the Face. A heavy impact injury, such as bumping heads or a direct blow to the face by a knee or helmet are the contributing causes of fractures of the face. A misguided elbow in basketball has also been the mechanical factor in this injury. The bones involved are the maxilla, zygoma, the zygomatic arch, and the temporal bones. These are located in the upper part of the head and face and are classified as upper-jaw fractures.

History will reveal the cause of the injury. Palpation will demonstrate the change in contour; possibly roughened ends of the bone may be felt, a slight depression may be felt, and point tenderness will be very evident. Inspection may or may not reveal swelling; comparison with the other cheek will reveal a difference, and the injury may be accompanied by a break in the skin.

Treatment of suspected fractures of the upper jaw is very simple on the level of the trainer. Apply ice and transport for medical attention. Athlete should be instructed not to blow nose, as swelling may become pronounced with this action.

Fracture of Lower Jaw. Diagnosis of fracture of lower jaw can be made by examination of the contour of the bone. The jaw bone (mandible) is immediately below the skin, and the outline may be traced with the fingers. Very often the teeth of the upper and lower jaws do not meet in normal position. A tender spot may be found as you palpate the jaw bone.

Treatment consists of immobilizing the jaw with a four-tail bandage and referral to dental surgeon for further treatment.

Disability varies with the degree of fracture and its location. Protective devices are available so that athlete may continue sports without too much loss of time. By necessity the athlete is on a liquid diet and this should be a governing factor as to the sport that the athlete can play with this condition.

Broken Nose. Nose fracture is the most common fracture of the face. The injury may result in fracture of the bones, cartilages, or a combination of both. Simple fracture may not be too obvious, but the more serious are easily observable. Again, swelling is immediate and generally profuse. Other symptoms are deformity and crepitus. History and inspection will help diagnosis. Palpation should be very gentle; crepitus may be felt quite easily.

Reduction of fracture should be done by a physician qualified to perform this treatment. Aside from the cosmetic value, the nose should be treated completely, since fracture may cause some impairment in breathing at a later date.

The athlete should be cautioned not to blow nose and advised to breathe through the mouth.

Disability depends on the severity of fracture. A simple fracture may be reduced readily, and with a protective mask, the athlete may return to duty in a few days. In the more severe type of fracture, it may be weeks before active participation is advised.

DISLOCATION OF JAW

In this injury the lower jaw is found to protrude forward in a majority of cases and the teeth of the upper and lower jaw do not meet. Dislocation may occur on one side or both. Review the anatomy of the jaw and you will note that the jaw is held in place by ligaments and muscles. Being a supple joint, injury is quite easily sustained by a direct blow to the jaw. The tissues are forced beyond normal limitations and a dislocation results. The blow can be a direct one or one that glances slightly to one side. The upper end of the jaw "slips out" of position, resulting in stretching of the ligaments and muscles. Symptoms are pain, overbite, and inability to move jaw.

Treatment consists of reduction of jaw bone. After reduction, a four-tailed bandage is used for immobilization, along with ice packs. Disability is from a few days to three weeks, depending on the injury and the sport.

Reduction should be performed by the team physician, since there is a possibility that other bone injury may be present. X-ray is used in diagnosis and should be taken before reduction.

To reduce dislocation, wrap both thumbs in gauze, place thumbs on back molars with fingers around lower jaw. Push down and backward, while pulling the jaw forward with the fingers. This is to be a steady traction rather than a jerking movement. When the jaw is

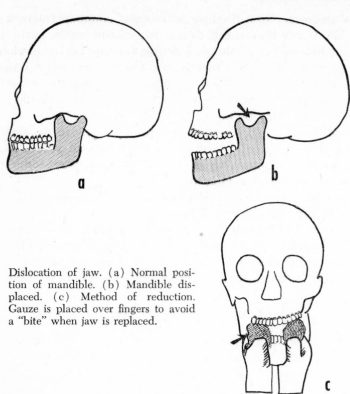

Dislocation of jaw. (a) Normal position of mandible. (b) Mandible displaced. (c) Method of reduction. Gauze is placed over fingers to avoid a "bite" when jaw is replaced.

reduced, it does so with a snap, and a bite may result if thumbs are not protected.

SYMPTOMS OF HEAD INJURIES

Head injuries require immediate medical attention. The trainer, therefore, must be able to recognize quickly the indications of such injury. The following symptoms demand fast action:

1. *Loss of consciousness.* This may be momentary or for a prolonged period of time. The longer the condition remains, the more damage to the brain will be evident.
2. *Blurring of vision.* The athlete will report a fogginess to his vision. He may also complain of seeing double or only half an object.
3. *Amnesia.* This follows all concussions, and if it persists, a more extensive examination is indicated.
4. *Vomiting.* This may or may not occur. It is the result of a severe injury and should be considered as a serious symptom if it occurs after the injury has supposedly quieted down.

5. *Headache.* This is a consequence of all head injuries. The length of time it lasts is a very important consideration. If headache persists, it may indicate a laceration to the brain or a more serious complication.
6. *Paralysis.* This is a very important symptom. The athlete should not be moved from the area without medical supervision if any paralysis is evident.
7. *Convulsion.* This is a very serious complication of a head injury. The athlete must be tended by a physician while in this state. Hold him loosely so that he will not hurt himself and apply a plug of some kind in mouth to prevent swallowing of tongue or the biting of tongue.
8. *Disorientation.* The athlete will look "foggy" and he will not know where he is or what happened to him.
9. *Rigidity or coma.* This is a very serious condition. Do not remove from area without medical supervision.
10. *Unequal eye pupils.* Pupils will react to light by contracting. When pupils are "fixed," enlarged, or abnormally small, they are evidence of injury to brain and are an important symptom of concussion.

HEAD INJURIES

An injury to the head is always a perplexing injury. Fortunately we do not see very many of them. All sports contribute their share, and for the number of athletes participating, the incidence is very low.

The unconscious athlete presents a very complex injury when seen on the field. He may be absolutely quiet or he may be in the process of a convulsion. Don't panic, but treat each symptom as you see it. If he is rolling and thrashing, quiet him so that he will not hurt himself. Check for air passages and be sure that breathing is adequate. Be prepared to apply a "plug" or something to keep mouth open for proper breathing. An oral screw, two or three tongue blades taped together, or a half-used roll of gauze will perform this function. If the athlete is in the process of vomiting, turn head so that it can be emitted. A head injury with any of the above conditions should not be moved from the playing field unless supervised by a physician, and then only on a stretcher.

By the time that you arrive on the scene the athlete may appear to be normal. He will wonder what has happened, who hit him, etc. His eyes will be normal, reflexes normal, and the answers to routine questions will be normal. (Questions such as time of day, the score, the place of the contest, the day of the week, the opponent, etc.) This type of injury should be further checked by the team physician before the injured man is permitted to play again. The time elapsed in this type of injury may be from a few minutes to the better part of the game. If all responses are normal, the athlete may continue to play.

The athlete who is still unconscious when you arrive on the scene presents a different picture. There will be more than a momentary unconsciousness and procedure will vary as to the treatment. These injuries are classed in three categories: mild, medium, and severe.

Concussion. A concussion is a blow to the head; so, any time an athlete has been hit on the head, he has had a concussion. There are all degrees of "hits on the head" and to put them in a single category would not be doing justice to the athlete or to the sport. The degree of concussion may be divided into three categories: mild, medium, and severe. Each injury should be handled as a separate condition and evaluation taken from the start. To say that an athlete should not participate with a history of three concussions does not present a true basis of disqualification. Sometimes one concussion may be enough to limit the athlete to nonparticipation in contact sports. Each individual is subject to varying degrees of injury, and therefore a concussion is a highly individualized matter and should be treated accordingly.

The first category, which is the largest, is where the athlete has been hit on the head, resulting in a momentary loss of consciousness. He may seem to recover immediately, but there is a period of disorientation which results. The recovery is usually uneventful; mental and physical faculties recover in a short time. In a concussion of this type a 24-hour observation period should be mandatory. We admit an athlete to the infirmary and an hourly check is made in this period of time. If all is well, the athlete is discharged from the infirmary and put on a noncontact disability. He may be able to run, etc., but will not be allowed to participate in contact drills. This disability usually lasts for one week, after which the athlete may return to full duty.

In the hourly check-up the following are observed:

1. Consciousness.
2. Pupil reaction.
3. Pulse.
4. Function of limbs, etc., and reflexes.
5. Headache.
6. Visual disturbances.
7. Nausea.

It is quite possible that the above symptoms may not be noted the first day but may occur at any time after the injury. Any of the above symptoms, when reported, should be immediately relayed to the team physician.

In the second category, a medium concussion, the athlete is unconscious more than a few seconds. The longer the recovery, the greater indication that there has been some damage to the brain itself. The athlete should be hospitalized and checked every hour. In this injury X-ray examination should be included.

Symptoms found in this injury are:

1. Nausea and vomiting.
2. Headache.
3. Grogginess.
4. Neurological findings, numbness, loss of function, etc.
5. Pulse should be steady.
6. Respiration may be labored and variable.
7. Blood pressure should be stable for at least 24 hours.
8. Drowsiness.
9. Pupils may be varied (one larger than the other).

The athlete should be kept still until all symptoms are clear, and then he should not be allowed to participate for at least one week; then light work may be started, gradually increasing the following week. Disability will be at least two weeks.

In the third category, the severe concussion, the athlete remains unconscious for a longer period of time. The longer the time for recovery, the more severe damage to the brain. Injury of this type may be associated with a fracture of the skull, and X-ray examination should be included in the routine examination. The athlete should be moved to the hospital for further examination, which should include the services of a neurosurgeon. In an injury of this type the athlete should be removed from the playing area on a stretcher. Do not attempt to roll him over or have him sit up. Keeping him still is of the utmost importance. Make sure that all airways are open so that breathing will not be interrupted. Also see that throat is clear in case the athlete chooses to vomit. Turning his head to the side will help to eliminate the above problems.

The symptoms in the second category may be found in a more severe state, and each should be checked out:

1. Nausea and vomiting.
2. Headache.
3. Grogginess.
4. Neurological findings.
5. Pulse.

6. Respiration.
7. Blood pressure.
8. Drowsiness.
9. Pupil reactions and size.

A severe concussion will have as a complication a skull fracture or neurological findings, and this type of injury results in a permanent disability of the athlete. He will not be allowed to participate in contact sports for the remainder of his time in college.

SPRAIN OF JAW

This occurs in the same manner as a dislocation but without the subluxation. (Subluxation is an incomplete or partial dislocation.) By being hit on the chin, the mandible (jaw bone) is forced beyond normal range of motion, and muscles and ligaments are stretched. There will be pain without loss of function. A slight deviation in the bite may be observed, owing to muscle spasm.

Treatment consists of ice packs for 24 hours. After that, heat and exercise is indicated. Applications of hot towels are very effective. The variation of the bite will leave as soon as the spasm is gone, usually in a day or two. No disability derives from this injury.

CONTUSIONS OF FACE AND HEAD

One of the most common injuries to the head is the bruise. We see this injury in all sports; none is exempt. With the introduction and use of the face mask in football, this injury has decreased in this sport. Hockey and basketball produce some of these injuries. Bruises about the head and face swell quite profusely and many times are quite awesome. Lips particularly are very prone to profuse swelling and, in turn, are very discomforting. Discoloration is also very common. It is interesting to note that very often the discoloration may not be at the direct site of the blow. Sometimes a jolt to the head will result in the "blacking of the eyes."

Hematoma is an organized mass of blood resulting from an injury to blood vessels. If, in an injury, the blood does not infiltrate the tissues, it will remain in a localized area and be visible to the eye and fluctuant to feel. When the blood is organized, it will absorb slowly. Blood usually remains in a liquid state but may clot as time goes by. Aspiration at an early date plus compression will hasten recovery. After the blood clots, an incision and drainage procedure may be needed.

Excellent results in treating this injury are attained by the prolonged use of ice. The circulation of the head is so complex and

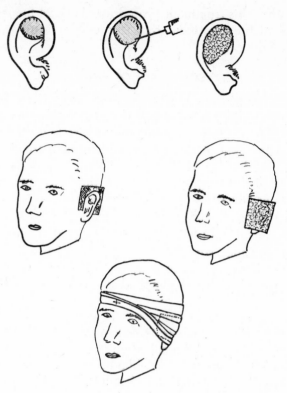

Hematoma as a result of bruise to ear. Aspiration is performed by the team physician. After aspiration, cotton soaked in collodion is placed in back as well as in front of ear, and a snug elastic wrap is applied.

profuse that bleeding, when it is started, may be hard to control. Treatments are designed to control the amount of hemorrhage in the area. Caution must be used in the application of heat or the bleeding may start again. Cold treatment applied in the form of cold, moist packs works very well. They are not only soothing but also very effective in the control of hemorrhage and in hastening absorption.

Protection must be afforded the athlete when he returns to his activity. Contusion of scalp should be thoroughly investigated. Very often such a condition may result in damage elsewhere in the skull. Observation must be the watchword in the first 24 hours.

Bruises to the scalp many times result in a hematoma; treatment consists of compression and ice. Pressure by means of a cold pack will spread the hematoma and hasten absorption. Ice in a towel, with manual pressure over the site, will be best applied by the athlete himself. This treatment is used for about 24 hours, and most times this is all the treatment that is needed. Results are usually rapid in this injury.

CONTUSION OF EAR

The contusion of the ear is often times referred to as a "cauliflower ear." The injury is caused by trauma, bruising, or by rubbing of the ear as in wrestling. A hematoma manifests itself between the cartilage and the skin of the auricle and forms a small lump. The mass, if left, will harden and become a permanent scar. Aspiration is the process of drawing off fluids from the body, performed by a physician under the strictest of aseptic conditions.

Treatment. If seen early, the use of ice and a compression wrap will help to control the hemorrhage and prevent further formation. The compression may squeeze the blood out of the area. If blood formation is evident, aspiration may be indicated. After aspiration, a compression wrap should be applied so that the ear will not fill up again.

To apply a compression wrap to the ear, apply cotton under the ear as well as on top of the ear, and then encircle the head with an elastic bandage. The use of a collodion pack after aspiration is very effective for compression. Apply collodion to the ear and then add strips of cotton so that the auricle is filled. Several applications of cotton and collodion may be needed. This compression should be applied for at least a week, and then protection applied to lessen the recurrence of the incident.

SCALP WOUNDS

Open wounds of the scalp and head area will bleed quite profusely. With this amount of bleeding evident, the wound takes on an important aspect and becomes very alarming. A very small laceration will bleed so that it will be completely occluded with blood in a very short time. Wounds of the scalp are very common and no sport is exempt. The wound may be very small or quite extensive. The bleeding that takes place will mechanically cleanse the wound.

Treatment. Control the bleeding by using a sterile gauze pad applied directly to the wound with pressure. When bleeding has stopped, the team physician will decide as to whether the wound will need suturing. If suturing is not indicated, apply an antiseptic and a sterile dressing to the wound. A dressing may be difficult to hold in place and therefore a collodion dressing may be indicated. A collodion dressing is waterproof and very stable.

Wounds that are sutured should also be dressed; again, the collodion dressing is indicated. To apply a collodion dressing, a small amount of collodion is needed plus sterile gauze. Cut a piece of gauze slightly larger than the wound, place on wound, and apply collodion to the dressing. The dressing will take a few minutes to dry, and the athlete may go back into action when it is firm. The athlete should not wash the area and should be careful in combing his hair, as the possibility of dislodging the dressing may occur.

When the dressing is to be removed, the use of acetone to soften the collodion may be used, being careful not to allow the acetone to get into the eyes.

ABRASIONS OF THE FACE

Very often abrasions of the face will be very dirty. Cleanse the wound with soap and water. Some abrasions may have to be cleansed with a small brush. Continual soaking in water or running a hot shower over the abrasion will help to cleanse the wound.

Treatment consists of the cleansing of the wound and the application of an antiseptic along with an ointment dressing. The ointment may be a bland ointment to keep the dressing from adhering to the wound or an antibiotic dressing in lieu of the antiseptic. Abrasions will ooze for a short period of time, and a dressing will help to control the oozing. After the oozing has stopped, the dressing may be discarded.

A controversy exists as to the application of an ointment to an abrasion. Many feel that the wound should not be dressed with an ointment, and others feel that it should be covered. Air exposure will dry the wound faster than the ointment, and an early scab formation is desirable. However, the wound will ooze and be very uncomfortable, and for this reason a dressing is indicated. After the abrasion has stopped oozing, then the dressing may be discarded. The application of a "stain" type of antiseptic to the face is unsightly and not desirable. The use of an antiseptic that is clear is a much neater means of handling the abrasion.

LACERATED TONGUE

This is caused by biting the tongue as a result of a blow to the head. Laceration may be simple to extensive. Small lacerations that do not present gaping wounds will heal without benefit of suturing. Wounds that are large and spread should be approximated by suture.

Treatment consists of keeping wound clean; this will include food particles as well as other matter. The irrigation of clean warm water will clean the wound nicely. Painting the tongue with tincture of benzoin is painful but very beneficial. Sucking on ice will lessen the degree of swelling of the tongue. Wounds heal very readily and the athlete may return to action in a day or two.

NOSE BLEED (Epistaxis)

The most common cause of nose bleed in athletics is a direct blow to the nose. Small blood vessels are ruptured and bleeding may be slight to profuse.

Pressure with a cold compress for a few minutes will usually stop the bleeding. The use of gauze plugs in the nostrils will give more pressure and compress the blood vessels so that bleeding will stop. If bleeding cannot be stopped by these methods, the athlete should be referred to the team physician for further treatment.

In packing the nose, the packs should be applied gently and with the course of the nostrils, not up the nose toward the head but straight back. These packs may be removed in a few minutes and the athlete may return to duty. He should be cautioned not to blow his nose because this will start the bleeding again. The use of a cool rinse will aid in comfort of the athlete on his return to action.

TEETH

Loose Teeth. Blows to the mouth will loosen teeth; when the teeth are disturbed, bleeding may result. Loosened teeth should not be treated; however, if crooked, they may be straightened and the athlete sent to dentist for treatment.

Many loose teeth will eventually tighten and serve as good teeth. This is a long process and immediate results are not to be expected. Athlete should be cautioned not to eat hard foods such as apples at this time.

The use of a mouthpiece fitted to the teeth will protect teeth from further injury. Thermal changes, hot foods, or cold foods or drinks may aggravate the condition, and the athlete should govern himself accordingly.

Broken Teeth. Unfortunately broken teeth result in a permanent loss; many may be prevented by the use of a mouthpiece. There are a number on the market that can be worn without any discomfort. This piece of equipment is a must in the prevention of injuries to the teeth.

An athlete with a broken tooth or teeth should be sent immediately to the dentist so that emergency treatment can be started. Very often the pain in a broken tooth may not start until later in the evening. At this time help is hard to get. Make a practice of sending this case to the dentist early.

NECK

When the neck is forced to go beyond its normal limitations and motions, an injury will result. Neck injuries are the result of a sudden whipping action of the head, a head-on blow, or a blow to the head which would cause a twisting action. Fractures, dislocations, and sprains are the result of these motions.

Fractures. Fractures of the neck are rare. They may occur with a dislocation or they may be an injury by themselves. They are caused by a severe torsion effect of the head, hitting head on, or by a blow to the head. In the more serious fractures of the neck, the athlete is unable to handle himself. If paralysis is evident, do not move the athlete without medical supervision. To do so may cause a very serious complication. The team physician will advise moving and the possibility of traction.

In the less severe fracture, where the athlete is able to move his limbs, complete immobilization of neck and spine should be performed before transportation from the area is attempted.

Symptoms of a fracture are pain, deformity, stiffness, point tenderness, neck "locked" in a fixed position, and the inability to move.

Splinting before removal is very necessary to prevent further damage. After splinting, move only one time, and then directly to hospital.

Dislocations. Fortunately, dislocations of the neck are very rare in athletics. When they occur, they are caused by the same mechanics as a fracture, and very often the two are found together. A severe wrench to the neck will cause a tightening of the neck, and immediate pain and stiffness will result. The neck will be fixed in a very abnormal position. The muscles on the injured side are very tight, whereas the muscles on the opposite side are very loose. Any attempt to move the neck will result in severe pain. The degree of dislocation will result in paralysis, or partial paralysis, or no paralysis at all. If paralysis is present, this is an indication that there has been damage to the spinal cord.

Under no circumstances should you move an injured player who shows evidence of paralysis except under the supervision of the team physician. Moving this type of dislocation is a very important step in the management of this injury. Do not handle any more than necessary. The athlete should be moved only once, from the area to the hospital, without a stop at the training room. Complete immobilization is indicated. The use of traction will be decided upon by the team physician. Transportation should be by ambulance *only*.

After ruling out the possibility of fracture or dislocation to the neck, the injury may be treated as strain of the muscles or intervertebral ligaments of the area. The history of the injury will greatly enhance the handling. The athlete will report a severe wrenching of the head and a resulting soreness in the muscles of the neck. He will pinpoint the soreness with his fingers. Inspection may or may not reveal a tilting of the head to one side. Palpation will reveal tenderness over the site and tightness of the muscles in the localized area.

Treatment. In the early stages, during the first 24 hours, the use of a collar will rest the neck muscles and offer much relief to symptoms. Along with the collar, mild heat and massage is indicated. Light exercises may be started when tolerable, usually on the second or third day. The athlete should not be permitted to resume

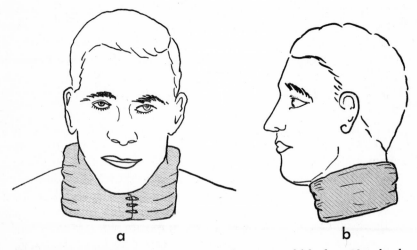

a   b

(a) Front view of collar for sprained neck muscle. A piece of felt about 18 inches long is enclosed in stockinette and pinned together with safety pins. The width of the felt varies with the length of the neck; usually a 3-inch width is sufficient. (b) Side view showing the fitting of collar for sprained neck muscles.

play until full range of motion has returned. The collar may be eliminated when the athlete is comfortable. The use of a towel or muffler wrapped around the neck while sleeping aids in relaxing the muscles of the neck. Disability varies in neck strains from a day or two to a week or ten days.

A collar may be fashioned by using a piece of half-inch felt about 3 inches wide and about 18 inches long. The felt is wrapped with gauze or inserted in surgical tubing. The collar is then applied snugly to the neck to hold the head firmly and in an extended position. The athlete is instructed to wear this brace at all times, even while sleeping.

Contusion of Neck. A contusion to the neck area is not a common injury, but when seen, usually does not present a serious problem. The blow will render the muscles stiff but will not cause any further damage to the tissues.

Treatment is symptomatic; heat and massage relieve the stiffness. The range of motion returns very rapidly, and the disability is not very long, maybe a day or two, and then full activity may be resumed.

Contusion of Throat. This is not a common injury but one that occurs upon occasion. A direct blow to the "Adam's apple" results in a very painful condition. The pain will be very acute, there will be spasmodic coughing, and possibly blood may be produced. Swallowing will be painful, and talking will be an effort. Palpation will reveal much tenderness. Treatment consists of the immediate application of ice to the area to control and lessen the degree of hemorrhage. The team physician should be consulted immediately to check air passages and prescribe further treatment.

In the mild contusion, after the application of ice, a Thomas collar is very effective for the splinting and resting of the neck. After the first 24 hours, heat will be very helpful in relieving symptoms of pain and hoarseness.

Chapter 9

Trunk and Back

ANATOMY OF SPINE

The spine is a very flexible column of bones, one placed on top of the other. Starting with the head and going down the back, the first 24 vertebrae are movable and are called the *true vertebrae*. The cervical vertebrae (neck), number seven, the thoracic (trunk), number twelve, and the lumbar (low back) complete the column with five. The fifth lumbar joins the pelvis at the sacrum, which is composed of five incomplete vertebrae fused together, while the coccyx (tail bone) is composed of four incomplete vertebrae and is the final portion of the spinal column.

A vertebra consists of a body composed of spongy bone placed one above the other and held together by discs of fibrocartilage. This construction allows for flexibility of the spine. Off the vertebra body may be found laminae, transverse processes, and spinous processes. The row of spinous processes can be felt by passing the finger down the back in the median line. The seventh cervical is easily seen and felt because of its prominence.

Cervical vertebrae have a cleft spinous process. The first cervical vertebra is called the *atlas* and is so named because it bears the weight of the skull. The second cervical vertegra is the *axis*, a strong process projecting upward and forming a pivot for the atlas to revolve around. Thoracic vertebrae have long transverse and spinous processes, and the bodies have articulations for the heads of the ribs.

The lumbar vertebrae are the largest and strongest in the vertebral column. The bodies are very thick, especially the fifth. The spinous processes of the lumbar vertebrae are almost square.

The sacrum is an irregular bone shaped like a curved wedge, with the base upward for its articulation with the fifth lumbar vertebra.

The coccyx, the terminal bone of the spinal column, is also wedge-shaped, with the base upward and joining the sacrum.

There are four normal curves to the spine: cervical, thoracic,

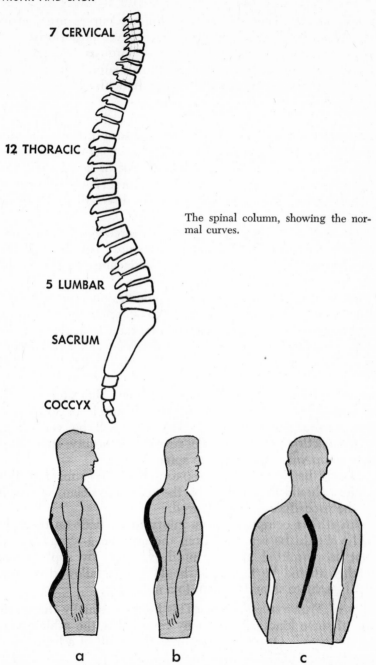

7 CERVICAL

12 THORACIC

The spinal column, showing the normal curves.

5 LUMBAR

SACRUM

COCCYX

a   b   c

Abnormal curves of the spinal column resulting in (a) lordosis, (b) kyphosis, (c) scoliosis.

lumbar, and sacral. The cervical and lumbar curves are convex anteriorly, while the thoracic and sacral are convex posteriorly.

Excessive or abnormal curves are called: lordosis (exaggerated anterior curve of the lumbar spine); scoliosis (lateral curve of the spine); kyphosis (posterior curve of spine, hunchback).

FRACTURES

Compression Fracture. A compression fracture of the spine is a very common injury in athletics, but it may occur as the result of a fall from a height, landing on heels or buttocks, or jack-knifing the spine (hyperflexion). Other causes may be a direct blow or a severe wrench of the back. Not too common is the direct dive or fall on the head or shoulders.

The nature of the injury is a crushing force that causes one vertebra to be crushed by the body of the next vertebra. If the crushing is severe, it may impinge upon and compress the spinal cord.

Any time an athlete complains of a hyperflexion type of injury to the spine, the injury should be X-rayed to eliminate the possibility of a compression-type fracture to the vertebrae. If neglected, the injury recurs and pain persists, and the athlete may suffer permanent disability. History will include the above with localized pain and spasm.

Palpation will reveal much tenderness over the site; pain is localized and is very distinct from the usual muscle or soft tissue pain. The surrounding muscles in the area will be very tight (spasm). Inspection may or may not reveal a deformity; sometimes an unusual lump will appear on the spine.

X-ray should be routine in all spine injuries. Treatment of this type of injury should be handled by the team physician, who will prescribe the procedures to be followed.

When an athlete complains of an injury to his back on the field or court, he should be removed from the area on a *stretcher* and should not be permitted to move until examined by a physician. The stretcher should be firm and should not be allowed to sag; motion of the athlete should be kept to a minimum.

Fracture of Transverse Process. This injury is usually the result of a blow of some kind. History may reveal that the athlete was "kneed in the back." Others may occur as the result of a bruise and a severe wrenching of the back at the same time.

There will be localized pain and motions of the back will be very limited because of pain and muscle spasm. These symptoms also prevail in an acute back sprain, but the localization of pain over the transverse process should cause concern, and the possibility of a fracture must be suspected. X-ray will reveal the fracture.

Treatment. Orthopedic surgeons, depending on the severity of the injury, have outlined as the best treatment:

1. Bed rest for about two weeks.
2. Strapping with adhesive tape for an additional month after being released from bed rest. The athlete may assume normal activities at this stage of treatment.

In bed rest, a firm bed is indicated. The use of a bed board is very effective. Bed boards are placed between the mattress and the spring, eliminating the "sag" of the mattress, which in turn relaxes the back muscles.

SPRAIN OF BACK

A sprain in the back area will involve the intervertebral ligaments and muscles in this area. The tenderness of the skeletal muscles may be felt on palpation, but the deep intervertebral tissues cannot be felt, and we must rely on the history of the injury to alert us in our methods of procedure. Functional tests, as outlined, will help considerably in localizing the condition. To say the athlete has a back sprain is not sufficient. The degree of pain, disability, etc., play a very important part in the proper handling of this condition. Questionable back conditions should be put into the hands of the team physician even before functional testing is demonstrated.

The mechanics of a back injury are very complete, and the athlete may recite in detail all the contributing factors. He may tell of a severe wrenching of back, of being twisted in a pile-up, tripping, being blocked, or blocking. In other words, he relates any motion that caused the tissues in the low back area to become overexerted.

Palpation will reveal muscle spasm (tightness of back) and acute pain on pressure. Joint areas may be painful, particularly the lumbar sacral or sacroiliac joints. Inspection may or may not reveal a deformity (list to one side). There may or may not be swelling.

Treatment. Mild cases (where pain is minimal and there is not too much discomfort) can be strapped (see page 166) for support, and rest on a firm surface for 24 hours may be sufficient. However, if pain persists, heat and massage will be very effective. Light exercise after treatment is also indicated.

Medium conditions should be treated with bed rest (mattress should be firm and not allow back to sag), heat, and massage. After acuteness has subsided, limited exercises should be started. Strapping, when up and around, is also very helpful.

Severe back conditions that manifest themselves with pain, disabilities, joint tenderness, or referred pains (back of buttocks, legs, etc.) should be handled with caution.

X-rays of back conditions may not reveal an injury to the bone, but they will rule out the possibility of any abnormalcy that may be contributing to the condition.

Treatment consists of bed rest, or the possibility of further management by traction or plaster of paris cast. These conditions should not be treated by any one other than the team physician. His orders must be followed to the letter in conditions of this type.

LOW BACK DISABILITY

One of the most perplexing problems in athletics is the low back disability. It is one of the hardest disabilities to evaluate. No attempt will be made to go into detail on chronic conditions of the low back area. Acute symptoms will be discussed on the level of subclinical conditions, and the more serious injuries will be described so that the trainer may be able to recognize and refer for proper management.

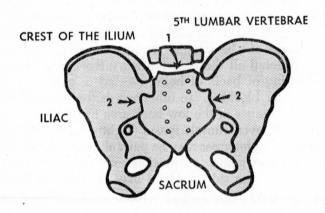

Areas involved in low back sprains. (1) Lombosacral joint. (2) Sacroiliac joint.

Functional tests for low back injury. The athlete stands erect with both hands at sides.

1. In standing position, compare both sides of back, look for tilt and obvious deformities (swelling, spasm, etc.).

2. With both feet planted, twist to right side and then left side. Athlete will advise of soreness and tightness, etc.

3. Tilt to right and then to left, with pelvis held firmly so that movement is in low back area.

4. With feet together, have athlete bend over to touch toes. He may need a little help, so place hand or arm under abdomen as he bends over. Athlete may or may not be able to do this, and this symptom should be noted.

5. In hyperextension of back, bend backward with feet together. The athlete will advise where the pain localizes in this position. Functional tests, as listed above, may be performed with some resistance from examiner for true evaluation. Caution must be observed, as the athlete may be injured to the degree that these tests should not be tried in the real acute period. Tests performed on a table will help to evaluate the specific muscles, etc., that may be involved.

Table tests. The following tests are recommended:

1. With athlete flat on back, lift extended leg as high as possible. Alternate and raise other leg. Symptoms of low back injury will show up in this test, and area of pain will be the tender point on this test.

2. With hands at side, lift both legs to right angle. (Should the athlete have trouble lifting one leg, this test should not be attempted.)

3. With hands behind neck, athlete should sit up. Legs may have to be held down in this test.

4. Rotation of hip, with knee flexed; the hip is rotated internally as well as externally.

5. Adduction and abduction of the leg is best done with resistance to establish strain in low back area.

6. In hyperextension of hip, move the athlete over to edge of table, hold leg off table, and let it hang. This will also localize pain and disability of low back.

These are normal functional tests for low back injury, and the interpretations will follow under the heading of specific back conditions. If history of injury indicates the possibility of fracture, these tests should not be attempted.

All these tests are to be used on ambulatory athletes, to help localize the injury and to facilitate proper treatment.

Low Back Sprains

Lumbosacral and sacroiliac. The pelvis provides a solid base through which the weight of the upper body can be transmitted to the lower limbs. The fifth lumbar vertebra attaches at the base of the sacrum and this is the lumbosacral joint. The two bones of the pelvis are attached to the sacrum and this is called the *sacroiliac* joint.

The fifth lumbar vertebra is connected to the sacrum by means of intervertebral ligaments and a capsule. There is also an intervertebral disc at this junction. Larger muscles of the body also support this joint, the psoas major, quadratus lumborum, etc.

In the sacroiliac joint, the two bones of the iliac are lined with a thin cartilage (as is both sides of the sacrum), and these are held together by very strong ligaments that are short and have a winding appearance. They attach between the bones in a variety of ways to hold the joint together.

Sprains of the back are the overstretching of the ligaments and the back muscles.

History. The athlete will recite the incident that caused the pain in the back area. He may have had a sudden wrenching of his back, lifting something off balance, or he may have met with too much resistance in a block or tackle.

Inspection may or may not reveal any swelling. There may be a list of the spine in the area, usually away from the side of the injury. By palpation, the exact source of the pain may be found.

There is a definite distinction between a sacroiliac sprain and a lumbosacral sprain, even though the symptoms may seem to be the same. Symptoms of a sacroiliac sprain are:

1. List of back (usually away from the affected side).
2. Muscle spasm (tightness of surrounding muscles).
3. Limitation of motion.
4. Tenderness in buttocks, thigh, and leg.
5. Local tenderness over sacroiliac.

Symptoms of a lumbosacral sprain are:

1. List of back.
2. Muscle spasm.
3. Limitation of motion.
4. Tenderness.
5. Local tenderness higher than in the sacroiliac.

In review, the above symptoms are very similar except for the last one, which is the localized area of the pain. The sacroiliac tenderness will be found directly over the sacroiliac joint, whereas the tenderness of the lumbosacral joint will be much higher over the joint of the fifth lumbar vertebra and the sacrum.

Functional tests must be tried to establish the true source of the low back pain. Flexion will have a tendency to aggravate the sacroiliac sprain, whereas hyperextension has a tendency to aggravate the lumbosacral sprain.

Mild conditions of these injuries may clear up in a few days with heat, massage, and strapping. If the condition should last more than the customary three days, a full work-up, including X-ray, should be made.

X-ray is indicated in back injuries to rule out any bony pathology such as congenital abnormalcies and also to help establish the condition of the disc space and bone structure of the lumbar vertebrae.

Treatment of Sacroiliac and Lumbosacral Sprains

Mild sprain. The athlete is ambulatory and feels normal when erect, but pain is present on lateral motion and flexion or extension movements. Heat and deep massage plus strapping for support are indicated. Heat may be of the deeper penetrating type such as diathermy, ultrasonics, etc., and should always be followed by massage and light exercise. The application of heat to the low back may have a tendency to tighten the back, and therefore massage and mild exercises are indicated to "loosen" the muscles.

Moderate sprain. Pain is constant and the athlete is very uncomfortable. Bed rest and the application of heat pad will enhance the relaxation of the low back. The use of a bed board for a firm support of the back is necessary. A board is placed between the mattress and the springs (a piece of plywood, door, etc.); this will allow the back to relax. Too soft a mattress will cause the reflex tightening of the back muscles as the body sinks into the soft surface, thus having a tendency to aggravate the condition. When symptoms subside, the treatment is the same as for a mild sprain.

Severe sprain. There will be much pain and discomfort; the athlete cannot get comfortable. Pain may radiate down the leg to where it is excruciating. There is inability to walk in any position; laughing, coughing, sneezing, etc., is very painful. Bed rest is indicated, and the possibility of traction must be considered. A complete work-up by the team physician to find the underlying cause of the severe injury must be made.

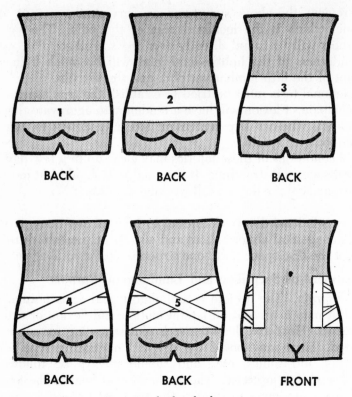

Strapping for low back sprain.

Disability in the sacroiliac and lumbosacral sprains vary from just a few days to a permanent disability. The possibility of a chronic back is always a problem, and every effort should be made to rehabilitate the back muscles, etc., before the athlete is allowed to return to full activity.

LOW BACK STRAPPING

Strapping is applied while athlete is standing with feet spread apart 18 inches for balance and comfort. This strapping may be applied over stockinette, T-shirt, or other like material. The spines of the ilium should be padded for comfort.

Step 1. The first strip of tape will start below the sacrum, and additional strips will be added toward the upper body. Start the first strip on the abdomen just beyond the pelvis and pull the tape snugly across the back and end in exactly the same position as the start except on opposite side of pelvis.

Step 2. Overlapping at least halfway, add additional strips to cover injured area (taping above and below area for maximum support). The size of the athlete and the extent of the injury will dictate the number of horizontal strips to use.

Step 3. Diagonal strips will be used to reinforce tape and add to support. Start at the front area, fix the tape, and then pull at a diagonal so that the tape will end at the upper position on the opposite side.

Step 4. Reverse the procedure and start at opposite side.

Step 5. Two diagonal strips going each way will be sufficient.

Step 6. Apply anchor strips to the ends of the tape to prevent rolling and slipping.

Three-inch elastic tape is excellent for this strapping. Tape used for diagonal strips may be 1½ or 2 inches regular adhesive. This same tape should be used for the anchors.

CONTUSIONS OF BACK, BUTTOCKS, AND KIDNEYS

Contusions of Back. The large muscles of the back are subject to much bruising. The pain will be severe on onset, gradually diminishing. The muscles become very stiff, and thus loss of motion is involved. The presence of hemorrhage is quite evident by the degree of swelling. The injury will be very painful on motion but at rest is fairly comfortable. The history will reveal a kick or blow to the area which caused the athlete to cease playing. This is the more severe type of contusion, whereas the injury that shows up after the athlete has "cooled off" is the minor type of bruise.

Due to the location of the muscles of the back, a thorough examination must be made to eliminate any bony injury. In the upper back, the ribs and vertebrae must be considered, and in the low back area, the kidneys and the transverse and spinous processes must be eliminated in the examination.

Treatment. This consists of the application of ice packs to lessen and control the hemorrhage. Strapping for compression is very helpful if it can be tolerated. After the hemorrhage has been controlled, the use of heat and massage is very effective in alleviating the pain and stiffness in the back. Full range of motion and complete function must be attained before the athlete should resume activity. Disability is from a day or two to two weeks.

Contusion of the low back over the spine is quite prevalent in all sports. It is characterized by a large hematoma that is very obvious. Treatment consists of ice to control the hemorrhage. Compression is most important and is best accomplished by applying a felt pad slightly larger than the area involved and strapping very snugly. Remaining off the feet as much as possible will help. Aspiration has been very beneficial in clearing up this lesion. Repeated aspirations may be needed, and the compression strap should be continued until the area is normal. Disability varies from a few days to a week or ten days. The recurrence of this injury is quite prevalent, and a pad must be worn for protection against repeated trauma.

Contusion of Buttocks. Due to the large area of muscle and the profuse blood supply to the area, a contusion of the buttocks causes quite a lot of concern. We have seen quite a few of these lately and they have been very troublesome. The persistence of the hemorrhage over a period of days has made the injury one that is hard to manage except by bed rest. The application of ice and compression has not been too satisfactory. The inability to secure proper compression has been the big deterrent in this injury. The use of girdles and elastic bandages have not been very effective. As of late, the admission to the infirmary for a few days has been the answer, along with the application of ice to the area. With the recurrent hemorrhaging, we have been very hesitant to apply heat at any time in the treatment of this condition.

Recovery time is from ten days to about three weeks. Proper padding must be used to eliminate the possibility of the injury recurring.

Contusion of Kidney. The kidneys are situated in the posterior lumbar region extending from the tenth rib to within 2 to 3 inches of the crest of the ilium. The main source of injury is a direct blow to the low back, with a history of being kicked or blocked in the region.

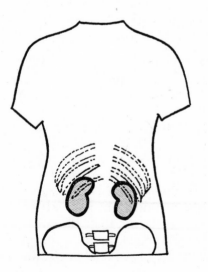

Location of kidneys. Injuries of the low back must first be checked for possible injury to the kidneys. Kidneys are located between the crest of the ilium and the lower ribs.

The athlete will complain of pain over the kidney area, and the urine specimen may show true blood. The description of the urine resembling "grape juice" is not uncommon.

In contusions of the low back, this injury should not be eliminated until a urine specimen has been examined.

Treatment must be undertaken by the team physician. Complete bed rest and medications, as ordered by the physician, must be carried out to ensure complete recovery. Disability varies from ten days to a full season.

ANATOMY OF TRUNK

The trunk includes the thorax, abdomen, and pelvis. The bones of the thorax are the sternum, ribs (24 with 12 on each side of the body), and the 12 thoracic vertebrae. The sternum (breast bone) is placed in front of the thorax and is about 6 inches long; it is a flat bone. The sternum is divided into three parts: the manubrium (upper part), the body (middle), and the terminal end (the xiphoid appendix). The lateral borders of the sternum give attachments

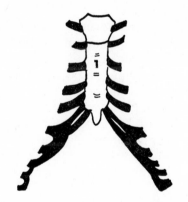

Cartilage of ribs as they attach to the sternum. (1) Black, filled-in area shows amount of cartilage that attached ribs to sternum.

to the clavicle (collar bone) and the first seven ribs. The xiphoid appendix gives attachments to some of the muscles of the abdomen.

The ribs are a series of elastic arches and are composed of bone and cartilage. The posterior head of the ribs attaches to the vertebral column and the shaft extends around the body. The first seven ribs, or "true ribs," attach by means of cartilage to the sternum. The remaining five are the false ribs. The eighth, ninth, and tenth are connected in front, each to the one above. The eleventh and twelfth ribs are not connected and are called *floating ribs.* The inner surface of the rib is grooved at the lower border; this groove accommodates the nerves and blood vessels. The 12 thoracic vertebra have already been described.

Fracture of Sternum. A fracture of the sternum is very rare, but it may occur as a result of a direct blow to the sternum. History will reveal details of mechanics; pain and limited breathing will result. X-ray will confirm this type of fracture.

Inspection will reveal some swelling, and if the fracture is displaced, a deformity will be evident. The athlete will tend to tilt his head toward his chest and will feel pain when his head is held normally. Palpation will reveal much tenderness, and if a displaced fracture is present, the fragments may be felt.

This injury should be recognized and then turned over to team physician. Treatment is usually bed rest with support, if there is no displacement. Fractures with displacement should be sent to hospital and treatment handled on that level.

If fracture is suspected, the athlete should be removed from the field on a stretcher. The stretcher should be firm, and the athlete should lie on his back.

Rib Fractures. Rib fractures are not uncommon in athletics and are usually caused by direct trauma such as a severe blow to the chest, either by knee or elbow, or as a result of being piled on. On occasion, falling on a ball will cause this injury.

The athlete will complain of pain on breathing, especially "deep breathing," or forced breathing. Injury will cause the athlete to tilt his head forward to lessen the pain, and he will also tend to breathe very shallowly. Pain will be very localized, so much so that the athlete can outline the area with his finger. Swelling may occur as a result of damage to the soft tissue surrounding the area. If there is a fracture displacement, an obvious deformity will be evident.

In palpation the course of the rib can be traced, and if the athlete is not too fat, the fracture line can be felt. By placing one hand on each side of the fracture on the rib, slight pressure may be exerted, and the fracture may be demonstrated by pain and crepitus.

X-ray will reveal the fracture in most cases. Because of the superimposed tissues of the chest and the nature of X-ray, many rib fractures may not show up on the initial picture. X-rays taken about two weeks later will reveal calcium formation over the site and diagnosis of fracture may be made at this time. Rib injuries are best treated symptomatically; if there is severe pain, even with a negative film a fracture must be suspected and the injury treated accordingly.

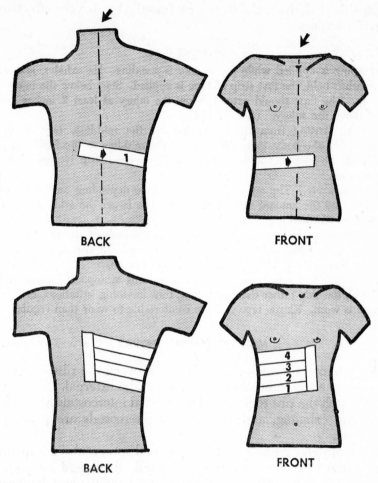

Rib strapping. Arrows point to mid-line. Strapping, to be effective, must extend beyond mid-line in front as well as in back.

Treatment consists of adhesive strapping of the area. Taping should start beyond the mid-line of the front and back of the injured side. Taping above and below the site will give excellent support. The length of disability time involved is about one month. The use of elastic adhesive has lessened the problems of tape irritation, but a "rib belt" is most effective for support over a long period of time necessary to heal a rib fracture.

Disability for football and contact sports is longer than for non-contact sports and the usual time is from four to six weeks.

Local heat daily in the form of infrared, etc., is very effective in relieving soreness.

STRAPPING RIBS

Strapping is applied while the athlete is standing. He exhales, and while the breath is held, the first strip of tape is applied. Start below the injury and work up. The tape should extend below the injury at least 2 inches and as much above the injury. (See p. 171)

Strip 1. Starting from the back, beyond the mid-line, tape is pulled snugly around the body, extending beyond the mid-line in the front.

Strip 2. Overlapping at least halfway, the second strip is applied in the same manner.

Strips 3, 4, etc., The number of strips will be dependent on the extent of the injury and the amount of area covered. The larger the athlete, the more tape will be required.

Anchor strips are then applied to the exposed ends of the tape. The use of anchor strips will keep the tape from riding and will also seal the ends so that they will not roll when clothing, etc., are put on.

Elastic adhesive tape is recommended for this strapping because it will move with the skin rather than against it, thus lessening irritations, etc., when the tape is worn. Elastic tape is more comfortable to wear than regular tape.

MUSCLES OF THE THORAX

The intercostal muscles are situated between the ribs. There are two sets: one the internal, and the other, the external. Their function is to pull the ribs together. The internal intercostals are primary muscles in exhaling, and the external intercostals are primary in inspiration.

These muscles are subject to bruises and sprains and are involved in all injuries of the ribs. When injured, there will be pain on motion of the ribs either in exhaling or inhaling; point tenderness will be quite prevalent immediately after the injury.

Treatment consists of strapping of the area, being sure to tape above and below the site of the injury. Strapping should extend beyond the mid-line of the front and back. The purpose of the strap is to limit the excursion of the rib and allow rest to overcome the spasm of the muscles. The immediate application of ice will help to lessen the discomfort; then follow with heat to the area. Disability depends on the amount of discomfort and is usually a day to weeks.

The diaphragm is a dome-shaped muscle that separates the abdomen from the chest. It is the principal muscle in respiration. It is not a common muscle to be injured, but we do see numerous cases of the "wind being knocked out." This does not necessarily mean that there has been an injury to the muscle itself. Any injury that affects breathing for any time should be seen immediately by the team physician to establish degree of injury and determine which specific muscle is affected.

"Wind being knocked out" was discussed as a separate injury in Chapter 6.

Contusion of Chest. If we eliminate injuries to the ribs and clavicle, we shall find that most of the contusions of the chest manifest themselves on the sternum. The sternum is a large flat bone and very thick, susceptible to bruising quite readily in football but not seen too often in other sports. The treatment is symptomatic and response is very slow. If treated as all bone bruises with heat and protection, the athlete may continue to play, provided there is no limitation of motion and the pain is not disabling.

Simple linear fractures are seen and the treatment consists of rest and heat. Strapping and other means of immobilization do not seem to produce results in this injury. In order to strap effectively, the adhesive must be pulled very tight. The discomfort in breathing makes this appear to be a hindrance rather than a help. However, if taping is indicated, it must be carried out.

ABDOMEN

Bones of the Abdomen. The five lumbar vertebrae have already been described. The pelvic girdle is composed of two hip bones, one sacrum, and one coccyx. The hip bone is composed of the ilium, ischium, and the pubis. The ilium is the highest part of the hip bone and wings out and becomes broad and flat. The upper border is called the *crest of the ilium.* The pubis is the front part of the hip bone. It has a body and two branches called *rami.* The body joins the ilium and the rami join the ischium and the spinal pubes. The two pubic bones join at the mid-line in the front to form the symphysis pubis.

The ischium is the lowest part of the hip bone and has a sharp spine called a *tuberosity,* upon which the trunk rests in the sitting position.

The pelvis is held together in the front by the symphysis pubis and the sacrum in the back with the coccyx attached to the sacrum. This is called the *pelvic girdle.*

Contusions of the Abdomen. Pain in the abdominal area must be regarded as serious, particularly if there is a history of a blow to the area. Pain and rigidity of the abdomen will be present. Some of the cardinal signs include vomiting, pallor, high pulse rate, and shock.

The athlete should be kept quiet and shock precautions should be taken. Transportation should be supervised by the doctor.

FRACTURES OF PELVIS

The pelvis is a very strong series of bones that supports the spinal column and transmits the weight of the upper body to the legs. It also affords protection to the abdominal organs and acts as an attachment for muscles of the leg and upper body. The pelvis is composed of two innominate bones (made up of the pubis, ilium, and the ischium) and the coccyx and sacrum.

Fracture of the pelvis is very rare in athletics. Fractures that do occur usually are the results of a very severe blow to the pelvis. An associated fracture with a severe contusion to the crest of the ilium is found on occasion. Complications of fractures of the pelvis must be suspected. Therefore any severe injury to the pelvis should be referred to the team physician as soon as possible. Damage to abdominal organs may be associated with this injury, and excessive moving will aggravate the condition or cause complications.

In suspected fractures of the pelvis, the immediate treatment should be for the prevention of shock. Keep the athlete as warm as possible and make him as comfortable as you can. Remove him from the area on a stretcher and move him directly to hospital and not to the training room.

Fracture of the Crest of the Ilium. This is an injury caused by a severe blow to the crest of the ilium. The athlete will tell you that on blocking, he was "kneed" on the hip. He may or may not be able to stand on his leg without pain. Deep breathing, laughing, or coughing will produce much pain in the area. The athlete will also pinpoint the site with his finger.

Inspection may or may not reveal any swelling or deformity. Palpation will cause much pain, and any attempt to feel for the deformity will not be possible because of the pain. X-ray is indicated to confirm this fracture.

Treatment. The team physician will advise bed rest and the possibility of a cast. Some of these fractures may be managed by the application of a firm belt or by adhesive strapping. The treatment will be prescribed by the team physician, and his orders must be carried out in detail.

HIP INJURIES

Dislocation of the Hip. Dislocation of the hip is a very rare injury in athletics. There are two types of dislocations: the anterior (forward) and the posterior (backward). Most of the dislocations seen are the posterior type and are quite often complicated by a fracture of the acetabulum. The head of the femur is thrust through the capsule as a result of an adduction and rotation action. The deformity will be very obvious. Pain will be severe and the loss of function of the leg will be noted. The athlete will be seen in a typical position, that is, with the leg flexed in an externally rotated position. This dislocation should not be reduced without the benefit of an X-ray, since the possibility of fracture may be a complication and should not be reduced by anyone other than the team

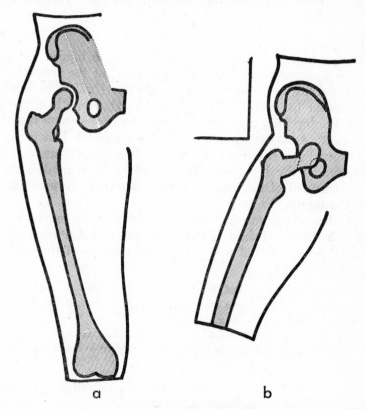

a   b

(a) Normal hip, showing position of the head of the femur in the acetabulum. (b) Dislocation of hip. Head of femur is out of the acetabulum and the leg is externally rotated. Note typical "step" effect when hip is dislocated.

physician. Immediate treatment consists of splinting and making the athlete comfortable for travel.

After reduction the athlete must be kept immobilized because too early ambulation may cause complications at the joint and render permanent damage to the area.

Fracture of the acetabulum. The acetabulum is a very deep cup that accommodates the head of the femur. It is situated on the side of the pelvis and is rimmed with a very thick border that acts as the attachment for the ligaments of the hip joint. The acetabulum is lined with a cartilage and a fossa (hollow) gives attachment to the ligamentum teres, the strong ligament of the hip joint.

Fractures that occur at the acetabulum are usually a complication of a dislocated hip. X-ray will confirm.

Treatment is given by the team physician, who will establish the degree of injury and prescribe treatment for the reduction of hip and fracture.

Hip

Sprain of hip. A hip sprain is not a common injury. However, a few are seen from time to time. The head of the femur is well rounded and fits into a very deep acetabulum (hollow in pelvis for head of femur to insert). There is also great strength in the ligaments of the hip joint and the large muscles of the thigh that overlay the joint. A severe wrench of the hip while the foot is planted on the ground or a slipping motion (wet floor) may cause a counter joint-motion of the hip joint. There will be local tenderness and some impairment of motion. History will reveal the incident that caused the injury.

Inspection may or may not reveal anything. (The joint is so deep that swelling will not show.) Palpation will reveal tenderness over the hip joint. Functional tests include all motions of the hip.

On table, flat on back:
1. *Flexion.* With knee stiff, lift leg to a right angle.
2. *Extension of hip.* Move athlete to edge of table and let leg hang off table and toward the floor.
3. *Rotation.* Flex knee, hold leg, and move foot inward and outward.
4. *Adduction.* Hold leg from body and ask athlete to bring leg into body.
5. *Abduction.* Move leg out from the body.

Resistance may or may not be needed to establish the extent of the injury and the exact location.

Treatment of hip sprains. The immediate application of ice and a compression spica bandage is indicated. In severe sprains of the hip, bed rest or the use of crutches may be necessary. Heat and passive motion should be started on the day after the injury and gradually increased to active exercises. Sprains of the hip respond rapidly if not forced.

Contusion of Hip. Because of the prominence of the femur at the hip joint, it is a very vulnerable area for contusions. Hitting the ground, floor, or ice is usually the cause of this injury. Most sports provide protection for this area, but often the trauma is severe enough to go through the pad. The blow results in a bone bruise that is quite painful. Like all bone bruises, hip contusions are slow to respond to treatment. In an acute condition, the immediate use of ice will be very effective. On the next day the use of a mild heat and limited exercise should be started. When normal activity of leg is recovered, the injury may be padded for protection and the athlete may resume. Disability extends from a day to about ten days.

The tendons of the abductors and the extensor muscles of the hip are often bruised. Unlike bone bruises, they respond quite readily to normal treatment. The application of ice for 24 hours is followed by heat and massage. Activity at this time will depend on the degree of the injury, but usually jogging and walking may be tolerated, and this in turn will enhance the recovery of the injury.

Greater Trochanteric Bursitis. A severe injury to the greater trochanter may involve the bursa in the hip area, along with the tendons and muscles that are also involved in a contusion of the hip.

The bursa involvement is very painful and is self-limiting. The pain will also increase the loss of function, and the athlete will have to be sidelined. Treatment consists of the immediate application of cold packs. This may be continued for a day or two, together with the use of crutches for rest. After the symptoms cool off, the use of heat is very effective. Mild exercises, passive to start and then gradually going into active exercises, are recommended.

Disability varies with the athlete and the degree of the injury. Some athletes may return in a day or two; others may take weeks.

GROIN INJURIES

Groin injuries may occur in any sport at any time of the year. Most groin injuries, however, are seen in early football practice where the change of direction is emphasized. Linemen "pulling out" and backs twisting on one leg are likely to suffer an injury of

the adductors of the thigh. The injury may be close to the attachments or a little lower in the muscles themselves. There may be a
tearing of fibers, either slight or rather extensive. With the tearing
of fibers, there will be damage to blood vessels, resulting in a
hematoma that will manifest itself in a hard area just below the
attachments of the muscles. This is usually not a serious injury but
very self-limiting.

We direct our treatment to the history, inspection, and palpation.
History will usually show a sudden change in direction and the
athlete will report a slight pain to a severe jolt. He may be able to
continue work-outs because he will compensate by keeping both
legs close to each other and changing body mechanics to eliminate
the strain on the affected leg. He will tell you that he feels very
little as he runs straight ahead but has pain when he veers. Inspection may or may not reveal any change in contour of the leg. Palpation will reveal a tightness in the adductor group of muscles and
some tenderness on pressure.

Functional tests for "groin strains." With the athlete on his back,
keep leg stiff and raise the leg to a right angle to the table. In same
position, lower the leg. (These tests may be done with the examiner
offering a little resistance.)

Now, with the athlete flat on his back, abduct the leg (separate
from body). Then, with leg to side, adduct the leg (bring back to
normal). These two tests may also be given with some resistance.

As the athlete goes through the tests, he will be instructed to
point with his finger exactly to the point of pain. From this the
diagnosis may be made. If he should use his hand and describe the
full area of the leg, he may only be "stiff and sore," rather than
sprained.

Treatment consists of controlling the hematoma. This is accomplished by the use of a compression spica bandage or strapping
with elastic adhesive. The spica compression bandage procedure
consists of applying cotton to the area and wrapping snugly with an
elastic bandage. The leg should be elevated by placing pillows or a
blanket under the lower leg rather than under the knee. The application of an ice bag to the area should be continued overnight, and
after the injury has been reviewed, functional tests are again tried
and progress noted. If there are no alarming symptoms, the athlete
may be allowed to work out. The work-out consists of a long warm-
up, stressing the necessity of running straight ahead and walking
the turns. As the injury "loosens" up, he can start to run slight
turns, gradually sharpening the turns and increasing the speed.

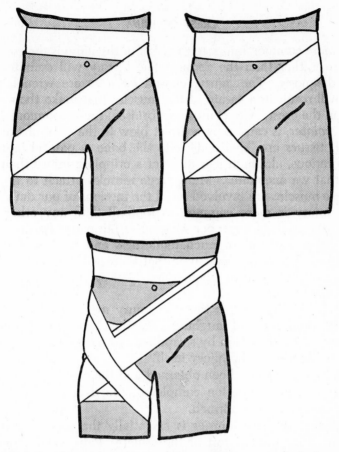

Spica as applied to the groin area. To start the strapping, wrap completely around the upper thigh; then cross the abdomen and go around the waist; then pull elastic down across the diagonal strip and repeat. Pressure should be applied to the groin area to support the adductor group of muscles. When a "hot pack" is applied, cotton is used to cover the ointment used as a counterirritant.

This injury responds very well to this type of work and the length of disability is usually from one to three days. The use of the hot pack is indicated in this injury, and the spica may be used for a few days until the athlete feels that he can do without. Heat on the second day is very effective, but caution should be used so that the hemorrhage is not disturbed and started again. In the more severe injury, the routine treatment of ice, elevation, and compression is continued for another 24 hours. After this time the injury is reviewed and the preceding program is instituted.

CREST OF ILIUM

The more common injury to the crest of the ilium is the contusion, or bruise, rather than the sprain. The history will definitely help in the diagnosis. The injury, caused by a severe wrench of the trunk, will result in a sprain of the muscles that make their attachments on the crest. The contusion (bruise), more commonly called the *hip pointer,* is caused by a direct blow to the crest of the ilium. The soft tissues are "smashed" onto the bone, a painful injury but not too serious, although it is more of a crippling injury than many others that we encounter. Many large muscles attach to the crest, and these muscles are involved in all the motions of our daily life.

This injury is more common in football than any other sport, usually as a result of improper wearing of hip pads. Because of the impact, there will follow much tenderness and limitation of function. As in all bruises, we assume that there will be damage to the blood vessels, resulting in a hematoma. The symptoms are the same as the sprain.

A particular incident is that the injury may be aggravated by sneezing, coughing, and laughing. Treatment is symptomatic, i.e., lessen the range of motion by strapping and reduce activity according to the dictates of the injury itself.

After the history has been obtained and the ensuing examination of inspection and palpation completed, the diagnosis of a sprain or contusion can be confirmed.

Treatment of these injuries is essentially the same. Immediate treatment is for the comfort of the athlete. Pain and limitation of motion manifest themselves quite readily in these injuries. Strapping with adhesive tape for compression and support is first; then the application of ice bags to the area will control hemorrhage and lessen the pain. Bed rest for the first day or two is very beneficial. The application of ice packs to this injury is carried out for the first two or three days, with the strap remaining on at this time. When the acute discomfort has subsided the use of heat is indicated. This injury may be treated effectively with any of the modalities. The most effective heat that has been applied is the hot shower. Results with this type of heat, plus limited motion in the shower, have been very beneficial and have contributed to excellent recovery from this lesion.

The "hip pointer" is slow in response and is self-limiting during the recovery period. This injury cannot be pushed without aggra-

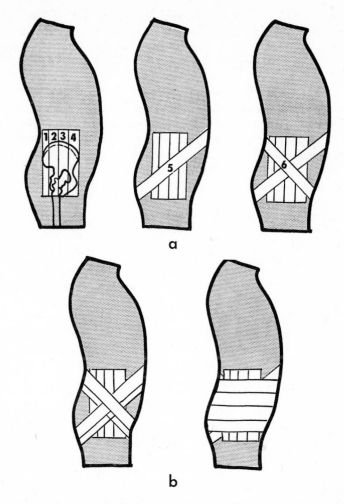

(a) Strapping used to support the injury to the crest of the ilium: shows crest of the ilium and the degree of coverage necessary for full support. (b) Completed strapping.

vating the original condition. The usual time of disability is from one week to three weeks. When the athlete is ready to resume activity, especially football, he should wear a specially constructed pad under his hip pads to prevent further aggravation in the early recuperative days.

Instruction in the proper wearing of hip pads will prevent many of the contusions that occur in this area. The tendency is to wear the hip pads below the crest, thus making the prominence of the bone a vulnerable target. It should be noted that if the hip pads are worn low, the pants will be out of position, and this will move the thigh guards from their protective position. Thus the thigh becomes susceptible to "Charley horses."

TAPING THE CREST OF ILIUM

The athlete stands feet together, with a slight tilt of the injured side toward the tape so as to shorten the muscle area of the injured side. (See p. 181)

Step 1. Apply at least six strips of tape vertically over the affected side, overlapping each one about halfway. The injury site should be completely covered with adhesive tape so that the vertical strips may vary in number.

Step 2. A diagonal strip, starting from the opposite buttock, is pulled across the injured site to beyond the mid-line of the abdomen.

Step 3. A diagonal crisscross strip is applied by starting on the upper border of the opposite hip and pulling across the first diagonal strip, ending on the lower part of the abdomen beyond the mid-line.

Two of each of the above are sufficient.

Step 4. Horizontal strips are applied by starting beyond the mid-line of the back and pulling around the hip, ending beyond the mid-line of the abdomen. Use as many of these as needed to completely encase the vertical and diagonal strips.

Anchor strips may be applied to the ends of the horizontal strips to prevent rolling of tape ends.

INJURIES TO THE COCCYX

Falling hard on the ground or floor or a severe kick to the coccyx may cause an injury. Although a rather uncommon injury, we have seen a few fractures of the coccyx. The possibility of a dislocation of the coccyx is always present in a severe type of injury. Fortunately most of the injuries to the coccyx are in the contusion (bruise) category.

In the case of a suspected fracture or dislocation, X-ray should be utilized. In the case of a fracture or dislocation, the team physician will carry out diagnosis and treatment. Treatment consists of the reduction of the condition, followed by bed rest for about three weeks.

Contusion of the coccyx is quite common, and the treatment consists of heat and rest. Symptoms disappear slowly, but the athlete may be able to participate in sports if he has adquate protection to eliminate another bruise to the area. Sitz baths or whirlpools are very effective modalities in this condition. The severe pain may leave after the first few treatments, but the residual pain may stay for a while, as in all bone bruises.

MUSCLES OF BACK, TRUNK, AND GROIN

Rectus Abdominus. This is a slender flat muscle that runs in the front of the abdomen. Its origin is the crest of the pubes, and its insertion is the cartilages of the fifth, sixth, and seventh ribs. The action of the rectus is to flatten the abdomen and the flexion of the spinal column. To help this action, the internal and external obliques are accessory muscles.

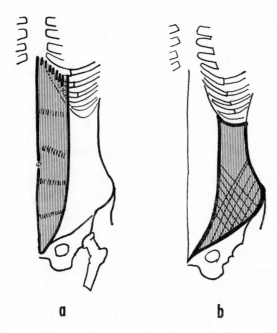

a   b

Rectus abdominus (a). Internal and external obliques (b).

External Obliques. This muscle covers the abdomen from the rectus abdominus to the latissimis dorsi in the back. The origin is the anterior half of the crest of the ilium, the upper portion of the thigh, and the linea alba (mid-line of the abdomen). The insertion is the surfaces of the eight lower ribs. The action is flexion and rotation of the trunk.

Internal Obliques. The internal obliques are under the external obliques. The origin is the lumbar fascia, the anterior two-thirds of the crest of the ilium and the upper end of the fascia of the thigh. The insertion is the cartilages of the eighth, ninth, and tenth ribs and the linea alba. The action of the internal obligues is flexion and rotation of the trunk.

The Diaphragm. The diaphragm is a dome-shaped muscle that separates the thoracic cavity from the abdominal cavity. It originates from the lower end of the sternum and costal cartilages of the lower ribs, and the transverse processes of the upper lumbar vertebrae. Its insertion is from all the fibers of the origin which converge into a central tendon. The diaphragm is the principal muscle in respiration.

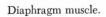

Diaphragm muscle.

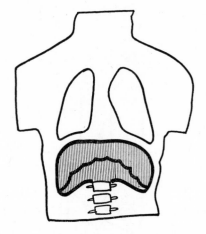

The Trapezius. The trapezius is a flat, triangular muscle located at the upper part of the back and is very superficial. It originates at the base of the skull and extends down the back to the twelfth thoracic vertebrae. It inserts at the outer border of the clavicle, the spine of the scapula, and the top of the acromion. The two muscles form a trapezium or diamond-shaped quadrangle. The trapezius acts to pull the head backward and sideway, with the shoulders stationary. With the head held stationary, it will elevate the shoulder girdle. The two acting together will draw the shoulders back. It is also a climbing muscle.

The trapezius is injured quite frequently because of its location and the fact that it is so superficial. Strain of this muscle is quite common and results in a stiff neck. A strain may be caused by blocking with the head when the neck is not "bowed," or in wrestling, when a head hold is not easily released and a strain is caused in trying to "break the hold." It is a muscle that is very close to the surface and therefore infrared heat, hot towels, or even a "hot shower" followed by massage will give much relief. Active exercises after treatment will enhance the "looseness" of this muscle. Athletes with a strain of the trapezius may do well to wear a muffler to keep the muscle warm and dry.

Contusions of the trapezius are common injuries in football, especially the insertion at the acromion process. They are usually caused by poorly fitting shoulder pads that are not adequate to deflect a "blow" received at the point of the muscle. This injury is a rather painful and disabling bruise, but after the full range of motion of the arm and neck has been attained, it can be padded to prevent aggravation. Proper fitting of shoulder pads will prevent many of these injuries.

The Rhomboids. The rhomboids are parallelogram in shape and lie under the middle portion of the trapezius. They originate at the spinous processes of the vertebrae (seventh cervical to the fifth thoracic) and insert on the vertebral border of the scapula. The action of these two muscles is to hold the scapula inward (adduction) and to rotate the scapula laterally.

Sprains and strains of these muscles are uncommon but are very likely to occur in baseball as a result of throwing "too hard too early." Pain is very definite and quite easily defined by the athlete. Fortunately this pair of muscles is easily treated. Heat and massage for a few days is usually sufficient to effect a cure. Strapping with adhesive tape is sometimes used to rest these muscles, and if the strain is severe, a sling may also help.

Latissimus Dorsi. The latissimus dorsi is a very broad muscle situated in the lower half of the back and is immediately under the skin, except for a small space where it is covered by the trapezius. Its origin is the six lower thoracic vertebrae and all the lumbar vertebrae, the crest of the ilium, the sacrum, and the lower three ribs. It inserts on the humerus at the upper portion. The actions are to lower the arm, rotate it medially, and draw the arm back.

Contusions and strains are common injuries of this muscle and treatments are symptomatic, i.e., pain, tightness, and loss of function. Applications of mild heat, massage, and exercise are very helpful to injuries of this muscle. Strapping with adhesive tape may afford some relief. Contusion of the latissimus dorsi at the crest of the ilium is very painful, and this is covered in the description of the crest of ilium injuries. This muscle is primarily regarded as a back muscle, but because of its attachment on the humerus, it must be included in the shoulder area.

The injury is sometimes the result of rowing. Pain will be in the back area, extend up into the shoulder, and manifest tightness at the attachment of the humerus. This is a broad and powerful muscle of the back but thins out at the upper attachment. Treatment consists of heat and massage and mild exercise. In an oarsman, the use of a single shell for light work for a day or so proves very effective. Keeping the shoulder warm, by means of a sweat shirt, etc., is very necessary to prevent "tightening" after the work-out. The use of a "hot shower" is excellent hydrotherapy after the practice session.

Levator Scapulae. The levator scapulae is a small muscle on the back and side of the neck and underlies the trapezius. It originates from the transverse processes of the first four cervical vertebrae and inserts on the vertebral border of the scapula. It raises the scapula or inclines the neck to the side. It is a muscle very important to the support and development of the neck and is injured as a result of "head butting" or severe wrenches of the head. Pain is typical of a sore muscle accompanied by a limitation of motion of the neck. Many "stiff necks" are attributed to this muscle being in spasm.

Treatment is symptomatic, using heat and massage with exercise to promote normal range of motion. Injuries to this muscle may be stubborn, but perseverance will win out. The athlete is instructed to keep his neck warm, using a towel or muffler to eliminate "drafts" to the area. Very little disability is found when this muscle is injured, and they very often "work out." Treatment is essentially the same as the strain of the trapezius, and the athlete should not return to action without proper protection to the injured part. Disability extends from a day or two to a week.

Erector Spinae. This is a very large and thick mass of muscle that is situated on each side of the spine. The origin is the crest of the ilium, back of the sacrum, the spinous processes of the lumbar, and the lower three thoracic vertebrae and the transverse processes of all the thoracic vertebrae. Its insertion is the base of the skull, the transverse and spinous processes of the vertebrae, and the angle of the ribs. The action of this muscle is, as its name implies, to hold the body erect. With variations of function, lateral motion and flexion of the trunk is permitted.

Gluteus Minimus. This is the smallest muscle of the gluteal group. Its origin is the lower part of the outer surface of the ilium and the margin of the greater sciatic notch. The insertion is the anterior border of the greater trochanter. The action of the gluteal group is to abduct the thigh when the leg is extended.

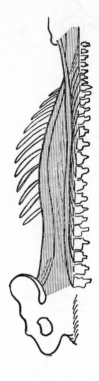

Erector spinae.

Gluteus Medius. The gluteus medius is a short, thick muscle, situated on the side of the ilium, that helps to make the rounded contour of the hip. Its origin is at the outer surface of the ilium near the crest. The insertion is the lateral surface of the greater trochanter. The action of this muscle is to abduct the thigh, with the leg in extension and also to help rotate the thigh medially.

Gluteus Maximus. A very large and fleshy muscle of the buttocks. Its origin is the posterior portion of the crest of the ilium, lower part of the sacrum and coccyx, and the sacrotuberous ligament. Its insertion is at the gluteal tuberosity of the femur and the iliotibial band of fascia lata over the greater trochanter. The action is controversial, but the literature states that this muscle extends the thigh, assists in abduction, and in lateral rotation of the hip.

Adductor Brevis. The adductor brevis is a very short muscle that underlies the adductor longus. It originates on the outer surface of the inferior ramus of the pubis. The insertion is the upper half of the linea aspera (ridge on the femur). The action of the adductor brevis is to adduct the thigh and assist in rotating and flexing the thigh.

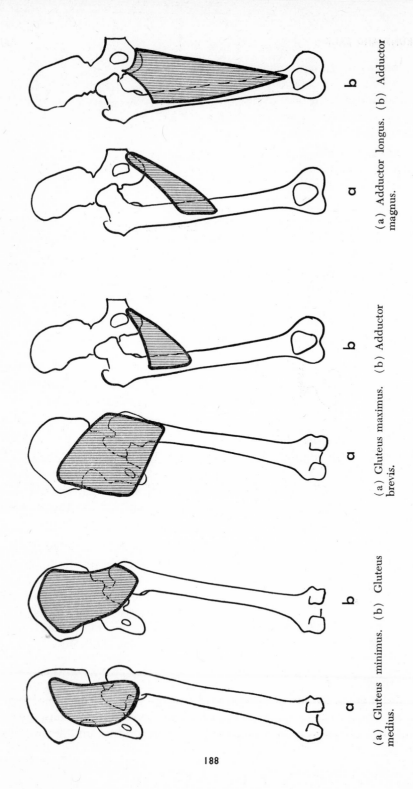

(a) Gluteus minimus. (b) Gluteus medius.

(a) Gluteus maximus. (b) Adductor brevis.

(a) Adductor longus. (b) Adductor magnus.

Adductor Longus. This is a fan-shaped muscle on top of the adductor brevis. Its origin is the front of the pubis, and its insertion is the middle half of the linea aspera (ridge on femur). The action of the adductor longus is to adduct the thigh and assist in rotating and flexing the thigh.

Adductor Magnus. Adductor magnus is one of the largest muscles of the body and is situated on the medial side of the thigh under the gracilis. The origin is the front of the pubes and the tuberosity of the ischium. The insertion is the linea aspera (ridge on femur) and the adductor tubercle. The action of the adductor magnus is to adduct and flex the thigh; the lower part aids in extending the femur.

Psoas Major. The bulk of this muscle is in the abdomen and cannot be seen or palpated as most structural muscles are. The origin is the transverse processes of all the lumbar vertebrae, and the insertion is the lesser trochanter of the femur. The action is to flex the thigh and to flex the vertebral column on the pelvis.

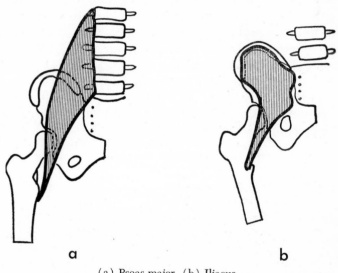

a   b

(a) Psoas major. (b) Iliacus.

Iliacus. This joins with the psoas major to flex the thigh. The origin of the iliacus is the upper two-thirds of the iliac fossa, the inner lip of the iliac crest, and the base of the sacrum. The insertion is the lateral side of the tendon of the psoas major and the body of the femur just below the lesser trochanter. The action is to flex the thigh and tilt the pelvis forward.

Chapter **10**

Shoulder

ANATOMY

The shoulder includes the clavicle (collar bone), scapula (wing bone), humerus (bone in upper arm), sternum (breast bone), and the surrounding soft tissues; namely muscles, tendons, ligaments, bursae, and capsule of the joint.

The shoulder joint is a free-moving, ball-and-socket joint. The joint is formed by a well-rounded head of the humerus and a shallow and small glenoid fossa. The capsule is loose owing to the range of motion in the joint. The ligaments do not hold the joint per se, but the burden falls on the surrounding muscles in the area. The muscles are the deltoid, pectoralis major, latissimus dorsi, teres major, and minor, supraspinatus, subscapularis, and the infraspinatus. There are several bursae in the shoulder area. (Bursae are sacs of fluid underlying moving parts.)

When diagnosing the shoulder, history, inspection, and palpation are used in that order. After the history has been established, the athlete strips to the waist and either stands or sits. Inspect both shoulders by comparing the injured with the "good shoulder." Any abnormality should be noted. Bone structure should be examined

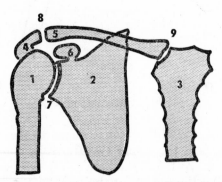

Bones of the shoulder. (1) Humerus. (2) Scapula. (3) Sternum. (4) Acromion process. (5) Clavicle. (6) Corocoid process. (7) Glenohumeral joint. (8) Acromioclavicular joint. (9) Sternoclavicular joint.

very closely for any change in contour before any functional tests for other injuries started. The examination should be systematic, starting with the clavicle and checking both ends; namely, the acromioclavicular joint and the sternoclavicular joint, scapula, the spine and body of the scapula, and finally the humerus. After the examination of the bones, functional tests should be performed to establish the extent and location of the "soft tissue" damage.

FRACTURES

Clavicle (Collar Bone). This is a rather common site of fracture in the early age groups, very common in the prehigh school and high school athletic programs, and reducing in frequency on the college level. The clavicle is very close to the skin, and by feeling all sides of the bone, any abnormality can be readily noted. Compare it with other side at all steps of the examination.

The frequency of fracture to this bone is readily attributed to its location and function. It is the only means of connection between the shoulder and the chest. A common cause of this injury is a fall on the outstretched arm or elbow or by direct blow over the bone itself. The most common site of a fracture to this bone occurs in the middle third. As mentioned above, the location will of necessity cause the bone to "bend," and when forced too far, a fracture will result. The middle third of this bone is where the compound curve exists. In the older age group, the fracture will be oblique; in the younger groups, the fracture will be of a "greenstick nature" (that is, one side of the bone will bend and the other will break).

In a complete fracture there will be an overriding of the ends, owing to the function of the clavicle, which will result in an obvious deformity. The athlete will hold his arm to his side and tilt his head toward the affected shoulder. Pain will be evident on touching the fracture site.

No attempt should be made to reduce this fracture. The injured side should be splinted by means of a sling and the strapping of the arm to the side, and the athlete should be sent to the team physician for treatment.

Scapula. This is a very rare type of fracture. Because of the many parts of the scapula, we shall discuss them one at a time.

Body of scapula. This injury, most times, is due to indirect causes such as falling on arm or the point of shoulder. There may be a fracture in the lower portion of the scapula. Upper parts are

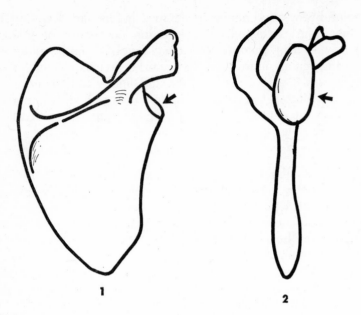

1   2

Scapula from the back (1) and from the axillary border (2), showing the location of the glenoid fossa.

very rarely affected. The scapula will fix itself in an attempt to raise the arm upward; the pain will be very noticeable, even to the point of preventing the full range of motion, and will be felt very deep. Feeling the fracture or deformity will be very difficult, and X-ray is indicated to complete the diagnosis. If fracture is suspected in the scapula, the affected arm should be placed in sling and the athlete sent to the team physician.

Spine of scapula. The very prominent portion of the scapula is easily palpated. There may be very little if any displacement, but the feeling of motion and crepitus is quite evident. Treatment is the same as for fracture of body of scapula.

Acromion process. In reviewing the anatomy of the scapula, the spine of the scapula turns in and forms the acromion process. This forms the top of the shoulder and is exposed to all direct contact that the shoulder makes. Also, force transmitted up the arm will cause injury to the acromion process. The acromion is so strong that rarely is it fractured; injuries that may cause the fracture of the acromion will also result in fractures of the clavicle, dislocated shoulder, or an acromioclavicular dislocation. This portion of the scapula is also close to the surface and very often the fracture may be felt. X-ray is necessary to pick up the small fractures that may occur. A sling must be used and conservative procedures taken by the trainer so that the athlete can be transported in comfort to the team physician.

Coracoid process. This is a very deep-seated process and cannot be felt. A fracture of the process does not occur as an injury in itself, but it is usually associated with other injuries in the shoulder joint. The coracoid process acts as the attachment for many strong muscles in the shoulder, and the spasm as a result of the injury will keep the broken fragment away from its base. X-ray is indicated to complete diagnosis. First aid is the same as in other shoulder fractures.

Glenoid fossa. This is the shallow cup in which the head of the humerus articulates to make the ball-and-socket joint. Falling on the outstretched arm or directly on the point of the shoulder is the cause of this fracture. The humerus is forced into the fossa, thus causing damage. This fracture may be of the small chip-type or a severe comminuted derangement. Fracture must be suspected when there is pain and crepitus on rotation of the humerus. Chip fractures of the glenoid may occur as a result of a dislocation of the shoulder joint. These are impossible to diagnose without X-ray.

Humerus. The humerus is a bone in the upper arm that articulates with the glenoid fossa to form the shoulder joint. A fracture to the humerus may be caused directly by falling on the arm, a direct blow to the humerus, or indirectly by falling on the outstretched

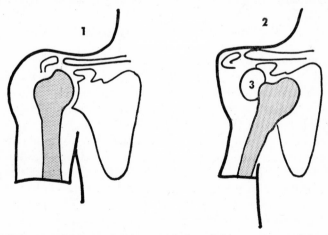

Humerus. (1) Normal position. (2) Out of glenoid fossa, as in a dislocation. (3) Glenoid fossa.

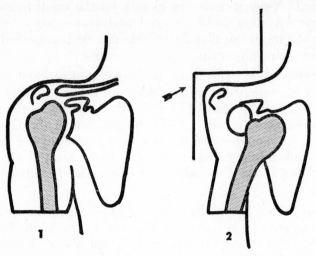

Humerus. (1) Normal position of head of humerus in glenoid fossa. (2) Head of humerus out of glenoid fossa in a typical dislocation. Arrow denotes typical "step" in dislocation.

hand. In the upper third of the humerus there are many parts of the bone that may be affected. To go into detail here would not be practical. Fractures of the shaft of the humerus are not so common as fractures of the upper part. We see a few such fractures, but they are not common. The diagnosis of a fracture is usually obvious, and it should be splinted with the arm in full extension, after which the athlete should be sent to the team physician.

DISLOCATION OF SHOULDER

A dislocation of the shoulder joint is defined as a complete displacement of one articular surface from the other. A partial dislocation is where the displacement is incomplete; the term *subluxation* may be used. Some athletes may have hypermobile or unstable joints which tend to subluxate in certain motions.

Dislocations appear more in the shoulder than at any other joint in the body. The reason may be the construction and the full range of motion of the joint. In athletics the shoulder is subjected to more counter joint motions than any other large joint in the body. The glenoid fossa is very shallow, and with the large head of the humerus, they do not make a perfect match. The soft tissue (ligaments and capsule) are comparatively loose. Also, the joint occupies a prominent place on our body and thus is exposed to more incidences of injury in which the head of the humerus is forced out of the capsule and away from the glenoid fossa.

The position of the head of the humerus after it leaves the normal position establishes the type of dislocation. If the head is in the front of the body, the dislocation is anterior and vice versa, namely, posterior (back), downward or upward. The anterior dislocations occur more frequently than do the posterior. A dislocated shoulder results in the tear of the capsule; the ligaments of the joint and the muscles around the shoulder are stretched and in some injuries are torn.

The history reported by the athlete will help in the establishment of the injury. There will be much pain, loss of function, and a very obvious deformity. There will be a flattening of the deltoid muscle area, and on palpation, you will be able to put your hand into the hollow formed by the absence of the head of the humerus from the capsule. The arm will appear to be longer because of the position of the humerus. The athlete will hold his arm in partial abduction and will tilt his head toward the injured side.

The clothing must be removed to establish a complete diagnosis. In football it is advisable to cut the jersey rather than try to pull it over the athlete's head. Cut close to the seam so that the jersey can be sewn back and used again.

After the diagnosis has been established, the quicker the reduction, the easier the athlete will feel. Many schools will not permit the trainer to reduce a dislocation. If so, with the injury as it exists, the athlete's arm should be put in a sling, with arm held to side by elastic bandages, and moved to the hospital for further treatment.

X-ray is used as a diagnostic procedure. Although the dislocation is obvious, the X-ray will rule out the possibility of any other bone pathology.

The incidence to fracture associated with a dislocation is not too common, and as a result many colleges will permit their trainers to reduce the dislocation immediately. This is often performed right on the field without taking time to remove the athlete to the training room.

Methods of reduction vary, but we shall mention just two.

Kocher's Method. Perhaps the most popular and the least traumatizing of all methods is the Kocher method.

Step 1. Flex elbow to a right angle and press closely to side.

Step 2. Holding the forearm at the wrist and elbow, slowly rotate the arm outward as far as it will go.

Step 3. While the arm is in this position, move the arm upward and across the chest.

Step 4. With the hand on the opposite shoulder, rotate the arm inward, slowly moving the hand downward.

At this point the head of the humerus will snap back into place. The motions described above should be done slowly without jerking. Slow, steady traction rather than fast jerking maneuvers are used.

Foot in Axilla. This method is used by team physicians all over the country and is very effective.

Step 1. Athlete is flat on back.

Step 2. Operator removes shoe and places foot under the arm of the athlete.

Step 3. Grasp the forearm of the athlete and apply gentle traction. The arm will be slightly abducted. As the muscle spasm relaxes, the arm can be brought in closer to the side.

Step 4. At this point the operator will rotate the arm inward; a very sudden and dramatic click should take place at this time, with the head slipping into position.

Should either of these methods fail to reduce the dislocation, the athlete should be sent to the hospital, where it may be necessary to use an anaesthetic in the procedure.

Treatment of Dislocation. The damage that results from dislocation is all in the soft tissue. We shall classify this as a series of sprains in the shoulder area. Start with the capsule, ligaments, and the muscles that surround the joint.

The shoulder is strapped with the routine strapping and a sling is worn along with a binder (elastic wrap to hold the arm immobile). The strapping will give the injured tissue support and will hold in close approximation for better healing. It will also serve as a compression bandage for the limitation of swelling. An ice cap should be applied over the shoulder joint to lessen the effusion. This strapping should be kept on for three days. The ice caps should be applied for the first 48 hours, after which the tape should be removed and heat and massage applied daily. After the treatment, the shoulder should again be taped and placed in sling, with the elastic bandage around the arm to prevent too much motion. This procedure is carried out for two weeks, and then passive motion is applied to the shoulder. It will not be necessary to strap the shoulder, but it is advisable to continue the use of the sling. As the passive exercises increase the range of motion, active exercises may then be substituted. Motions to avoid include full abduc-

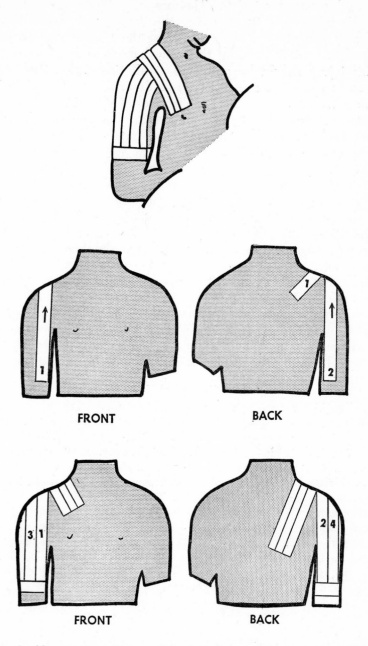

FRONT   BACK

FRONT   BACK

Routine shoulder strapping. For acromion clavicular separations, a piece of felt cut 2 by 2 inches square, or a 3-inch circle may be placed on the distal portion of the clavicle.

tion and external rotation. The use of weights as well as the shoulder wheel may be started in the third week. Full rehabilitation will take at least six weeks, and the athlete should not be allowed to participate until this time has elapsed.

This injury should be protected at all times when the athlete returns to activity, since this type tends to recur. The use of the shoulder harness (see p. 204) is effective. This can be bought from sporting goods dealers or may be made by a brace maker. Using 4-inch webbing, the chest is encircled, snugly but not too tightly; otherwise, breathing will be limited. The webbing may be held in place by shoulder straps. A similar piece of webbing is used to encircle the upper arm. A chain is used between the chest band and the arm band to limit the range of abduction of the arm. The arm should be limited to a range approximately 20 degrees short of shoulder level. The purpose of this harness is to prevent full abduction, since it is very unlikely that a shoulder will dislocate if it cannot reach full abduction. Some team physicians permit the use of a dog collar catch that can be unhooked at times. Unhooking on offense, in the case of an end, is very essential, and it is felt that with the athlete being under control, he will be able to keep his arm tensed to a point where he will be less likely to suffer a recurrence. On defense, the moves are so unexpected that the danger is high, and therefore the chain should be fixed at all times.

SHOULDER STRAP PROCEDURE

The shoulder strap is applied as the athlete stands with arm of affected side hanging at side. The arm should remain in this position while taping. The principle of this strapping is to pull the shoulder up, and this should be accomplished by the tape and not the athlete's own power. (See p. 197)

Step 1. Start the first strip about 2 inches above the crease of the bent elbow. Fix the tape on the arm and pull snug. The arm should be pulled upward to take the strain off the muscles. This strip of tape should run parallel with the arm and as close to the outline of the arm as possible. (Do not cross over axillary space with tape, as arm will then be fixed to side.) Extend tape over the shoulder and down to the lower portion of the scapula.

Step 2. From the back side of the arm, a similar strip runs parallel with the outline of the arm. Pull the arm upward and run the tape over strip 1, ending about 2 inches below the clavicle.

Step 3. Overlap strip 1 at least halfway.

Step 4. Overlap strip 2 at least halfway.

Step 5. Keep alternating until arm is completely enclosed in tape.

Step 6. Start the full anchor strip on the back side, just below the border of the scapula, and pull over the shoulder onto the chest, ending at the nipple line.

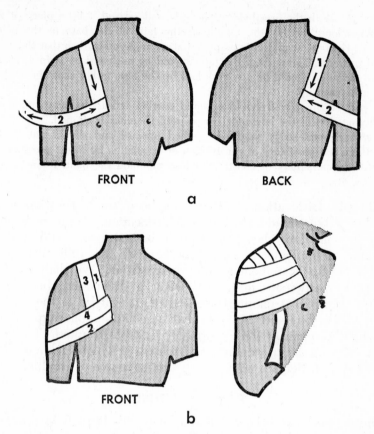

FRONT   BACK

a

FRONT

b

(a) Shoulder cap used as routine strapping, steps 1 and 2. (b) Steps 3 and 4.

Step 7. Overlap strip 6 at least halfway and continue with same procedure until shoulder is covered.

Step 8. Anchor strips should be applied to the ends of the strips that cross over shoulder.

Step 9. The lower end of the arm taping should be encircled with a strip of tape; however, do not apply tightly, as constriction will result. This is just an anchor and in no way adds to the support of the injury.

Shoulder Cap Procedure

This strapping is applied with the athlete in the standing position. It is considered by many trainers as a routine strapping for all shoulder injuries.

Step 1. Using a piece of tape approximately 24 inches long, place tape on top of shoulder close to neck and pull the ends downward in the front and back. The front strip should end just above the nipple line, and the back end should extend to approximately 1 inch below the scapula.

Step 2. With the arm held at the side and relaxed, take a piece of tape 18 inches long and lay the middle of the tape at the base of the deltoid muscle. The tape should then be pulled at an angle upward so that the arm is pulled upward. The ends of the tape should be anchored on strip 1. Action of arm elevation should be accomplished by the tape rather than the athlete's pulling his arm up.

Step 3. Strips across shoulder should overlap at least halfway and should be alternated with the horizontal strips until shoulder is capped.

The horizontal strips should be pulled upward and should not be flat, since there is a possibility of constriction of circulation by direct pressure. Be alert for the possibility of constriction by examining the hand for numbness, blueness, etc.

Chronic Dislocations. There has been some question as to whether a boy should play after a dislocation. Many orthopedic surgeons will allow a boy to continue if he is strapped with adhesive tape and an appliance of some type is used. It is difficult to make a hard and fast statement about this condition. We shall allow an athlete to participate in football after a dislocation, but should several recurrences manifest themselves, it will be to the best interests of the boy and the team that he consider some type of surgery for the repair of the abnormalcy that has resulted. There are many sports in the curriculum at all schools in which such a disabled athlete can participate without a potential source of trouble.

FUNCTIONAL TESTS

Inspection. The athlete stands erect with head held normally, feet together, and hands at his sides. Look at the injured shoulder and compare with other side. A change in contour may indicate a fracture, dislocation, or severe swelling. Compound fractures, where bone fragments are exposed, are very obvious. Should there be an obvious deformity, do not proceed further in your examination but immediately call the team doctor.

Palpation. Most of the bones of the shoulder are immediately below the surface of the skin and can be readily felt. Any abnormalcy felt but not visible should be noted and respected. A false joint or abnormal motion may be felt. Avoid any unnecessary roughness in handling any injury. By grasping bone on each side of the injury site, gently bend to and fro. You may feel a false joint or hear a grating sound. Do not proceed further if this is found.

Rule out the possibility of the more serious injuries before other tests (listed below) are started. Sprains and contusions of the shoulder may be localized by passive motions first and then active

motions with slight resistance. In the progress of the examination
the athlete will be able to point with his finger to the exact location
of the injury and the motion that causes the pain. From this a definite diagnosis can be made. To say that an athlete has a shoulder
injury is not complete or satisfactory. A definite diagnosis should be
made before any treatment is started.

General procedure in inspection is as follows:

1. Raising arm sideways to shoulder level, test for function of the deltoid
muscle. (The supraspinatus will perform this function for the first 10 degrees
and the deltoid the remainder of the way.) Middle fibers will perform most
of this function, with the anterior and posterior fibers as accessory muscles.

2. Lower arm from horizontal position. This will be easy, since gravity
enters into the picture, but with resistance from the trainer, this procedure
should locate the source of injury if it is in the latissimis dorsi, pectoralis major,
or teres major.

3. Extend the arm, stretching it backward. Muscle tested will be posterior
and middle third of the deltoid, infraspinatus, and the teres minor.

4. Flex the arm and swing forward. This tests the anterior deltoid,
pectoralis major, and the coracobrachialis.

5. The athlete rotates his arm, raising it to shoulder level, with elbow
bent as in throwing; the forearm is moved downward, thus rotating the
shoulder interiorly. Muscles tested will be the subscapularis, pectoralis major,
latissimus dorsi, teres, and the accessory muscle, anterior deltoid.

6. Rotate the arm as above but externally. Muscles tested in this movement will be the infraspinatus, the teres minor, and the accessory muscle,
posterior deltoid.

ACROMIOCLAVICULAR DISLOCATION

This dislocation is commonly called a *separation*, or "knocked
down shoulder." The acromion and clavicle that form this joint are
located directly under the skin and are frequently injured because
of the location. The ligaments that hold this joint intact may be
stretched or torn. The action that causes the separation is a fall
on the outstretched hand or elbow. In recent years many cases
have been caused by a direct blow to the point of the shoulder,
through either blocking or falling on the point of the shoulder. We
divide this injury into three categories: mild, moderate, and severe.

Mild. When the condition is painful but without any displacement or tearing of the soft tissue, the injury is mild. This will manifest itself in a very painful joint with some swelling. The use of
functional tests, as outlined, plus palpation will confirm the injury
to this joint. The clavicle, which is immediately below the surface,

can be held firmly with the fingers and gently moved up and down, and in some injuries forward and backward. Compare with the other joint. The degree of motion plus the amount of deformity will help to place injury in one of the three categories.

The immediate application of a strap and ice with a sling will help considerably during the first 24 hours. X-ray is indicated in mild as well as severe injury. On the second day the joint will feel better to palpation but will remain swollen. The same treatment continued for another day will do wonders. The application of heat between strapping will be very effective for the complete recovery of this injury. Infrared heat, hot towels, etc., are easily applied and work very effectively because the injury is immediately below the skin and all heat applied to the surface will help this condition. When all the soreness is out of the area, the athlete is allowed to go back to participation. This is usually after a period of three to six days. Padding for protection is indicated. This type of pad consists of cutting a hole in a piece of sponge rubber and taping it over the injured area, with the tender part encircled by the sponge rubber.

Moderate. Soft tissue is stretched or even slightly torn. The acromion ligament is most frequently involved, but the other ligaments are sound. There is usually a slight displacement and much swelling and tenderness over the joint. The tip of the clavicle will be well pronounced, with the weight of the arm pulling the acromion down. The range of motion will be affected, primarily abduction of the arm. X-ray should be taken to establish final diagnosis.

With the partial tearing of the ligament, it will be necessary to keep the joint quiet for a longer period of time than in the mild case. The treatment will be the same as in the mild case but will have to be carried out for a longer period of time. In strapping this moderate type of acromioclavicular injury, a piece of felt ½ inch thick and cut 2 inches by 3 inches is placed on the end of the clavicle. This helps to approximate the joint. Adhesive tape may have a tendency to bridge over the "site," and the use of felt to mold to the contours of the shoulder will enhance the direct compression needed to treat and strap the injury properly. We are inclined to use infrared heat on this injury. Our results with this modality have been very satisfactory. The injury will be strapped daily and a sling will be used. The length of time that this joint is strapped is usually ten days. In this period, passive exercises are used to a limited degree. Active exercises are started on or about

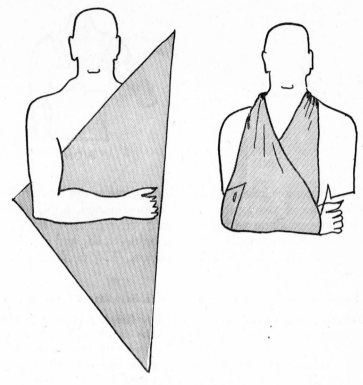

Application of a sling.

the tenth day. There will be atrophy of the muscles in the shoulder and arm, and the athlete will not be allowed to go back into action until this has been overcome. The length of time lost due to this type of separation is usually from three to six weeks.

Severe. The ligaments that hold the joint intact have been torn and there will be much displacement. The clavicle will be displaced as much as 1½ inches. This is an injury that is very obvious to the trainer because the amount of deformity can be readily observed. Do not attempt to reduce the displacement, but place the arm in a sling and send the athlete for immediate medical treatment.

Surgical procedures are indicated in an injury of this type. The conservative treatment, as mentioned in the moderate type of injury, has failed to give adequate results, and surgical intervention is now the procedure followed. However, the conservative treatment used is the application of a modified Watson-Jones strapping and a sling. This strapping is worn for a period of about four weeks,

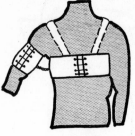

Restrictive harness to avoid recurrent dislocation.

FRONT

with the strapping reinforced from time to time as the tape stretches. After this time, if the joint remains approximated, applications of heat and massage along with passive and active exercises are started. There will be much atrophy in the shoulder area, and much work must be done to overcome this condition. The disability time of this injury is about three months.

STRAPPING FOR ACROMION CLAVICULAR SEPARATION (SEVERE)

The athlete stands with arm at side and elbow flexed. A piece of ½-inch felt 2 inches square is placed on the distal end of the clavicle, and another piece of ½-inch felt is cut 2 by 4 inches and applied under the elbow. (See p. 206)

Step 1. Start the tape on the back side of the affected shoulder; pull at a downward angle over the felt applied to the distal end of the clavicle. Con-

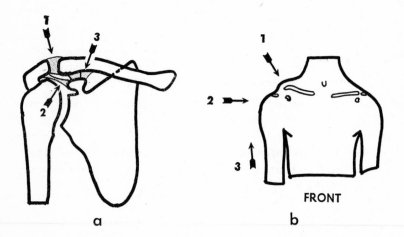

a   b

FRONT

(a) Ligaments of the acromioclavicular joint. (1) Acromioclavicular ligament. (2) Coracoacromial ligament. (3) Coracoclavicular ligament. (b) Acromioclavicular separation. (1) Position of clavicle and deformity. (2) Force that may cause separation. (3) Direction of humerus when falling on outstretched arm elbow.

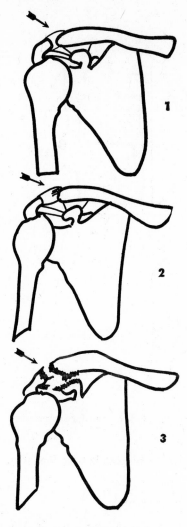

Acromioclavicular separation. (1) Mild injury; tissues are stretched but not torn. (2) Medium injury; tissues are slightly torn. (3) Severe injury; tissues are completely torn.

tinue the tape along the upper arm around the elbow (2 by 4 felt pad will be held in place by this strip), up the back of the arm, crossing the shoulder, with the felt pad ending on front of chest.

The felt pad must be under the distal end of the elbow in line with the humerus for a direct upward push of the shoulder. If tape is applied forward on the forearm, the elbow will flex with the movement, and loss of pressure will result.

Step 2. The second strip is applied by overlapping at least halfway (preferably three-quarters). The use of more strips will be governed by the severity of the injury and the amount of support needed. The arm may be fixed to the side by the use of a horizontal strip completely surrounding the

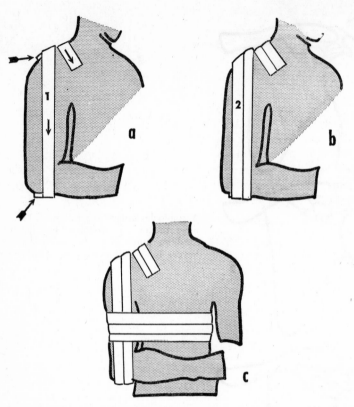

Strapping for moderate to severe separation. Large arrows indicate felt for compression.

body. Do not pull too tightly. This strip is not for support but for limitation of motion.

STERNOCLAVICULAR DISLOCATION

This dislocation is a rather uncommon injury in athletics, but it is wise to be aware of its possibility. It may occur by falling on the arm or by falling directly on the point of the shoulder. We have seen two of these caused by a direct blow to the inner end of the clavicle. The displacement may be backward or downward, but most displacements are forward. The clavicle will manifest itself in the form of a pronounced lump on the breast bone, with a fair amount of motion. When this injury occurs, there is damage to the soft tissue from stretching of the ligaments or the extensive tearing of all the soft tissue. History is usually vague, with reports

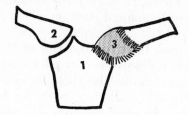

Sternoclavicular joint. (1) Sternum.
(2) Clavicle. (3) Sternal clavicular
ligament.

of pain at areas other than this point. Very often the pain is referred up into the neck. On examination the deformity is obvious,
even if it is slight. The clavicle is directly beneath the skin, and it
can be readily seen as well as easily palpated. Along with the visible
condition, an X-ray should be taken, to eliminate any further bone
pathology.

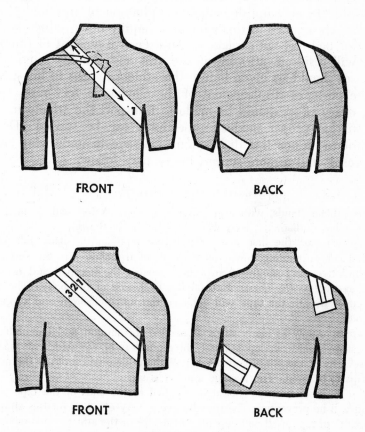

FRONT   BACK

FRONT   BACK

Strapping for sternal clavicular separation or sprain.

The treatment of an anterior (or forward) displacement is designed to compress the clavicle back to its normal position. This is best accomplished by applying a piece of felt approximately 3 inches square, or a 3-inch circle at least ½ inch thick, on the end of the clavicle. By using adhesive tape (elastic adhesive is very effective), this is held in place by pulling the tape across the shoulder over the pad and extending around the side and anchoring on the back. Several strips should be used. A sling is also used to immobilize the arm on the affected side. The treatment is designed to hold the joint immobile and allow the soft tissues to heal. If removed too soon, the clavicle will tend to slide forward. The immobilization is usually applied for three weeks. After three weeks, the arm may be taken out of the sling and light exercises permitted. It may be well to note that the deformity will always remain in this joint. This is due to the amount of scar tissue formed and the fact that it is almost impossible to accomplish complete reduction of this injury. The more severe injuries in this joint may require open reduction (surgery) or bed rest with traction. An excessive amount of time in a sling will result in atrophy of the arm and shoulder, and active exercises should be given before the athlete returns to his sport.

The posterior displacement of the clavicle is very rare, and if seen, every effort should be made to transport the athlete in comfort so that proper medical procedures can be started. Do not attempt to reduce this dislocation. Damage to underlying tissues may result and a more serious injury may follow.

STERNOCLAVICULAR STRAPPING

The athlete stands, with arm hanging at side. A felt pad, ½-inch thick and 3 inches in diameter, is applied over the site of the injury. (See p. 207)

Step 1. Start the first strip of adhesive tape on the back side of the affected side, extending down the back about 6 inches. Fix the end of the tape and then pull snugly at an angle, crossing the felt pad and extending down and across the chest. End on the back side of the body. The larger area covered with the tape will enhance the immobilization and support of this joint.

Step 2. Apply as many strips as needed for support and immobilization. Each strip should overlap at least three-quarters of the width of the tape. The severity of the injury and the size of the athlete will indicate the number of strips to be used. The average number is six.

Step 3. Anchor strips should be applied to the ends of the tape so that rolling will be prevented. Elastic adhesive is very effective for this strapping. The width of tape used will depend on the size of the athlete. A 3-inch width is used regularly and seems to be the best allround size.

SPRAIN OF SHOULDER

A sprain of the shoulder is a very common injury to the athlete. All sports contribute their share of this injury. A sprain in football caused by arm tackling, baseball pitcher throwing too hard too soon, the fencer lunging beyond normal—all are examples of how the shoulder can be sprained. To say a shoulder is sprained means nothing. Time must be taken to establish the full extent of the injury. History, inspection, and palpation must be put to practice to establish the final diagnosis. A sprain to the shoulder joint may include all the ligaments as well as the larger muscles that surround the joint.

The athlete will help in his history by using hand or finger to localize the pain. The depth of the pain will also be described by the athlete. A sprain, as we have already mentioned, is the partial tearing or separating of fibers in the ligaments of the joint. Along with the sprain of the ligaments, there is damage to the overlying tissues; namely, tendons and muscles. The tendons of the smaller muscles are closely allied and form part of the capsule. We cannot lose sight of the fact that the nerves in this area may be also involved. When this type of injury occurs, we have an increase of joint fluid and hemorrhage resulting from damage to the blood vessels. We must try to limit the overproduction of fluid and the hemorrhage that results from the sprain.

The immediate application of a compression strap and the use of ice must be made as soon as possible. The more swelling, the longer the period of absorption, and this will in turn extend the disability time. Use ice for several days, accompanied by adhesive strapping for compression, and the sling for support. Be careful not to start heat too early, so that recurrence of hemorrhage will not be the result of too early and too vigorous treatment. After the 48-hour period, apply heat and exercise (active or passive, depending on the severity of the sprain; active exercises as soon as possible). As mentioned before, use the shower in an injury to the shoulder. The shower is applied directly to the shoulder for 5 minutes, allowing the area to become pleasantly red. When the skin is red, instruct the athlete in active motion, starting with arm swinging forward and backward. All motion is governed by the tolerance of the athlete. Then abduction is started, followed by complete circumduction. In starting, the athlete may only have a 10-degree range of motion in all directions. This should not be forced, but as the athlete continues this treatment, the tissues will relax and thus allow more freedom of motion.

Circumduction of the shoulder can be accomplished easily by having the athlete bend over, letting his arm swing by partially swaying the upper body. If this treatment is not available, hot towels are very effective. At this stage of repair, again apply the compression wrap and sling. The next day the same procedure takes place. When full range of motion is reached, eliminate the wrap and sling and encourage as much activity as possible. Resistance exercises are started at this time, i.e., weights, push-ups, etc. (Incidentally, start the push-ups by having the athlete stand 2 feet from a wall and do the push-up from this position before full body weight is allowed on the arm.)

The use of massage is quite beneficial in all types of shoulder sprains. Strapping may be continued when the athlete returns to full activity. This depends on the degree of injury and the sport involved.

STRAIN OF SHOULDER

Shoulder strain is a very common injury and not relegated specifically to any sport. The degree of strain will vary from intensive pain and loss of function to just plain soreness. The incidence may be the result of a countermotion or just plain overexertion. There may or may not be damage to the tissue fibers, depending on the severity of the activity. Functional tests are referred to for final interpretation of injury.

Treatment of a mild strain will consist of overnight rest with the arm in sling. Ice packs may be used to alleviate the pain and "cool off" the injury. Very often this is all that is needed in a mild strain.

In the moderate-to-severe type, strapping with routine shoulder strap, sling, and ice bag for 24 to 48 hours is required. After this time, heat and massage are indicated. As soon as heat is applied, either active or passive exercises should be started. The strain of the shoulder will respond readily to gradual exercise after the acute pain (first 48 hours) has subsided. Stiffness from lack of exercise may disguise the recovery of this lesion. Stretching is a vital procedure in the treatment of all sprains and strains. Specific exercises will be handled separately later in this chapter.

The disability time for a strain is from overnight to three or four days. The need to continue the use of strappings will depend on the sport and the individual.

CONTUSIONS TO SHOULDER

Acromion Process. The acromion process is a very painful and disabling injury in the early stages. This is quite prevalent in foot-

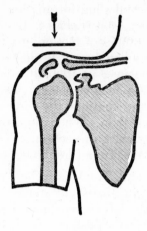

Typical swelling over the acromio-clavicular joint. Arrow points in direction of blow.

ball but not too common in other sports. It is caused by a direct blow to the shoulder, very often through the shoulder pads on a hard block or tackle. This is a self-limiting injury, since the pain will guide the range of motion in the arm. The acromion process is a very important attachment for the shoulder muscles, and we must consider that these tissues, as well as the bone, are bruised.

The immediate treatment consists of the application of ice to the area. Use a routine shoulder strap and the sling. This procedure is carried out for the first two days. On the third day the strapping will be removed and the injury inspected. If the swelling has subsided and the amount of pain diminished, use heat and active mo-

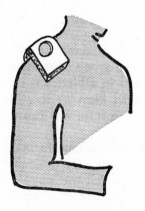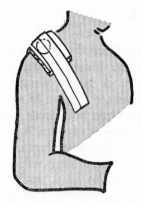

Sponge rubber with hole cut for protection of a contusion of the acromion process.

tion. If not, continue the strapping, ice, and sling for another day. Infrared heat is very effective in this injury, as it is close to the skin.

Starting with passive exercises, in all ranges of motion, graduate to active motion as soon as tolerable. The hot shower is most effective in this injury, as the athlete will be in a position to exercise the arm after it is warm, thus hastening the healing process. Do not strap the injury after the first few days, but continue the sling until the arm can be held at the side without pain. When the athlete returns to play, he should wear a pad for extra protection.

Length of disability of this injury averages from three to ten days.

Contusion to Soft Tissue—Muscles and Tendons. The larger muscles are quite susceptible to bruise in almost all sports. The deltoid, trapezius, pectoralis major, and the latissimus dorsi are most commonly affected. The athlete will give the history of the force and will point with his finger or whole hand to the extent of the area. In all acute bruises of the area, use ice and compression for the first 24 hours. A sling in this case, even though the athlete does not like to wear it, is very effective. Use the sling overnight, and on the next day start active exercises. If function returns with limited exercise, allow the athlete to work on a schedule that is within his bounds. Very often the injury will not deter the athlete from all his drills, and in this way the motion tends to promote healing in the injured muscle.

Contusions of tendons are not as likely to respond to this treatment, since the circulation is limited in this type of tissue. Use the sling for longer periods of time and limit the amount of activity to the joint. Use heat earlier in the tendon injury than in the muscle injury.

BURSITIS

A bursa is a sac filled with fluid that underlies moving tissues (i.e., tendon over bone, or tendon over a group of tendons) to prevent friction. Most bursitis encountered in athletics is of the traumatic type. A severe wrench or a hard blow to the area of the bursa will cause the sac to swell. This, in turn, will cause pressure, and the pressure will cause pain.

The diagnosis of bursitis is a very difficult one to make. Functional tests include abduction of arm (extremely difficult but with a little help the athlete will be able to go all the way). Touching the small of the back with the affected arm is either extremely painful or impossible. The area may be warm to the touch, indicating inflammation. X-ray may show the distended bursa or cal-

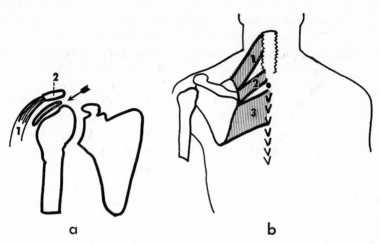

(a) Bursa. (1) Deltoid muscle. (2) Acromion process. Arrow indicates the subdeltoid bursa. Note its extension under the acromion. (b) Rhomboids. (1) Levator scapula. (2) Rhomboid minor. (3) Rhomboid major.

cium deposits from previous injuries. On pressure of the area, crepitus may be felt.

Once the diagnosis is made, the treatment consists of rest, by means of a sling, and either hot or cold packs. Some cases respond beautifully to heat. Others will react violently to this modality. Conversely, the same has taken place when cold packs have been used. Try both and find the one that is tolerable to the athlete. After pain has subsided, continue with sling and include abduction and rotation exercises for the restoration of movement in the shoulder area.

Injections of medications are best left in the hands of the team physician. X-ray has been recommended as a means of treatment. This also should be decided by the team physician.

TENOSYNOVITIS OF LONG HEAD OF BICEPS

Review the anatomy of the biceps tendon, the sheath, and the position and action of the muscle. This condition is many times confused with bursitis and tendinitis. Diagnosis is difficult and history is very important. Pain is persistent, even at rest. There may or may not be obvious swelling at the site, caused by overlying muscles. This condition may be either "wet" or "dry," the "wet" being from the overproduction of synovial fluid in the sheath; the "dry" is the failure of enough fluid to lubricate the tendon. Both conditions are caused by irritation, either from excessive use of the tendon, or trauma, such as contact with a hard object (i.e., helmet, etc.). During the course of the activity, a dull soreness will prevail. As soon as the athlete stops and is cooled off, the condition will set up a continuous ache. The motion of the arm and shoulder will be minimized because of pain.

Treatment consists of a good history, inspection, and palpation. Inspection will not usually reveal anything of consequence. Palpation will show tenderness over the area of the biceps tendon and a general tightness in the upper arm. In functional tests the athlete may not be able to go through the normal functions of the shoulder because of intense pain and tightness. Abduction and rotation of the shoulder joint will be limited.

Treatment will consist of much rest and support. Both are best accomplished by shoulder strapping and a sling. The immediate use of ice is indicated in the early stages but may aggravate the condition on the second day. Extensive physical therapy measures should be taken; any modality of heat will help in early recovery. Diathermy, ultrasonics, etc., are helpful. Length of disability varies with the condition from a week to months.

INDIVIDUAL SHOULDER MUSCLES AND THEIR INJURIES

The rhomboids, the latissimus dorsi, the levator scapulae, and the trapezius muscles have been described in Chapter 9. Other muscles affiliated with the shoulder and sometimes involved in shoulder injury are described in subsequent paragraphs along with treatment of injury to them.

The pectoralis major is a flat muscle situated directly under the skin over the front of the chest. It originates at the sternal half of the clavicle (collar bone), the sternum, and the cartilages of the first six ribs. Insertion is at the bicipital groove of the humerus. The pectoralis adducts the arm, draws it forward, and rotates it inward. Injuries are not common to this muscle, but when they happen, they are inclined to linger on.

Complete rest is indicated. Forcing the pectoralis major to function against its will may result in a rupture of this muscle. Unfortunately we have seen too many ruptures of this type, all of which could have been avoided by simple rest and progressive treatments of heat and massage until symptoms had been eliminated. The more serious of these injuries have occurred in discus throwers who insisted upon "working out the soreness," the result being a partial rupture of the muscle. When handled properly, this muscle will respond beautifully, as its circulation is excellent.

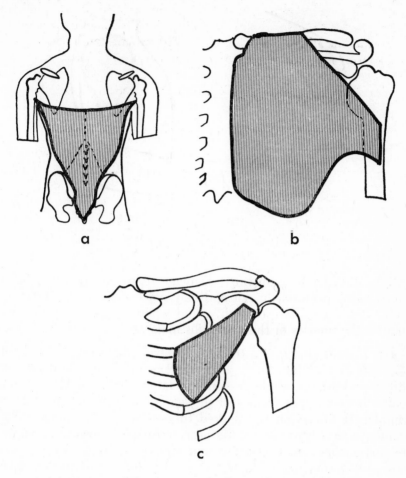

(a) Latissimus dorsi. (b) Pectoralis major. (c) Pectoralis minor.

Much success in treating this injury has been attributed to the use of the routine shoulder strap (allowing the vertical strips of adhesive to extend below the nipple line and across the sternum) and a sling. The purpose of these two steps is to take as much strain off the muscle as possible. By eliminating the weight of the arm, the pectoralis is allowed to relax in complete rest.

The pectoralis minor is located under the pectoralis major on the front part of the chest. It originates on the outer surface of the third, fourth, and fifth ribs and attaches to the corocoid process of the scapula. Its action is to depress the point of shoulder and also

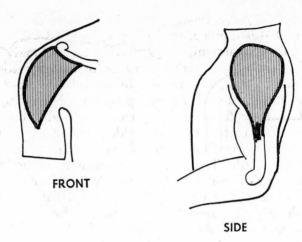

FRONT

SIDE

Deltoid (front and side view).

to draw the shoulder forward. Damage to it may be included in injury to the pectoralis major and may not be seen as an injury by itself. It is a very rare disability, and when seen, it is treated the same as the injuries of the pectoralis major.

The deltoid muscle is a triangular muscle that covers the shoulder. It is divided into three parts: anterior third, middle third, and posterior third. It originates on the lateral third of the clavicle (collar bone), upper surface of the acromion, and the spine of the scapula. It inserts on the deltoid tuberosity of the humerus. Its primary action is to abduct the arm (raise arm upward). Injuries are not uncommon; contusions and strains are seen in all sports. Injury to any one of the three portions interferes with all the movements involved in the elevation of the arm. The inability to elevate the arm presents a serious problem to the athlete, and in many cases it renders the athlete unable to participate.

Contusions and sprains of any portion of the deltoid are treated symptomatically. Rest, support, heat, and massage are most effective in this region. Support with the routine shoulder strapping or the shoulder cap are indicated, as is the use of a sling for the first 24 hours. In football the most common injury to the shoulder is a strain of the deltoid (anterior third) from "arm tackling." The force of the runner against the outstretched arm results in a stretching of the deltoid, thus inducing a strain. Blocking with the shoulder in an awkward position often results in a contusion of the anterior third of the deltoid.

These injuries, even though different in incidence, are treated similarly; that is, strapping, ice, and a sling for the first 24 hours. After this initial treatment, the use of heat (preferably moist) is very effective, along with active exercises for the restoration of motion. The hot shower has proved to be most effective in this injury. The heat of the water and the light pounding of the droplets gives a very relaxing condition to the muscle involved. Also, the heat allows free active motion of the shoulder joint so that active exercises may be performed under the shower. Simple movements are stressed at first, gradually going into free-swinging exercises. When the athlete is being treated by other methods, he must remain inactive. As a result, he feels that the treatment has "tightened him up," and there will be more pain on motion than previous to the "heat treatment." The shower allows for heat and motion at the same time. After the shower treatment, the use of massage is very effective to loosen further the muscles that also surround the joint.

Instruction in the proper way to wear the shoulder pads, plus coaching the athlete in the rights and wrongs of tackling, will help to eliminate these conditions found in the deltoid muscle.

The rotators of the humerus present a group of three muscles; namely, the *infraspinatus, subscapularis,* and the *teres minor.* The infraspinatus and the teres minor originate at the scapula and insert at the tuberosity of the humerus. The subscapularis originates on the interior side of the scapula and inserts on the lesser tuberosity of the humerus. The first two named are known as the *outward rotators* of the humerus; the last, as the *inward rotator* of the humerus. All these muscles act to hold the humerus in the socket.

The most common injury to this group is strain. The mechanic of a strain in this area is forced rotation of the arm, either inward or outward. A common cause of this injury is "arm tackling" or a similar action. The pain is pinpointed by the athlete and rotation of the arm causes pain over a very localized point in the joint. The athlete complains of pain deep in the joint. He says that he cannot touch it with his fingers but will point with one finger to the location. Routine strapping and ice are very effective in early treatment, followed by heat and active motion on the next day. This injury is often confused with a strain of the anterior deltoid, but it does not respond as readily. Disability varies with the sport, from a few days to weeks, and is very exasperating at times, especially in a pitcher. Certainly, an athlete should not try to force this injury in work-outs. Gradual increase in motion should be emphasized because the tendency to recur is very prevalent.

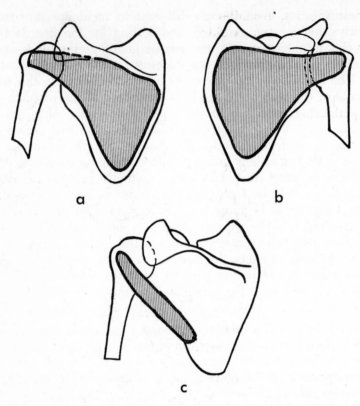

The rotators. (a) Infraspinatus. (b) Subscapularis. (c) Teres minor.

Very often in the dislocation of the shoulder, there will be a rupture (tear) of the rotator cuff. Some surgeons believe that a rupture of the rotators is the specific underlying cause of the dislocation of shoulders. Care of this injury must be complete, and the athlete should be symptom-free before returning to full duty.

The supraspinatus is a small but very powerful muscle that underlies the trapezius. It originates in the supraspinous fossa and inserts on the greater tuberosity of the humerus and the capsule of the shoulder joint. The action of the supraspinatus is to help abduct the arm along with the deltoid and also to hold the humerus in the glenoid cavity.

Injury to the shoulder joint, dislocation, etc., will involve this particular muscle, as will strains of the rotators. Pain will be deep and accentuated on abducting the arm. Treatment of acute injury should include strapping of the shoulder and the application of ice.

Heat may be started after 24 hours, followed by light exercise. Overexertion should be avoided, as this injury is very persistent and is easily aggravated in the early stages. It is a very disabling injury to a pitcher, weight thrower, etc., and treatment should be slow and deliberate.

The teres major is a small, round muscle that runs along the axillary border of the scapula. It originates on the scapula on the dorsal surface of the inferior angle. Its insertion is on the bicipital groove of the humerus. The action of the teres major is to adduct the arm and medially rotate the humerus. It also draws back the arm.

Common injury is a strain, seen more in baseball than in any other sport. Immediate treatment consists of ice and a sling for support. Early heat applications and gradual exercises are very effective, and the response is rather dramatic if not forced. Disability varies with the degree of strain and may be from one day to three or four.

Injury to the teres major, and in some degree to the teres minor, has been advanced as the true "Glass Arm" so often reported in the newspapers. Others have advanced the theory that the long head of the biceps, which sits in its own little hollow, is the true "Glass Arm." The mechanics of the biceps injury is that the small ligament holding the tendon in place has stretched and does not hold the tendon in its proper location. Constant irritation causes pain, pain in turn causes ineffectiveness, and thus the pitching career is ended. From personal experience we cannot deny or confirm these reports, but we feel that they should be mentioned as a matter of record.

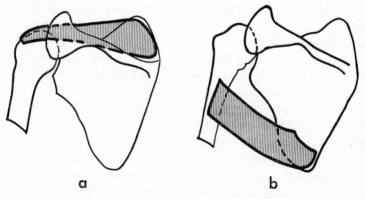

a   b

(a) Supraspinatus. (b) Teres major.

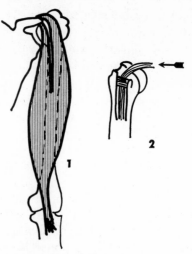

Biceps brachii. (1) Biceps. (2) Long tendon of biceps and transverse ligament.

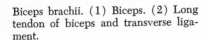

Biceps brachii is a very prominent muscle of the upper arm and has two tendons for its origin. The long head originates on the top of the glenoid fossa (this tendon passes over the head of the humerus and blends with the capsular ligament of the shoulder joint); the short head originates from the corocoid process. The insertion is on the bicipital tuberosity of the radius. The action of the biceps is to flex and supinate the forearm. The tendon of the long head of the biceps is very slender and lies in the bicipital groove of the humerus. The tendon of the long head is enclosed in a special sheath, which is lubricated with synovial fluid. The tendon is held in the groove by a transverse ligament.

Injuries to the upper end of the biceps (shoulder) are often confused with injury to the middle portion of the deltoid, the biceps being deeper. Pain and findings must go below the surface of the skin to fall in this category. Inflammation of the tendon sheath has been discussed earlier in this chapter; injury to the belly of the muscle will be found in injuries to the upper arm.

Contusion of the long head of the biceps will also result in other injuries; namely, contusion of deltoid and the humerus itself. Treatment is symptomatic; heat and rest for a short period of time will bring excellent results. Strapping, etc., is applied as described in the paragraph on the deltoid muscle.

The serratus anterior originates on the outer surface of the upper ribs and resembles the fingers of the hand stretching over the ribs. Its insertion is the vertebral border of the scapula. The action is to abduct the scapula and raise eight ribs in the chest. A direct injury is very rare and functional loss with "winging" is uncommon because of the peculiar anatomy of the long thoracic nerve, although occasional direct contusion to this may occur along its exposed course. Most injuries are usually associated with injuries of the ribs. These may affect the action of the arm by limiting the abduction of the humerus, and in turn, disguise an injury to the

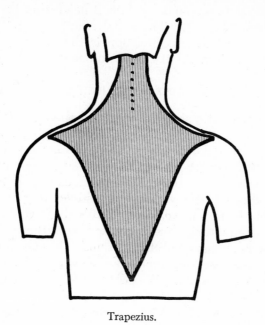

Trapezius.

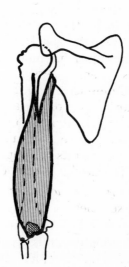

Triceps.

anterior deltoid. Treatment is symptomatic, i.e., pain and limitation of motion. Heat and exercise will help to overcome this injury. Disability is very short or not at all.

The triceps muscle is located on the back of the arm and has three separate places of origin. The origin is (1) long head from the tuberosity of the scapula, (2) lateral head from the lateral surface of the humerus, and (3) medial head from lower posterior portion of the humerus. Its insertion is the olecranon process of the ulna. The action of the triceps is to extend the arm.

SHOULDER REHABILITATION

The shoulder is not a simple joint to rehabilitate after an injury; it is one of the most difficult on which to obtain results. In comparison to an ankle or a knee, where daily chores help, the shoulder is a most sedentary part of the body. The student may at some time of the day carry his books or laundry, and at other times the only exercise that he does with the shoulder girdle is to feed himself. With this in mind, we must always be concerned with the amount of atrophy that manifests itself and then try to devise means to overcome this condition at times other than at a practice session. Some exercises for "home work" will be listed as well as rehabilitation exercises that can be used in the training room or on the field.

To increase range of motion in the shoulder, the *pendulum exercise* takes first place. With the athlete bending over to touch his toes, he allows his arm to swing to and fro. Gravity has a very important role to play in this exercise. By gradually twisting his trunk, the arm will "float" in the breeze without discomfort, thus increasing his range of motion.

Shoulder shrug is a very mild form of exercise that may be done at any time and will help to lessen the degree of atrophy. Deltoid setting, without moving the arm, contracting of the deltoid, and then relaxing continued until muscle is slightly tired is also helpful. Walk the wall with the fingers by facing it with elbows bent and placing the palms of the hand flat on the wall. Attempt to grasp the wall with the fingers, moving the arm upward. This exercise should be done to the point of tolerance. When height is attained, walk down the wall as well as up for better control.

Push-ups may be attempted from the same position described above. The athlete stands approximately 2 feet from the wall with arms extended at shoulder level; the body will dip toward the hands, and then with effort the starting position can be assumed. Should this prove too much of an effort, the athlete may move closer to the wall.

By using a wand, all motions of the shoulder may be tried, as the "good arm" will carry the load, with the injured arm moving forward, thus increasing motion. The wand is gripped with both hands separated about 24 inches. Raise the wand overhead so that all motions of the shoulder joint may be included in the exercise. These are a few exercises and they will suggest others to you. At the point of full motion, add resistive exercises to the program. Resistance builds strength faster than exercises without resistance; the types of exercises are numerous, so only a few will be mentioned.

General Exercises

1. Hanging from a high bar, plus pull-ups.
2. Push-ups, either on the floor or between two chairs as dips on the parallel bars.
3. Pulley weights, if they are available, may be used in many variations. Weights are also recommended at this stage, starting off with a light weight and then building up to heavier weights.
4. Presses and lateral raises are very good for the deltoid. The variation of the angle of lift will benefit various parts of the deltoid muscle.

For the baseball player with an injured shoulder that has become very weak, the simulated throwing motion with the weight is a

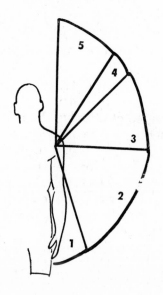

Shoulder adduction. (1) Supraspinatus. (2) Deltoid. (3) Trapezius and serratus anterior. (4) External rotation of humerus. (5) Deltoid.

recommended exercise. The average of the weight is about 5 pounds, and the number of throws start at 20 and build up gradually from work-out to work-out. The best results from this program have been obtained on a three-day-a-week basis rather than every day.

Chapter 11

Arm

UPPER ARM

Fractures. The humerus, the long bone of the upper arm, is divided into three categories: the upper end, the shaft, and the lower end. The upper end is at the shoulder joint and the lower, or supracondylar, at the elbow joint.

The cause of fracture to the humerus is direct (such as a blow, etc.) or indirect (such as falling on the outstretched hand with transmission of the force up the arm to the humerus). Some fractures are the result of a severe sprain, where a part of the bone is pulled off with the mechanics of the muscle tear. These fractures are hard to see or feel and X-ray must confirm findings. Fractures of the upper and lower end of the humerus fall in this category, and suspected fractures must be X-rayed for final diagnosis. Fractures of the shaft of the humerus occur in athletics, and the bone may be palpated to feel any abnormality. Fractures may be transverse, oblique, or spiral, and these may be comminuted as a result of the indirect force. There may or may not be a deformity, but pain and tenderness will be apparent. Point tenderness over the site will also be apparent. In suspected fractures of the humerus, splint and transport for medical services. The use of a sling, if arm is splinted in flexion, is vital. However, suspected fractures of the humerus may be splinted with the arm in full extension, with the arm in splint strapped to the side.

STRAINS

Long Head of Biceps. Because of its location and functions, the long head of the biceps is subject to many conditions that may be classified as an injury only because of the disability.

Dislocation of the long head. This is an injury that does occur but which is fortunately very rare. It may be the result of a dislocation, partial dislocation, or overstretching of the arm. The biceps tendon is located in the bicipital groove and is held in place by a band that overlies the tendon. The band is stretched or torn and the tendon leaves its groove. The deformity will be obvious, since there will be an unnatural hollow in the upper part of the arm. The symptoms are loss of function, pain, swelling, and deformity.

Treatment consists of the immediate application of ice and the use of a sling. The team physician should be seen at this time. The tendon should be replaced and strapped into position, using the shoulder cap or routine strapping with additional support over the tendonous groove. The continued use of the sling is also recommended.

Strain of the Biceps. The mechanics of a strain to the biceps is the forcing of the muscle to do more than it is capable of doing. The symptoms are soreness, inability to function properly, pain, point tenderness, and possibly swelling.

Treatment consists of the application of ice and sling. Depending on the severity of the strain, the use of whirlpool on the next day, with exercise, may be started. If the pain has not subsided, the continuance of cold for another day will help alleviate the condition.

The disability is from a day or two to about two weeks.

The biceps flexes the arm, and to strap this injury would be very difficult. However, the use of the cinch strap to prevent hyperextension of the elbow will help to limit the range of motion of the biceps muscle.

CONTUSION OF UPPER ARM

One of the more common injuries is a bruise to the outside of the upper arm. It is very common in football but is found in all contact sports. Soreness and swelling are evident, but limitation of motion depends on the severity of the bruise. History will reveal the incident, while palpation will produce pain. Inspection may or may not reveal swelling.

Treatment. The immediate application of ice and compression controls bleeding. The next day, depending on the severity of the injury, heat may be applied. Moist heat, whirlpool, hot soaks, hot shower, etc., are very effective forms of heat for this injury. If the bruise is very swollen, the continuance of a sling should be indicated. In severe bruises the use of a sling during the acute stage is very beneficial. In mild cases the use of a "hot pack" and a protective pad may be all that is necessary.

Myositis ossificans. This is a complication of a severe bruise to the upper arm. Calcification of the hematoma results in the production of a very hard mass. Treatment by diathermy and ultra sonics, etc., has helped resorb the calcium. A protective pad is very necessary to prevent further aggravation of this injury. The possibility of surgical intervention in this condition must be handled by the team physician and the athlete. They, in turn, will make the decision. Surgery, however, is not recommended until the injury has "cooled down," usually about two years after the incident of injury.

INJURIES TO FOREARM

There are two long bones, the ulna and radius, and many muscles in the forearm. The muscles may be divided into two categories: the *flexors* and the *extensors*. These muscles are superficial or deep. The *ulna* is a long bone and is sometimes referred to as the *continuation* of the humerus. It is superficial and can be palpated all the way. There is a narrowing in the upper third that presents the weakness of this bone.

The *radius,* a long bone in the forearm, is thicker at the wrist end and narrows at the elbow. The radius is slightly curved and lies on the outer surface of the ulna when the hand is palm up. When the palm is down, the radius lays across the ulna.

Between the ulna and the radius is the interosseus membrane, which fills in the space and holds the bones together. The membrane also acts as a shock absorber for blows transmitted upward from the hand.

Functional tests for the forearm are the same as for the elbow: flexion, extension, pronation, and supination. Palpation of these bones is accomplished rather easily, as they are both close to the surface. Palpation should be gentle and is best accomplished by laying the arm on the table and using both hands to feel the bones gently. By gently squeezing both bones together, the pain site may be established. Inspection may or may not reveal a deformity; swelling may be dramatic or not at all. X-ray is of utmost importance in the diagnosis of bone injury to the forearm.

Fractures of the forearm are an occasional injury seen in athletics. Do not attempt to manipulate the fracture; splint as is and send for further treatment. Splint the forearm with a cotton-padded board in flexion; wrap securely with an elastic bandage and place arm in sling; send to proper facility for repair.

The forearm is a frequent site of fractures of the arm. There may be a fracture to one or both bones.

Ulna. The ulna is located on the little-finger side of the forearm and is not a frequently injured bone. The ulna is very close to the skin, and the bone may be felt for any change in shape, etc. The fracture may be the result of direct blow or a very severe torsion action of the elbow or wrist. Pain at the site will be present, and there may or may not be any deformity. Loss of function may not be involved. In a suspected fracture of the ulna, apply a splint and a sling, and transport the athlete to a medical facility.

Radius. The radius is located on the thumb side of the forearm, and its fracture is common. The fractures are usually found in the lower end of the radius, usually in the lower half. The radius may be traced by palpation and any abnormality felt. Pain will be present over the fracture site, but there may not be any loss of function. In a suspected fracture, splint, apply a sling, and send for medical attention.

Ulna and radius. A fracture to both bones of the forearm is very common, more so than a fracture to any one bone of the forearm. This may be caused by a direct blow to the area or by falling on the outstretched hand. There may not be any displacement of the bone fragments, but there is usually an abnormal bow to the forearm. Pain and tenderness will be present, and loss of function will be noted. Treatment consists of splinting, putting in a sling, and transporting to the team physician or hospital facilities.

Sprains and strains of the forearm are uncommon. History will reveal that the athlete has been using the forearm excessively and therefore the arm is sore. Inspection and palpation may reveal a tender area and not much else. Treatment is symptomatic: usually rest, mild heat, and massage for a day or two. The athlete should be cautioned to go a little slower in his work-outs. Persisting pain in the area may indicate a tenosynovitis, or a tendinitis, and should be examined by the team physician for a complete diagnosis. Treatment for both conditions is rest and heat and mild therapeutic exercises. Diathermy and ultrasonics have produced good response in these injuries.

Contusion of Forearm. This is a very common injury and occurs more to the ulna side (little finger) of the forearm than the radial side (thumb side). The arm, when placed in a position of protection, reveals the ulna side of the forearm and thus makes this the vulnerable area. Sometimes a severe blow will result in a fracture of the ulna. If suspected, all treatments should be designed along the fracture treatment level (i.e., splint and sling). When fracture is ruled out, the result of the blow will be a bruise to the area. When feeling the forearm, it will be noted that the bone is exposed. Most

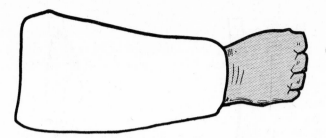

Forearm pad used to protect the lower arm in football, hockey, and lacrosse. Made of sponge rubber or plastic foam covered with an elastic material. Very light and comfortable to wear.

of the bruises are "bone bruises" that occur on the ulna side of the forearm. History will reveal the incident, palpation will reveal local tenderness, and inspection may or may not reveal swelling.

Treatment of contusion of forearm consists of immediate application of ice and compression. After the first 24 hours, heat may be started. The use of a pad for protection may be applied, and the athlete may return to activity. Usually in a contusion of the forearm where there is no swelling, the athlete may participate without losing any time. Where there is profuse swelling, there will be a loss of function to the hand and forearm, and the athlete should not participate until full range of motion has recovered. The use of hot soaks, whirlpool, etc., are very effective means of resorbing the swelling that results from this type of bruise.

Other contusions of the forearm may be treated the same way and response is usually rapid in this type of injury.

With the introduction of the face masks in football, the forearm bruise is now quite prevalent. Prevention by the use of a forearm guard is essential. They are made of sponge rubber or a similar product and are enclosed in an elastic covering to hold in place. This pad is very effective in the prevention of forearm injuries.

MUSCLES OF ARM

Brachioradialis. This muscle is situated on the outside of the arm and gives rise to the rounded contour of the elbow area. The origin of the brachioradialis is the lateral supracondylar ridge of the humerus, and its insertion is the lateral side of the styloid process of the radius. The action is to flex the forearm for action in pronation and supination, depending on which way the hand is turned.

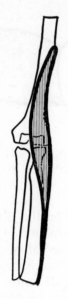

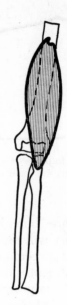

Brachioradialis.   Brachialis.

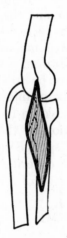

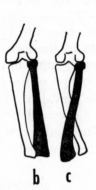

The location of the supinator muscle (a). The forearm in supination; the radius is parallel to the ulna (b). Pronation; the radius is crossed over the ulna (c). A simple form of explanation is that when the palm is up, the hand is in supination (therefore able to hold soup). When the palm is down, the hand is in pronation.

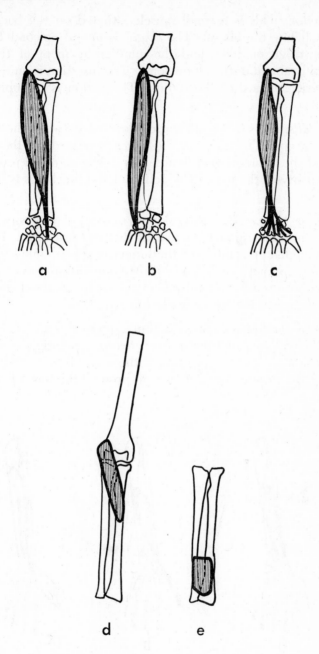

Pronator teres (a). Pronator quadratus (b). Flexor carpi radialis (c). Flexor carpi ulnaris (d). Palmaris longus (e).

Supinator. This is a small muscle situated on the back of the arm just below the elbow. The origin is lateral epicondyle of the humerus, ridge on ulna, and the annular ligament of the radial collateral ligament of the elbow joint. The insertion is on the lateral and anterior surface of the radius. The action is to supinate the forearm.

Brachialis. This is a small muscle located between the humerus and the biceps. The origin is the lower two-thirds of the anterior portion of the humerus, and its insertion is the coronoid process and the tuberosity of the ulna. The action of the brachialis is flexion of the elbow.

Pronator teres. The small skinny muscle that crosses over in front of the elbow joint is known as the pronator teres. Its origin is at the medial epicondyle of the humerus, the common tendon of the flexor group, and medial side of the coronoid process of the ulna. The insertion is on the lateral side of the radius in about the middle third. The action is to pronate the forearm.

Pronator quadratus. This is a thin, square sheet of muscle that crosses the wrist on the front of the forearm. The origin is the lower part of the ulna, and its insertion is the lower fourth of the lateral border of the radius. The action is to pronate the forearm.

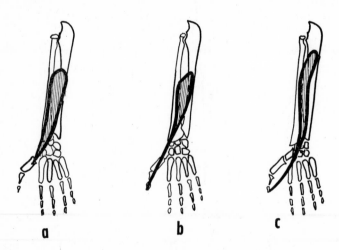

Abductor pollicis longus (a). Extensor pollicis longus (b). Flexor pollicis longus (c).

Flexor carpi radialis. This is the long muscle that lies under the skin and has its origin at the inner condyle of the humerus. Its insertion is at the anterior surface of the base of the second metacarpal. The action is flexion of the wrist.

Flexor carpi ulnaris. This muscle is on the ulna side of the forearm, and its origin is the inner condyle of the humerus and the back of the ulna. The insertion is on the hamate, pisiform, and the base of the fifth metacarpal. The action is flexing of the wrist and assisting in adduction of the wrist.

Palmaris longus. This long slender muscle on the ulna side of the forearm has its origin at the inner condyle of the humerus. Its insertion is the annular ligament of the wrist. The function is to flex the wrist.

Abductor pollicis longus. This deep muscle of the thumb has its origin at the posterior surface of the ulna and the middle third of the posterior surface of the radius. The insertion is the radial side of the first metacarpal. The action is to abduct the thumb and wrist.

Flexor pollicis longus. This is the only flexor muscle of the thumb that is in the forearm; all others are in the hand. The origin is the anterior surface of the posterior portion of the radius, and its insertion is the base of the distal phalanx of the thumb. The action is to flex thumb.

Extensor pollicis longus. The origin of the extensor pollicis longus is the posterior surface of the middle third of the ulna. Its insertion is base of the second phalanx of the thumb. Its action is to extend the last phalanx of the thumb.

Chapter 12

Elbow

ANATOMY OF ELBOW

The bones that form the elbow joint are the humerus, ulna, and radius. The true joint is formed by the lower end of the humerus, which flattens in its lower third where the borders change and form the condyles. On the condyles will be found a projection called the *epicondyles*. The epicondyle is more prominent on the inside of the elbow joint than on the outside. The medial condyle articulates with the olecranon process of the ulna, and the smaller condyle articulates with the head of the radius to form the joint.

The upper end of the ulna thickens and forms the hollow cup in which the medial condyle of the humerus articulates. The olecranon process is immediately below the skin and is readily felt on palpation. The radius articulates with the humerus by means of a slightly concave flat head that unites with the neck of the radius and forms the shaft. This joint is well supported by a strong ligament that binds the radius to the ulna. The stability of the joint is dependent on the humerus sitting in the olecranon and the strong ligaments that hold the ulna in approximation with the humerus. The capsule is very thin and is reinforced by the lateral ligaments. The lateral ligaments are helped in the stability of the joint by the

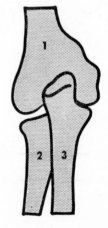

Bones of the elbow joint. (1) Humerus. (2) Ulna. (3) Radius.

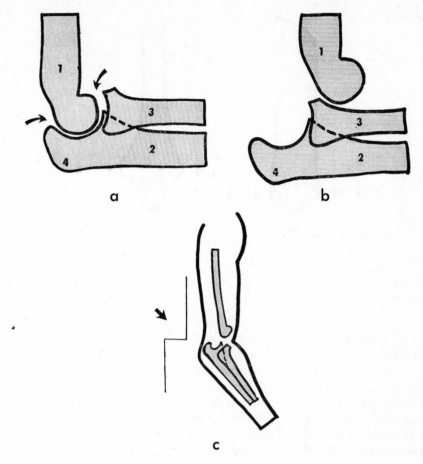

(a) Side view of elbow. (1) Humerus. (2) Ulna. (3) Radius. (4) Olecranon process.
(b) Dislocation of elbow, showing humerus out of the olecranon process. (3) Dislocation of elbow, showing typical "step."

larger muscles of the arm, which run on the front and back side
of the joint.

The elbow joint is a hinge joint, motions being to bend the arm
(flexion) and to straighten the arm (extension). It may be said that
the elbow area has two joints, one between the ulna and humerus;
the other, the radius and ulna. The radius rotates and revolves
around the ulna. The action is to turn the palm of the hand downward (pronation); in this motion the radius lays across the ulna.
When the palm of the hand is up (supination), the radius and ulna
are parallel.

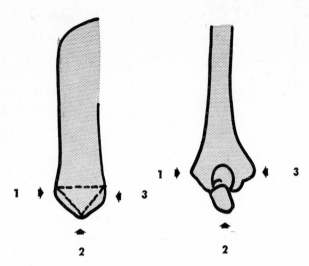

Elbow as seen from the rear. The three points of the triangle that are evident in a normal elbow. Any deviation of the triangle suggests an injury to the bone. (1) Lateral epicondyle of the humerus. (2) Olecranon process. (3) Medial epicondyle of the humerus.

In front of the elbow, just below the skin, are the main veins that drain the blood from the forearm. The main artery is deep and divides into the radial and ulna arteries. The median nerve lies next to the artery, where it becomes the ulnar and radial nerve for the forearm. The musculature is divided into two categories, flexion and extension. Muscles that flex the elbow are the biceps, brachialis, and coracobrachialis; the triceps is the extensor muscle of the arm. The origin of the extensors and flexors of the wrist and fingers will be found at the joint margins.

FUNCTIONAL TESTS FOR ELBOW

Functional tests include:

1. Extension of elbow with or without resistance tests the triceps muscle.
2. Flexion tests the biceps, brachialis and coracobrachialis.
3. Pronation (palm down) tests the pronator teres and pronator quadratus.
4. Supination (palm up) tests brachioradialis and short supinator.

Rotation will help to elicit pain of the injured lateral ligaments of the elbow. Test should be performed gingerly at first; resistance may be applied later.

Examination of the elbow joint should include the exact history of the incident that caused the injury. The athlete will spell out all that has happened, including such things as "popping" or "crunching." Inspection compares the injured member with the other elbow. Examination should include all views of the elbow joint. The amount of swelling should be noted. When palpating, look for the three bony prominences: the olecranon and the two epicondyles of the humerus. When the elbow is flexed, these three points will form a perfect triangle. If swelling is profuse, slight pressure will be squeezed aside and the point felt. All the bones of the elbow are close to the surface, where they can be felt for abnormalities.

X-ray of the elbow joint should be a routine procedure, as the joint is very complex and its structure results in many bony problems that cannot be diagnosed without the benefit of X-ray.

FRACTURES IN THE ELBOW AREA

An elbow injury that shows any deformity at all is a candidate for the fracture squad. Those that do not have a deformity, although history would indicate such, should not be subjected to any functional tests as listed previously. Inspection of the extremity will reveal the deformity. However, if there is not a deformity, gentle palpation starting from a nontender area and progressing toward the joint will reveal tenderness or an irregularity that may be felt and not seen. This must be suspected as a fracture and regarded a such until the team physician tells you otherwise.

The immediate concern of the trainer is to transport the athlete for further attention. In fractures or suspected fractures, the athlete may prefer to hold the injured extremity. He can do this better than you can with a sling. If there is intensive pain on the least amount of motion, a splint should be applied before the athlete is transported.

If the involvement is in the humerus, a full splint in extension should be applied. If the lower arm is involved, a splint in flexion is necessary. Splints should be made of something firm, covered with cotton, and wrapped loosely over the suspected fracture site. The use of a sling, when possible, will aid in the comfort of the injured athlete.

Treatment of fractures of the elbow will not be discussed in this book.

DISLOCATION OF ELBOW

The incident causing a dislocated elbow is a fall on the extended arm or a severe counter joint motion, such as hyperextension or a twist of the arm that involves an unusual motion of the joint. The dislocation may be backward, forward or lateral. One of or both the bones in the forearm may be involved. The commonest dislocation seen in athletics is the backward type.

History, inspection, and palpation used to diagnose this injury will greatly help the trainer. First, the athlete will tell you the action that caused him to have much pain and loss of function in the elbow joint. On inspecting the injury, a very obvious deformity will manifest itself in an unnatural depression of the upper arm just above the joint. There may or may not be swelling when seen early. There will be a definite loss of function, the arm being held in one position and the elbow being unable to flex. Compare the injured member with other arm and note the physical changes. Palpation will reveal a hollow that your hand will feel as well as see. The three points of the triangle will not be normal to the touch. X-ray will be required to complete the diagnosis.

Reducing dislocations of the elbow is not in the realm of the trainer. These should be handled by the team physician only, or his referral. Treatment by the trainer consists of first aid in the form of a sling, ice to control the hemorrhage, and providing for the comfort of the athlete. The arm should be held closely to the side and as much weight as possible eliminated from the forearm.

After the reduction, the elbow will be kept at rest for a short period of time (varying with the degree of discomfort and amount of swelling), usually about five days, at which time heat, gentle massage, and exercises are instituted. The exercises are passive, progressing to active as soon as such can be tolerated. While treatments are given, the arm will be wrapped with an elastic wrap and held in a sling. After two weeks the elastic wrap is removed, and the sling is discarded the following week. Total time of immobilization is about three weeks. However, this does not mean that the athlete is ready to resume activities. Extensive resistance exercises should be employed to develop normal strength of the arm, including the shoulder and the neighboring joint, the wrist. Full period of disability is about two to three months.

The athlete should not be permitted back to play until full range of motion is recovered and strength is regained. The use of a "cinch or halter" type of strapping is applied to prevent hyperextension when the athlete returns to action.

SPRAIN OF THE ELBOW

After a sudden wrench of the elbow, the athlete will complain of pain in the elbow joint which may radiate on motion, especially pronation (palm down) or supination (palm up). The twisting of the joint may be lateral or anterior, or posterior (usually hyperextension). In full flexion or full extension, the condition may also be aggravated. Injuries to the elbow joint must be examined carefully to be sure that there is not an accompanying fracture or dislocation.

History will reveal that the athlete fell or that his arm was caught and a counter joint motion resulted. The pain may or may not be too severe when the arm is at rest, but motion aggravates the condition. He will carry his arm by grasping the wrist with his other hand and he will not care to let it go.

Inspection will reveal swelling in the front, in the back, or completely around the joint. This swelling must be examined so that it will not be confused with the change in normal contour, which could suggest bony pathology. The swelling may be palpated gently so that an examination of the bone can be made and detection made of abnormal changes that cannot be seen. Tenderness will be localized by gentle pressure, and the exact site of the injury can thus be located.

Immediate treatment consists of compression (care must be taken so that pressure will not be put into the fold of the elbow, thus constricting blood vessels) ice, and rest in sling. Ice packs should be applied to the elbow joint for at least 48 hours, after which the application of heat and massage plus limited exercises may be started. Sprains of the elbow joint are slow to respond, and at best there will be much discomfort along the recovery trail. Many physicians will aspirate the joint of the elbow, as the release of pressure from the distention results in less pain and discomfort. Limitation of motion is always present no matter how slight the injury.

Whirlpool baths are very effective, as the athlete can perform active exercises while the arm is immersed. Work-outs should not be discontinued because of this injury; running calisthenics, etc., are very helpful in the over-all condition of the athlete. For the work-out, use a counterirritant hot pack on the elbow (which is removed for the shower) and then an elastic support applied overnight. The use of the sling may be discontinued as the recovery progresses. The prolonged use of support in the elbow joint delays the return of active motions, and may result in an excessive formation of scar tissue, which in turn will cause a limitation of motion.

Depending on the severity of the sprain or strain, the disability will vary with the sport. The use of constrictive strappings can be beneficial in some types of sports but it would have detrimental effect in others.

A common injury to the elbow, even though it is a sprain, should be considered separately; namely, the hyperextension sprain.

This injury is caused in football by arm tackling and in basketball by being caught between two players. The arm is forced to go beyond its normal limitation in extension, and the soft tissue of the joint is stretched or torn. Swelling may or may not be present, but there will be pain and a definite loss of motion. The history is usually enough to make a diagnosis, but all facts should be investigated by normal procedures. Immediate treatment consists of compression, ice, and rest in sling. On the second day, the injury is re-examined and range of motion observed. At this time there may be a definite tightening of all the tissue around the joint, thus making it immobile. Ice and compression, along with the sling, will be carried on for another day. On the third day, if swelling has usually reduced, heat may be applied along with massage, which should be light and above and below the injury. Active exercises may be started, being careful not to force the joint either in extension or flexion. The sling may be discarded after this treatment and exercises for the shoulder and hand may be started. Progressive resistive exercises must be started so that full recovery of normal strength may be accomplished. These exercises may be started as the range of motion increases, which is usually five to seven days after injury.

As full range of motion is acquired and swelling and pain disappear, the athlete may assume his normal activities. When he returns to the sport, the use of the "cinch or halter" should be used daily. Depending on the sport and the degree of injury, the length of disability will vary from a few days to a couple of weeks.

CONTUSION OF ELBOW

This is a very common injury, seen more in recent years since the introduction of the new type of blocking techniques in football. It is caused frequently in hockey from hitting the boards and occurs in basketball when falling on floor. It manifests itself in immediate swelling, and sometimes gives the impression that it is continuing to swell while you are looking at it. Pain will be intense, gradually easing in a little while. Contusions of the elbow will involve both the bone and soft tissues.

Contusion of Soft Tissue. Swelling is rapid and pain turns to a dull ache that will disappear when the joint is at complete rest.

Immediate treatment is to control the hemorrhage by the use of a compression wrap and an ice bag. Pressure, where there is localized swelling, can be increased by applying a piece of felt or sponge rubber over the area before wrapping with an elastic wrap. The use of a sling will give complete rest overnight and lessen the pain. On the next day there may be negative findings as a result of the above treatment, and the athlete may go about his activity, using only a sponge rubber pad. However, if pain and swelling are present, continue the treatment for another day and then heat; "hot pack" and exercise may be started without danger of complications. Disability lasts from one day to three or four. Contusion of bone is a frequent condition seen in athletics. Treatment is the same as contusion of soft tissue but the injury lasts much longer. Irregularities of the bone must be watched for, and X-ray should be routine in all severe bone contusions around the elbow.

Hyperextended Elbow Strapping

Strapping is applied while the athlete is standing. The elbow is held in a flexed position.

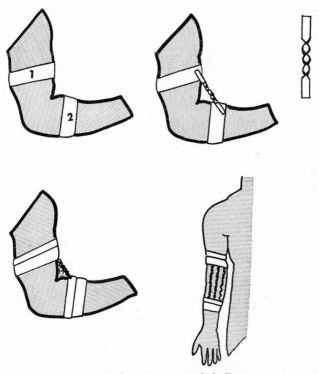

Strapping for a hyperextended elbow.

Step 1. Place an anchor strip around the upper arm, approximately 6 inches from the joint line or point of elbow. The anchor strip should not be applied so tight that it constricts the circulation or the lateral motion of the biceps muscles. Use 1½- or 2-inch tape for anchors.

Step 2. Place an anchor strip 6 inches below the elbow joint or point of elbow. Apply so as not to constrict the muscles, etc., of forearm.

Anchor strips are applied so that the strips to be used for limitation will have something to adhere to that will be firm.

Step 3. Using 1-inch tape, strips about 8 inches long should be cut. Twist the strips so that they resemble a spiral with the ends of the strips remaining flat. Apply the flat ends to the anchors at the forearm and upper arm. The limitation of motion and the range of extension may be controlled by the length of these strips.

Step 4. Apply as many of these strips as needed. Depending on the extent of the work to be done, the strips may vary in number from three to six.

Step 5. After applying the spiraled strips, anchor them in the same manner as strips 1 and 2. The use of double strips may be indicated for football, etc.

Place a small piece of cotton under the tape in the crook of the elbow to lessen the possibility of irritation from the tape over the joint area.

Fixing the tape with an elastic wrap will enhance the strapping and prevent tape from rolling while dressing. The elastic wrap may be removed after 30 minutes.

BURSITIS OF ELBOW JOINT

Olecranon bursa is located superficially under the olecranon process and is subject to much trauma. It is very common in sports where contact is indicated. Falling on the ground, as in football or on ice as in hockey causes the bursa to become inflamed and distended. The pressure of the swelling causes much pain and limitation of motion. When the bursa is full, it is very apparent to the eye because it manifests itself as a localized mass under the elbow joint. It may feel hot to the touch and seem extremely tight on pressure.

Treatment. Injury may not be seen until much time has elapsed; the bursa is a self-limiting sac, and when it is filled, the secretion will be stopped. However, even at this time, ice is used as the immediate treatment, along with compression. Placing a pad of sponge rubber over the bursa and then applying an elastic wrap may speed up the absorption of the fluid. (The elastic wrap must not be applied so as to constrict the circulation of the arm.) When the area has cooled off after the first 24 to 48 hours, heat may be started. Diathermy is very effective, as are ultrasonic waves. Wrapping with the elastic wrap for compression is continued until all the symptoms have disappeared. On return to active participation, a sponge pad should be used for protection, to overcome the tendency to recur.

Team physicians may prefer to aspirate the bursa. If this is done, recovery time will be shortened. The use of compression, etc., is also carried on with the aspirated bursa. Recurring bursitis may be a condition for which surgical intervention is indicated, particularly when all conservative methods fail to produce results.

Golfer's Elbow. From the constant pronation and supination of the elbow, such as in golf, baseball, etc., a very painful condition exists at the head of the radius or the external condyle of the humerus. There will be pain, point tenderness, and loss of function (weakness). Pain will be increased on the twisting of the forearm (pronation and supination). The underlying cause is the inflammation of the bursa located immediately below the tendon of the elbow and the overlying muscles of the forearm. The bursa is located so close to the attachment that a bone condition is suspected. The team physician may suggest X-ray to help in making diagnosis.

Treatment. If seen early, the application of ice and the use of a sling is indicated. However, most of these conditions are not seen until a later date, and the use of cold is not very effective then. The application of heat and rest is necessary for good results. This is an aggravating injury, and the disability is somewhat difficult to predict; some conditions respond in a few days but others may take months.

Very often the severe cases require surgical intervention to secure relief from pain and disability.

MYOSITIS OSSIFICANS

Myositis ossificans is a condition not often seen, but it may be suspected in a severe contusion of muscle. This is limited not only to muscle but to tendons as well, usually as a result of trauma to soft tissues. Calcium forms in the tissues and results in a very hard and firm mass. The most common site is around the elbow joint and particularly in the brachialis anticus muscle. If the formation is large, so as to limit function of the muscle, surgical intervention may be indicated.

Conservative treatment in the mild ossificans is the application of heat and prolonged rest. Very often a long extended rest will result in the resorbing of the calcium in the tissue. Diathermy and the use of ultrasonic waves have been mentioned in the literature as having a very good effect on this condition.

In long immobilization after severe elbow injuries, a myositis ossificans may develop to such a large extent that it blocks the joint. In this condition surgery may be indicated, but the timing must be established. Many surgeons will wait until the mass has fully formed or has "stopped growing"; this may be as long as two years.

Chapter 13

Wrist and Hand

ANATOMY

The lower 2 to 3 inches of the radius and ulna, plus the carpal bones (wrist), comprise the wrist joint. Review the long bones of the forearm, the ulna on the outside, and the radius on the inside (thumb side); they are held together by fibrous bands. The lower end of the radius articulates with the first row of the carpal bones and has a projection on this aspect that is called the *styloid process*. The ulna has its head, styloid process, and pit for the articulation of the first row of carpal bones.

The carpal bones are short and cubical in form. There are eight of these, arranged in two rows of four each. The proximal row (closest to long bones of the forearm) are the scaphoid, lunate, triquetrum, and pisiform. The distal row (closest to hand) carpal bones are the trapezium, trapezoid, capitate, and the hamate.

The scaphoid is also called the *navicular,* and the trapezium is often referred to as the *greater multangular,* while the trapezoid is known as the *lesser multangular.*

The names of the carpal bones express their general appearance:

Navicular (boat shaped)
Lunate (moon shaped)
Triquetral (triangular)
Pisiform (pea shaped)
Great multangular (many angles)
Lesser multangular (lesser angles)
Capitate (head shaped)
Hamate (hook shaped)

The two separate rows of carpals work as units, and they are bound together by transverse ligaments, capsular ligaments, and numerous fibrous bands. The joint has several synovial cavities.

The metacarpal bones (hand) are slender long bones that articulate with the distal row of carpals and the phalanges (fingers) and are bound together by transverse ligaments. The metacarpals are prevented from spreading by the deep transverse ligaments of the palm and their own ligamentous bands.

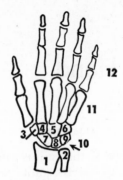

Bones of the wrist and hand. (1) Radius. (2) Ulna. (3) Greater multangular. (4) Trapezoid. (5) Capitate. (6) Hamate. (7) Navicular (scaphoid). (8) Lunate. (9) Triquetrum. (10) Pisiform (under triquetrum). (11) Metacarpals I, II, III, IV, V. (12) Phalanges.

There are 14 phalanges, two for the thumb and three for all the other fingers. These bones are held together by collateral ligaments, a loose capsule, and the tendons of the muscles of the hand and forearm. The motions of the fingers are simple flexion and extension; adduction and abduction are very limited.

Motions of the Wrist. The easiest and most common motions of the wrist joint are flexion and extension and adduction and abduction. By combining the above motions, circumduction is permitted. Rotation is minimal in this joint. The effect of rotation is due to the motions of supination and pronation of the forearm.

Thumb. The thumb has two phalanges and one metacarpal bone that articulates with the carpal bone of the wrist. There is much freedom of motion of the thumb owing to its location and construction. The metacarpal of the thumb is short and stout, and the capsule that holds this bone to the phalange is very thick and extremely loose.

The motions of the thumb are flexion and extension, abduction and adduction, circumduction, and a small amount of rotation.

FRACTURES

Colles Fracture. Fracture of the distal end of the radius is called a *colles* fracture, a very common fracture that results from a fall on the hand, severe wrenching of the wrist, or as a result of a direct blow to the lower end of the radius. History will reveal the incident.

Inspection may or may not reveal a deformity. Compare the injured member with other arm. Palpation will reveal tenderness over the lower end of the radius and a very definite loss of function.

Treatment consists of placing hand and forearm in a splint and a sling. Transportation to the team physician should be arranged so that X-rays can be taken and proper treatment started.

The colles fracture is the most common fracture seen about the wrist in athletics. However, fractures of the ulna are also seen, and procedure as outlined for fracture of the radius is used in all suspected fracture around the wrist area.

Carpal fractures. Owing to the location and forces applied to this group of bones, many fractures are seen. The frequency of these fractures warrant routine X-rays of all injuries to the wrist area. The so-called sprained wrist that does not respond to treatment is usually a candidate for the fracture squad. Very often fractures of the carpal bones are not seen until much time has elapsed from the time of the injury to the time of reporting. Many athletes feel that all they have is a "sprained wrist," and they do not bother to report the injury but force themselves to play with this condition. The complexity of the joint is such that the fracture may not show on the original film but will show at a later date when calcium has formed and a check film is made.

Suspected fractures of the wrist should be splinted and a sling applied. X-ray, etc., will confirm diagnosis and treatment by team physician will be instituted.

Fractures of the Metacarpals (Hand). These are caused by a direct blow to the bones, being stepped on, etc., or from indirect blows, i.e., punching with the hand or force transmitted to the metacarpals, resulting in a fracture. History will reveal the mechanics of the injury: severe blow or indirect force to hand.

Inspection will reveal swelling, deformity, and loss of function of the hand. Also, normal contour of the knuckles will usually be changed. Very often, due to the shortening of the bone as a result of the fracture, one knuckle may be shorter than normal, and

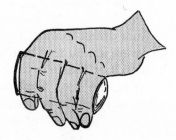

Method of splinting fingers and hand. A roll of gauze or elastic bandage is grasped in hand and wrapped in place.

a resulting deformity will be seen. Compare with other hand for a check of the normal contours.

Palpation may result in crepitus (bones rubbing together) and a change in shape of the bones' normal lines. Swelling may be felt and local tenderness will be quite evident.

Treatment consists of splint and a sling. Do not attempt to make hand conform to splint. If hand is partially closed, do not attempt to apply a straight splint but use a roll of gauze, etc., and wrap in place snugly but not too firmly. If hand is straight, apply a padded splint to palm and extend splint from the elbow to the ends of the fingers. A sling with the hand in elevation is very comfortable. Send the athlete to the team physician for further management.

Fracture of Thumb. More common than we like to see is a fracture of the thumb. Owing to its location and varied movements, a fracture is not a rare injury. There will be much pain, swelling, and false motion. History will reveal the incident that caused the injury.

Inspection will reveal swelling, and there may or may not be deformity. Palpation will reveal much tenderness and also the false joint and crepitus.

Treatment consists of applying a splint to the thumb and a sling, with the hand in elevation. The splint may be made by covering a tongue blade with cotton and gauze and applying directly to the thumb. Services of the team physician should be sought as soon as possible.

Phalanges. The most common type of fracture seen in athletics is the fracture of the fingers. Quite often, as in the wrist, these injuries are not apparent as soon as they happen. This injury is probably the most undertreated injury in athletics because of the insignificance of the digit in the mind of the athlete. Policies established in some schools require: (1) that all the sprains of the fingers be treated as fractures, and (2) that all finger injuries be X-rayed. Both requirements have their merits; the policy at Yale is to treat each case as it arises. X-ray may or may not be indicated.

Fractures of the fingers result from direct blows to the joint or to the end of the finger. They also result from direct trauma, such as being stepped on. Another cause is the severe sprain that results in a fracture. History will reveal the mechanics of the injury.

Palpation will reveal much tenderness over the site. Pinpoint tenderness may indicate a fracture. Crepitus will also be present if complete fracture has been acquired.

Inspection will reveal a change in contour of the bone; swelling may also be evident. Compare with other hand for normal contours.

Treatment should be in the form of a splint. This can be accomplished by cutting a tongue blade to size of finger, covering with cotton and gauze and strapping in position. Further management should be in the hands of the team physician.

DISLOCATIONS

Dislocations of the wrist and hand are not a common injury in athletics. Dislocations of the wrist and hand quite often occur as a complication associated with a fracture. Dislocations of all joints of the limbs usually manifest themselves in a very obvious deformity, and this should be respected. To go into detail about this injury is not the purpose of this chapter, and we advise the reader to splint "as is" and make arrangements for proper handling. The typical characteristics of a dislocation are:

1. Loss of function.
2. Deformity.
3. Swelling.
4. Muscle spasm.
5. Pain.

Splinting in a full arm splint and the use of a sling is the immediate procedure. As in all dislocations, the sooner the reduction, the more comfortable the athlete will be. Expediency in securing proper treatment should be the first consideration. Send the athlete to the team physician immediately.

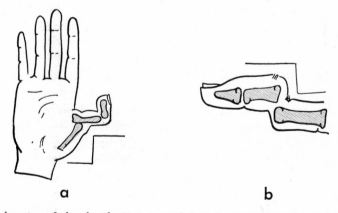

a   b

(a) Dislocation of the thumb. Note typical "step." (b) Dislocation of finger. Note typical "step."

Dislocation of Thumb. Owing to its location and the free range of motion, the thumb is often subjected to counter joint motions that will result in a dislocation. The condition will be very obvious, since the typical "step" will be present along with much pain, loss of function, and swelling.

History, inspection, and palpation should be carried out in this order. Treatment consists of reduction as soon as possible by the team physician. Owing to the complexity of the thumb, the soft tissue is usually torn, and healing is a very slow process. Much patience and hard work on the part of the athlete is necessary for a strong joint after the immobilization, etc., is removed. Early motion and exercise is necessary for complete recovery.

Dislocated Fingers. A rather common injury in sports and one that occurs mostly in the first and second joints of the fingers is dislocation. A dislocation between the metacarpal and phalange is not very common. The injury is a result of a counter joint motion, being hit on the end of the finger by a ball, causing undue stress, or severely wrenching the joint, such as catching the finger in a jersey, etc. History will reveal the cause.

Inspection will reveal a very obvious deformity; the more common condition seen is the backward displacement. Displacement to one side (lateral) or the other is also seen but not so commonly as the backward displacement.

The ends of the bones may be felt by palpation if the fingers are examined early; after swelling has taken place, palpation will be useless.

Treatment. A chip fracture is often the result of a dislocation of the finger, and with this in mind, X-ray should be indicated in all dislocations of the finger. Routine reduction of dislocations without X-ray is not indicated and may result in further damage to the finger.

If inspection is negative for fracture, and after dislocation has been reduced, the finger is placed in a splint for approximately ten days to two weeks. The splint should be straight and can be made from a tongue depressor. The splint should be padded with gauze, etc., and applied snugly with adhesive tape. Do not apply tightly because the possibility of constriction must be guarded against. Instruction of elevation by holding hand across chest should be explained to the athlete. Elevation of the finger will be most comfortable and the possibility of swelling will be lessened. After this period of time, the splint should be removed and active motion started. The use of hot soaks, whirlpools, etc., will help to loosen this joint and aid full recovery. After the splint has been removed, the finger should be strapped daily for participation in sports. Strapping consists of taping the neighboring finger to the injured one. The "good" finger will act as a splint for the injured one. For flexion and extension movements, two narrow strips of tape are used and are applied between the joints of the fingers. For full limitation, the fingers should be completely enveloped with the tape. This procedure should be carried out for about a month after the injury.

SPRAINS

Wrist. A complete history is a *must*. Particular attention should be paid to the nature of the injury, position of wrist at time of injury, what the athlete felt or heard, and the position of wrist when reported. Compare both wrists and note any visible deformity of swelling. Localized swelling will locate the injury, while over-all and extensive swelling will suggest a severe injury.

Palpation should be systematic, starting with the bones of the forearm, the bones of the wrist, and finally the bones of the hand. Tenderness over various parts of the wrist will designate site of the injury. Tenderness over bone may suggest a fracture and should be respected as one. In inspection, look for all landmarks (normal indentations or projections) and compare with the other wrist. Swelling should be palpated for texture, soft or firm, and whether it is bone or fluid.

Functional tests include motions of flexion and extension, adduction and abduction, circumduction and rotation. These should be attempted passively before active motions are instituted. Findings in each motion should be reported to the team physician.

If there is moderate swelling and not much tenderness plus good performance of the functions of the wrist, the injury is probably a sprain. As mentioned in Chapter 6, it may be wise to X-ray all wrist injuries. Negative findings will help all concerned. The athlete needs assurance, and quite often an X-ray will give him that assurance.

Treatment of sprained wrist. Moderate sprains should be immobilized with an adhesive strapping, and ice and elevation applied for the first 24 hours. If swelling is minimal, hot soaks and support by strapping may be all that will be needed for a few days. Wrist injuries tend to be slow in healing, and their recurrence is quite prevalent. The use of a strap may have to be continued for a prolonged period of time. The use of exercises is indicated early and should be repeated often during the course of the day.

Severe sprain of the wrist. The application of a hard splint for complete immobilization will greatly help this injury. The use of an aluminum splint or padded basswood is preferable to a plaster cast, as this allows for treatments during the recovery period. After the splint is applied, the use of ice and a sling with the wrist in elevation is used for the first 48 hours. After this time, mild heat and massage, with light passive exercises, are indicated. When the swelling and pain has subsided, active exercises are started. If active exercises can be tolerated, the splint may be removed and an adhesive strapping applied for support. Whirlpools and hot soaks are indicated in this injury. Diathermy, ultrasonics, etc., may be used, but excellent results have been attained by moist heat in this injury. Exercises are indicated as soon as possible.

Rehabilitation is long and arduous, and the results are not readily seen. A sponge-rubber ball, a little large than a hand ball and a little smaller than a tennis ball, should be carried by the athlete and squeezed at any time. The more exercise, the better; and the quicker the return to normal strength. The use of pulleys, springs, etc., are also helpful. The continued strapping while engaged in athletics should be carried out for an extended period of time.

HAND AND WRIST STRAPPING

Strapping for hand. The position of the hand should be normal. Fingers should be held in a semi-tightened position. The fingers should not be spread nor should they be clenched just in between. This is a complete tape procedure and individual strips are not used as in other procedures.

Step 1. Start with the tape on the back side of the wrist and pull under and across the palm of the hand and then back up to the wrist.

Step 2. Encircle wrist and then repeat as far as the tape will go. Do not force the tape; let it go where it wants to go. For a wrinkle-free strapping, the proper angles must be maintained.

Step 3. The number of strips applied will be established by the amount of support needed.

4. When crossing over the knuckles do not go too low, as this will hamper motion of hand.

Strapping for wrist. For strapping of the wrist the hand should be in a closed position but not firmly clenched. Individual strips of 1-inch tape should be used.

Step 1. Start the first strip as close to the hand as possible, and apply in a snug manner, completely encircling the wrist.

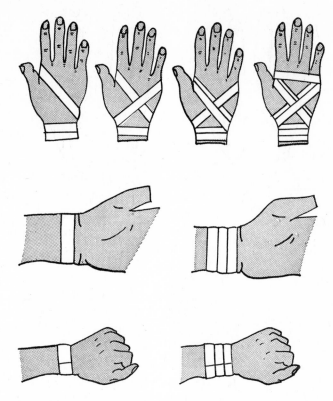

Strapping of the hand and wrist. Each view shows individual strips as applied. Individual strips will mold much better and give more support than a continuous winding of the tape. To wrap the hand and wrist, start at the wrist and cross over back of hand and again circle the wrist. The number of strips will depend on the severity of the injury and the protection desired.

Step 2. Overlap at least halfway and repeat as in step 1. Added strips are applied in the same manner. The number will depend on the amount of support indicated.

Thumb. Sprains of the thumb are very common and have a tendency to recur. Sports that require the handling of a ball are the producers of this injury. Daily handling of the ball after a sprain to the thumb is always a source of further irritation. Owing to its location and function, this is a very common condition to the thumb. The cause is usually hyperextension of the joint. Pain and swelling result. X-rays may or may not be indicated. However, pain and tenderness at the base of the thumb may indicate a fracture to the

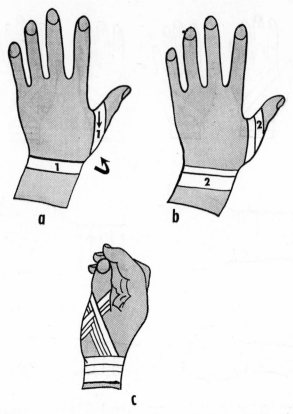

Strapping the thumb. (a) Strip 1 starts at wrist and goes under thumb. (b) Strip 2 overlaps strip 1 and also goes under thumb. (c) Completed strapping. Use as many strips as needed to support the thumb.

carpal bone (scaphoid), and X-ray will be needed to eliminate this possibility.

Treatment consists of compression strapping and the application of ice. If the strain is severe, elevate the hand in a sling for the first few days.

Whirlpool baths or hot soaks are very effective in the treatment of the sprained thumb. The use of protective strappings is indicated when the athlete is engaged in athletics. The use of a ball for exercise is very effective for the strengthening of this joint.

Fingers. Sports that require the use of a ball are the producers of injuries to the fingers. By being hit on the end of the finger or having a finger caught in jersey, etc., a sprain of a joint is produced. All sprains to joints of the fingers are painful but not often serious.

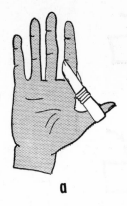

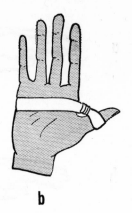

a

b

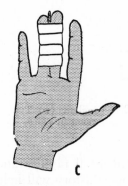

Various types of restriction for thumb and finger injuries. (a) Cinch strap for thumb. (b) Alternate cinch for thumb. (c) Immobilization of fingers by taping to neighbor.

c

A splint for a day or two will relieve pain, as will the application of cold packs to the area. After the first day or so, hot soaks will loosen the joint and help repair the injury. Swelling is prevalent, and it may be noted that when the finger is sprained, it will never again be the same size as before the injury. The fingers of baseball players are certainly good proof of this statement. However, with proper treatment and exercises, the swelling may be reduced to a minimum. Strapping the fingers together will protect them while playing, and continued use while not playing will greatly help healing and the return to normal.

CONTUSIONS

In contact sports such as football, contusions to the wrist and hand are quite common. The football player whose forearm hits a helmet or a mask, or whose hand has been stepped on, must be

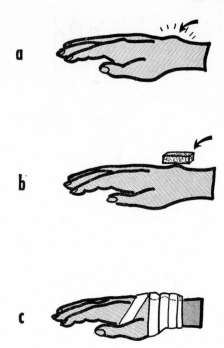

Pressure strapping for bruise of hand. Also used to compress ganglion. (a) Typical swelling. (b) Sponge rubber cut to size. (c) Sponge rubber strapped in place.

treated. Contusions of the wrist and hand will swell rapidly and will be painful for the first few hours. The proper history will help in the handling of this injury. The athlete will recite the blow that caused the injury, and further tests will help to diagnose the condition.

Inspection will reveal the exact spot and the degree of swelling. Inspection will also rule out any obvious deformity that indicates a more serious injury. Palpation will be effective in locating the exact site. The pain may be in the bone or in the soft tissue; palpation will reveal which is affected.

Contusion of the wrist should be treated by a compression bandage and ice packs. Elevation will be very helpful in hastening absorption of the swelling. Heat may be applied when swelling has stopped (usually 48 hours after injury) and active exercises have been started. The athlete may resume activity, using a sponge-rubber pad for protection against further trauma.

Contusion of the hand is a very common injury in football and can be most bothersome. The hand will swell readily and a hematoma (organized mass of blood) may be quite evident. Compression by means of cotton or sponge rubber should be used to force the hematoma to be absorbed. The immediate application of ice to stop the hemorrhage is indicated. Very often this procedure is all that is needed for the dispersement of the swelling.

Heat and exercise may be started when the swelling subsides. The early and vigorous treatment of a contused hand by heat and massage may result in the recurrence of the swelling. Caution should be practiced, and the delay in heating the area considered. The athlete may resume activity as soon as full motion has returned. The use of a pad for protection should be applied daily.

WOUNDS

Wounds of the hand and wrist are everyday occurrences, and they should be treated with respect. Most of the local infections treated in athletics are wounds of the hand. The reasons may be many, but neglect is the number one cause of trouble. All abrasions and lacerations, regardless of how minor, should be treated. An antiseptic dressing should be applied, and the wound should be redressed periodically. The proper protection against infection while playing must also be considered.

The tetanus toxoid protection is routinely practiced at Yale. All athletes are required to have the series, and when they have completed it, they are given a card to this effect. When an open wound is treated (especially one that has occurred on the athletic fields), this card is presented and evaluated by the physician. If indicated, a booster shot is administered.

Lacerations are viewed by the team physician, and if necessary, are sutured.

Abrasions are thoroughly cleansed with soap and water, after which an antibiotic ointment dressing is applied. This dressing is changed daily until the wound is healed. Proper padding and strapping is applied so that the athlete can continue participation in his sport.

MALLET FINGER (BASEBALL FINGER)

Mallet finger is caused by a forced flexion of the distal phalange while the extensor tendon is contracted. Most of these injuries are a result of being hit on the end of the finger by a ball, which causes the extensor tendon to be pulled away from the bone so that the distal phalange cannot fully extend. This results in a dropped finger, commonly called a mallet finger. History will reveal the force of the blow, etc.

Inspection will show that the distal phalange cannot and will not straighten. There may or may not be any swelling. Palpation will reveal that there is a tender spot where the tendon attaches. By passively extending the distal portion of the finger, it will be noted that as soon as it is released, the finger drops.

Treatment consists of immobilization of the finger in a splint. The length of time for immobilization will depend on recovery progress. This time is unpredictable, and often splinting will not be sufficient management of this injury. Surgical intervention may be indicated.

The athlete must be cautioned not to remove the splint at any time, for the less disturbance, the better. Frequent changes and the frequent testing of the injury results in slow progress. Once the splint is applied, leave it alone.

FINGERNAILS

Fingernails often present a problem to the athlete, especially when he fails to manicure them properly. Instruction must be given in the proper care of nails. In many sports, long fingernails are dangerous to the individual as well as to the opponent. Wrestlers must be cautioned that long nails may cause dangerous wounds, and therefore proper cutting is necessary.

Fingernails, unlike toenails, should be cut with the contour of the finger and should not extend beyond the end of the digit. Nails that extend can be broken off, and this will be painful as well as disabling. In sports where ball handling is essential, this injury is quite common. Treatment for a broken nail consists of immediate cleaning of the wound. Trimming the uneven edges, etc., is essential, after which an ointment dressing is applied. Antibiotic ointments are very effective in the management of broken nails where the skin has been torn. Protective dressing should be worn until the wound has healed.

Contusion of Nail with Hemorrhage. Blood forming under a nail is very painful and is usually the result of a contusion, i.e., being stepped on, placing hand in glove before ball, etc. By releasing the pressure, pain and discomfort may be relieved. By drilling a hole in the nail to release the blood, immediate relief is attained. The hole may be drilled by a regular nail drill or by the sharp blade of a knife (sterile conditions prevail). Heating the end of a paper clip until red hot and introducing it into the nail has met with much success. As soon as the clip hits the blood, it will cool off and will not burn the tissues. The heat will also sterilize the area. After the hole has been made, a dressing should be applied to keep wound clean. Ointment applied to the dressing will stop the blood from clotting and allow the wound to drain. Continue dressing until oozing has stopped.

Chapter 14

Upper and Lower Leg

THIGH

Fractures. The femur is the longest and strongest bone of the body. It is composed of the shaft and two ends, the upper at the hip joint and the lower end at the knee joint. The ends of the bone flare out and thereby become very large. The upper end at the hip is composed of the head and neck, and the femur at this point forms a seven. The lower end also flares out and forms two very well-rounded knuckles or condyles. Thigh fractures that occur in athletics are more likely to be in the shaft and the lower end of the femur. Fractures of the head and neck occur more in elderly people.

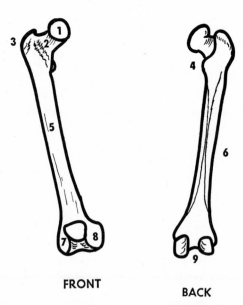

FRONT   **BACK**

Front and back view of the femur. (1) Head of femur. (2) Neck of femur. (3) Greater trochanter. (4) Lesser trochanter. (5) Shaft of femur. (6) Minea aspera. (7) Lateral condyle. (8) Medial condyle. (9) Intercondylar notch.

Fractures of shaft. The cause of fracture of the shaft of the femur may be direct or indirect. Direct causes are those that occur from a severe blow or kick; or as the result of a pile-up with the leg off the ground; or force applied to the thigh area, resulting in a stress on the bone and a break in the continuity. The indirect causes are those under the heading of a force transmitted through the bones of the lower leg and manifesting itself in a force to the thigh bone, such as jumping and landing on heels or severe muscular contractions.

In a fracture of the femur there will be much pain, and as a result of pain, the athlete will suffer a degree of shock. Care should be taken not to increase the pain by excessive movements, thus increasing the shock. Excessive movements may contribute to damage of other tissues and should be avoided. The symptoms of fracture of the shaft are:

1. Deformity: muscular contraction may cause the fragments to vary their normal position.
2. Loss of function of thigh.
3. Pain.
4. Point tenderness.
5. False joint.
6. Shortening of thigh (due to overriding of bone fragments).
7. Leg will be everted (foot turned outward).
8. Swelling due to damage of soft tissue.

The athlete should be splinted immediately. The splint used should be a Thomas splint or a long splint running from under the arm to the foot. Shock is a condition that will be present to some degree, and all efforts to prevent this complication should be made. Keep the athlete warm by using blankets, etc.

When applying the Thomas splint, the ring is placed around the leg and the leg wrapped securely in the frame. Traction is applied around the foot and ankle by means of a hitch which is tied to the end of the splint.

If a board or Thomas splint is not available, tying both legs together will act as an improvised splint. Remove the athlete from the playing area by a stretcher which is firm. Transportation to a hospital by ambulance is extremely important for the welfare of the athlete.

Upper end of thigh. This is not a very frequent fracture in the age group of athletics and is more common to the elderly. Symptoms are pain, disability of the hip joint, shortening of the leg, and swelling. The athlete will be flat on his back and will have his hip rotated outward and the leg slightly abducted. There will be loss of function of the leg and point tenderness will be found over the hip area. The fracture is usually so deep that the fracture line cannot be palpated.

Institute shock treatment immediately. Place the leg in a Thomas splint or a long board splint. Remove the athlete from the playing area on a stretcher and transport to hospital by ambulance. If splints are not available, strapping of both legs together will act as an improvised splint.

Lower end of femur. The lower end of the femur flares out and terminates in two condyles (rounded knuckles) that articulate with the tibia to form the knee joint.

Fractures are a result of a direct blow or torsion motion to the knee; or of indirect action such as falling from a height and landing on the feet. Fractures to the lower end of the femur may not be obvious; history of severe injury, etc., must be noted and a fracture suspected. Inspection may or may not reveal a deformity; swelling will be present and simulate a knee injury. Palpation will reveal point tenderness over the fractured site, and possibly the fracture fragments will be felt. Swelling will be felt all around the joint (posterior aspect as well as anterior). All symptoms of fractures should be applied, and any present should guide the trainer into the treatment for fracture.

Treatment consists of splinting in the Thomas or long-board splints.

Shock treatment is given immediately after splinting. The athlete is removed from the playing area on a stretcher and transportation to the hospital by ambulance is arranged.

Fracture of the femur should not be handled any more than necessary, owing to the location of the arteries, nerves, and veins. All are in close proximity to the femur and particularly the lower end, and therefore there is a possibility of injury to these important vessels.

Compound fractures. Compound fractures of the thigh should be handled in the same manner as a simple fracture except that the control of bleeding must be the first consideration in this injury. Proper splinting, etc., will not be very effective if the athlete is allowed to bleed to death. Manual pressure over the femoral artery or the application of a tourniquet will stop bleeding from a wound made by a compound fracture. A sterile dressing should be applied

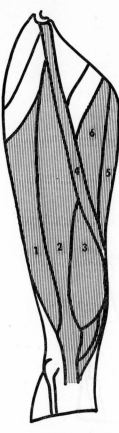

Muscles of the anterior thigh (front). (1) Vastus lateralis. (2) Rectus femoris. (3) Vastus medialis. (4) Sartorius. (5) Gracilias. (6) Adductor longus.

**ANTERIOR THIGH
(FRONT)**

to the wound, and after bleeding has been controlled, the splint may be applied. Extreme shock will be present and treatment for shock should be started immediately.

Strain. Strain, more commonly called *pulled muscle*, is also a very common injury to the thigh. Muscles on the front of the thigh as well as the back of the thigh are potential strain areas. When a muscle or tendon is forced to go beyond its normal limitation, it will strain; the degree of stress will establish the extent of the injury. Poor condition, improper warm-up, and fatigue are predisposing factors in this condition. A mild strain, where a few fibers are torn, to a severe strain, where there has been a tearing of many fibers is the usual extent of injury. A complete tear is very rare, but the possibility cannot be overlooked in the course of the examination.

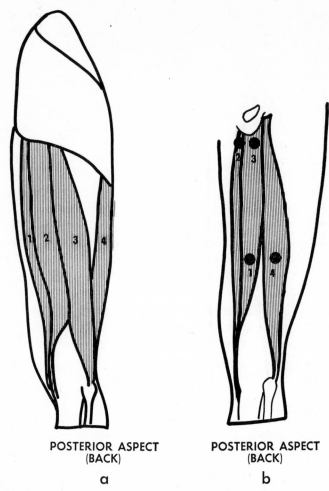

POSTERIOR ASPECT   POSTERIOR ASPECT
(BACK)   (BACK)

a   b

(a) Posterior muscles of the thigh (back). (1) Semimembranosus. (2) Semiten-
donosus. (3) Biceps femoris. (4) Vastus lateralis. (b) Most common sites of injury
to the hamstrings (in order). (1) "Belly" of the semitendinosus. (2) Attachment of
the semimembranosus. (3) Attachment of the semitendinosus. (4) "Belly" of the
biceps femoris.

A strain may occur in any part of the muscle: at its bony attachment, anywhere in the belly of the muscle, or at the aponeurosis
(where the muscle passes into a tendon).

Along with the tearing of the fibers, there may be damage to
blood vessels, which in turn will result in a hemorrhage. The amount
of pain will be determined by the severity of the injury and the
location of the muscle involved. A hamstring (back of leg) strain

is very painful, whereas the strain to the anterior group of the thigh is not so painful. The hemorrhage will result in a hematoma (localized mass of blood), and the initial step in the treatment of this injury is to control the amount of bleeding that takes place. The control is set up by the use of cold packs and a compression wrap.

In the hamstring strain, or "pull," there is usually an associated ecchymosis (black and blue) area. The discoloration may be at the site of the injury or considerably below. The old theory that the injury is better when the discoloration leaves is a fallacy and definitely should not be used as a criterion. The discoloration will change its location and its color over a period of a few days; this is due to the normal processes of the body. The injury is well when full range of motion and full strength is returned.

The muscles most commonly involved in thigh injuries are the biceps femoris, semimembranosus, semitendinosus, and the quadriceps extensors.

Treatment for Sprains and Strains. *History.* The athlete will complain of a pain in his thigh after he has run a race, sprint, or other form of exercise. If the athelete is able to complete his work and come to you with his problem, there is in all probability a mild "pull," or a strain. However, on the other hand, if the athlete is running and is suddenly forced to pull up because he has become lame, he will tell you that he felt something "pop" or that he has a burning sensation in his leg. This history will no doubt indicate that the athlete has sustained a more serious injury than a minor "pull." These injuries are treated the same way, whether the lesion is on the front of the thigh (quadriceps) or the back of the thigh (hamstring).

Inspection. Look at the thigh and compare with the other leg. Look for change in contour, which may indicate profuse swelling (hematoma); look for discoloration (black and blue), which may or may not show up immediately.

Palpation. Feel the thigh and compare findings with the other thigh. There will be a tightness, such as that seen in the contusion, which will be a spasm.

Functional test. The anterior thigh is tested, with the athlete on his stomach, and by gentle action applied to raise the heel to buttocks with knee bent. The degree of flexion will establish the severity of the injury. In flexing the knee, focus attention on the buttocks; as the area of pain is reached, the buttocks on the affected side will rise. Should there be a full range of motion, the degree of injury will be very slight; loss of flexion will establish the degree of injury to anterior thigh. If you cannot raise the leg to a right angle, there will be more than a mild sprain; stopping at less than a right angle will demonstrate a severe sprain. The same test should be made on the "good" leg for comparison.

The posterior thigh (hamstring area) is tested, with the athlete on his back, by grasping the ankle firmly with one hand and lifting the leg to full flexion. The other hand may be placed on the knee to prevent flexion of the knee. The degree of flexion of the leg will establish the type of injury involved. The higher the foot goes, the lesser the injury. In a severe strain, the leg cannot be lifted off the table at all.

Treatment. Immediate treatment consists of compression, elevation, and ice packs. This immediate treatment is aimed at the control of the hematoma which results in this type of injury. We assume that there is bleeding in every injury and treat it accordingly.

A severe injury should be placed in bed rest and seen immediately by the team physician. The moderate type of sprain is best treated by eliminating any weight bearing for the first 48 hours by means of crutches. The ice is continued for this length of time. Daily examinations are made, and as the hemorrhage subsides and the range of motion increases, have the athlete exercise the injured thigh, starting with mild exercises such as walking and leg swinging. Soft tissue injuries will respond better to activity than complete rest, providing the activity is not too strenuous. When normal walking is established and range of motion is progressing on a daily basis, start the athlete running and walking on a limited basis, gradually increasing to tolerance.

The use of heat is indicated after the first 48 hours, being very careful not to start too soon. Early use of heat may promote the hemorrhage and retard recovery.

Rehabilitation. Stretching exercises are started as soon as possible after full range of motion has been established. For example:

1. *Quadriceps stretching.* On stomach, reach back and grab ankle, and gradually pull heel to buttocks. *Do not jerk but pull evenly.*
2. *Hamstring stretch.* Spread legs 24 inches, bend over to touch toes, and stretch back of legs. The ultimate accomplishment in this exercise is to be able to place elbows on the floor.
3. *Hurdler's stance.* Sitting on ground with one leg forward and the other leg back, bend over and reach beyond toes; alternate with other leg forward.

4. Place heel on table with leg extended; reach over and grasp toes. The ultimate accomplishment is to have chest flat on thigh.

These exercises will suggest many more that can be added to the routine. However, the athlete should not be allowed to return to full activity until the limb is free of pain and a full range of motion reached. The particular sport involved plays a big part in how soon the athlete returns to the sport. His condition must be inspected and must be satisfactory before his return to full duty. It is questionable that strapping adhesive on the skin will give any support to a pulled muscle. The use of "hot packs" for work-outs seems to have greater beneficial effect than strappings.

CONTUSION OF THIGH

Injuries to the thigh are a very common occurrence in athletics, and they are not limited to contact sports alone. The most common injury to the thigh is the contusion or "Charley horse." This condition must be thoroughly diagnosed before any treatment can be started. In the case of a thigh injury, the history plays a very important part in the diagnosis. Pain in the thigh area may be very perplexing, and therefore the incidence to pain must be investigated. The athlete must describe in detail the circumstances that caused the injury. If the athlete, while running, felt a sudden pain in his thigh, this can be diagnosed as a "pull" in the area, whereas the athlete who received a "blow" on the thigh should be suspected as having a contusion or "Charley horse." The circumstance of injury is one way to differentiate between "pull" and "Charley horse." In other words, a "Charley horse" must be related to trauma from a blow rather than a strain or sprain.

After a full history has been attained, inspection and palpation are the next steps in making a diagnosis. With the athlete on his back, examine the anterior thigh; conversely, as he lies on his abdomen, examine the posterior thigh (hamstring area). Starting with the contusion, or "Charley horse," which is the most common injury to the front of the thigh, proceed step by step. Assuming the athlete has reported that he was hit on the thigh:

1. Compare the injured member with the other thigh; look for a change in contour of the thigh. The swelling may or may not be present but do not eliminate its possibility of later development.
2. When you palpate the thigh, you will probably feel that there is an abnormal tightness in the muscles. This is nature's means of splinting the leg for protection, commonly called a *spasm*.

3. Turn the athlete on his stomach, grasp his ankle with your hand, and gently bring his heel to his buttocks. This is the functional test for range of motion in the anterior thigh. The degree of flexion will establish the extent of the injury. If the leg cannot assume a right angle, then there is a more than average "Charley horse," which may be classified as moderate to severe. If the leg will go into full flexion, there will not be too much damage to the tissues, thus the lessening of spasm, and this degree of injury can be classified as a mild contusion.

4. Treatment consists of immediate compression, elevation, and ice packs.

Compression for Contusion of Quadriceps (Charley Horse). In a moderate to severe contusion of the thigh, it is very wise to have as much compression as possible. A layer of cotton and a snug elastic wrap applied above and below the site of the injury is very effective. However, excellent compression is better afforded by sponge rubber placed over the hematoma (swelling). A piece of sponge rubber ½ inch thick and 6 inches by 8 inches (depending on the size of the area to be compressed) is strapped to the thigh with elastic adhesive. In this procedure, do not encircle the thigh. After this is applied, a 4-inch elastic bandage is applied directly over the sponge rubber, starting at the knee and working up. In some instances it may be advisable to start below the knee and work up; this will completely compress the quadriceps (thigh) group of muscles. The leg is then elevated by placing pillows or blankets under the ankle rather than under the knee. Cold packs are then applied by using ice bags, held in place by an elastic bandage.

A massive hemorrhage, which will manifest itself immediately by forming an exaggerated curve to the thigh, is indicative of much damage to the soft tissues of the thigh and the blood vessels. This type of an injury should be put in bed rest as soon as possible, and the team phyician should prescribe further treatment.

Testing and Rehabilitating Thigh Contusion

Mild Contusion. Routine "Charley horse" cases may be treated with the foregoing procedures and sent home with instructions to continue the treatment through the next day. On the second day the leg is subjected to the same examination as the day before. History is reviewed, and inspection and palpation are again carried out, with particular emphasis being placed on the functional test.

If there is a full range of motion on the second day, assume the injury to be of a minor nature. Then apply a hot pack and have the athlete work out the "Charley horse." (Hot packs are applied in the same manner as the compression wrap; i.e., a counterirritant is applied to the skin, covered with cotton, and then wrapped with

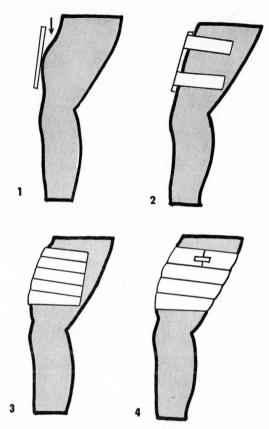

Contusion of the quadriceps (Charley horse). (1) Sponge rubber applied over the hematoma (arrow) for compression. (2) Sponge rubber held in place with elastic adhesive. (3) Complete coverage of sponge rubber with elastic adhesive. (4) Compression wrap of elastic bandage applied very snugly.

a snugly applied elastic bandage.) The athlete is assigned to work out the injury, starting with walking and then light jogging at distances of about 50 yards each time. As the injury "loosens up," ask the athlete to increase the jogging in distance and alternate this exercise with walking the same 50 yards.

When full motion is attained, speed and distances are both increased. This running is done on straightaways and turns, and change of direction is not permitted until the injury is fully without loss of function and devoid of tenderness. When the athlete has full recovered, he may be sent back to activity with a pad strapped to his leg to prevent a recurrence. The length of inactive time for a mild "Charley horse" will vary with the individual and may range from one day to two or three days. In the mild condition, the use of heat other than the "hot pack" is usually not necessary.

Moderate to severe contusion. In the moderate to severe injury, the same functional tests are again carried out on the second day. Should the loss of function and pain persist, continue ice packs, compression, and elevation for another day. On the third day, depending on functional tests, start physical therapy, *being very cautious not to start too early, as this may aggravate the condition so that increased hemorrhage will result.* Mild heat is applied either in the form of an infrared lamp or hot towels. The compression wrap is reapplied and the treatment repeated again the next day. Treatments should be continued until the lower leg can be flexed at greater than a right angle. At this time a hot pack may be applied, and the program as suggested for the mild contusion can be instituted. Again, the athlete should not be allowed to go into full activity until full range of motion has returned. The use of a pad for protection should also be used.

The length of disability time will vary from ten days in a moderate contusion to six weeks in a severe injury.

MYOSITIS OSSIFICANS

In the severe contusion to the thigh, a "Charley horse" that does not respond readily must be suspected as myositis ossificans. This is a laying down of calcium in the deep hematoma. It starts as small spicules of calcium and then increases over a period of time. The calcium is in the muscle and may be seen by area X-ray. Early X-ray may not show this condition, but films taken at a later time will reveal the calcium deposits. The first film, taken in about three weeks, may be negative, but the follow-up film in six weeks will very clearly outline the growth. The calcium deposits may interfere with the normal function of the muscle, and if so, surgical removal is indicated. The activity of the bone cells must be at a standstill before this procedure can be attempted.

A myositis ossificans that has "cooled down" and does not limit the function of the muscle is a handicap that an athlete can tolerate, but proper protection must be afforded so that the area can be protected from further contusions. A recurring contusion may start the process over again, resulting in the production of more calcium and a possibility of limitation of motion.

Treatment consists of rest and the application of heat to the area. Recommend modalities are diathermy and ultrasonic waves, or both. The literature mentions the possibility of using X-ray treatments for this condition. This is out of the realm of the athletic trainer and must be decided upon by the team physician.

Conservative approach is foremost in this type of injury; any effort made to hasten recovery will cause further disability. The best routine consists of rest, rest, and more rest. Heat is applied during this rest period.

LOWER LEG

Fractures. The tibia, the weight-bearing bone of the lower leg, is very large at the top, thins off, and then enlarges at the ankle. Fractures of the tibia do occur in athletics, either with an associated fracture of the fibula or as an injury in itself.

Upper end of tibia. The fracture may occur in one condyle or the other, or both. It is caused by severe wrenching and twisting of the knee. The joint will swell profusely, be very painful, and will disable the athlete. Loss of function of the knee joint will result. History will reveal the cause of the injury.

Inspection will show a very swollen knee. There may or may not be any deformity. Loss of function of the knee joint will be present. Palpation will reveal point tenderness over the fracture site.

Treatment consists of splinting in a comfortable position and transportation to proper medical facilities. If possible, posterior splinting is desired. Place splint in back of leg and wrap securely.

Shaft of tibia. Fractures of the shaft may occur at any level. The most common location is at the junction of the lower and middle third, and the fracture may be spiral, oblique, or transverse, and may also be comminuted. It is usually caused by a direct blow to the area, by being blocked, kicked, etc. The tibia is directly under the skin and any abnormality may be palpated. Pain and tenderness will be present. In a suspected fracture of the tibia, splint and send to medical facilities.

Fibula. The fibula is the nonweight-bearing bone of the lower leg. Fracture may occur at any place along the shaft, but the most common site is the lower third of the fibula. The athlete may be able to walk, inasmuch as the tibia will be bearing all the weight. The fibula may be palpated and the incidence of a deformity noted. Pain and tenderness will be present; point tenderness over the exact spot of the fracture will be very evident. The tibia acts as a splint for the fibula, and the use of an elastic compression wrap and crutches will suffice as first aid before transportation.

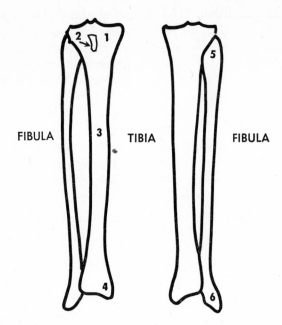

FIBULA   TIBIA   FIBULA

Bones of the lower leg (anterior), or front view; and posterior, or back view. (1) Upper end of tibia. (2) Tibial tubercle. (3) Shaft of the tibia. (4) Lower end of tibia (ankle). (5) Upper end of fibula. (6) Lower end of fibula (ankle).

A Potts fracture is one that is localized in the lower inch or two above the ankle. It is usually associated with a severe sprain history of the ankle. Very often the athlete will be able to walk. There will be pain, but usually the athlete will feel that this pain is the normal pain for a sprain. Tenderness over the site will be present, and there is usually severe swelling. This fracture is not easily recognized without the benefit of an X-ray, and in some cases it may be missed because this procedure was not performed. Treatment is the same as in other fractures of the fibula.

Stress fracture. Stress fractures are becoming more and more frequent. The cause is rather vague. It may occur by constant jarring, uncoordinated muscular action, fatigue, or perhaps a difference in the bony make-up of the individual.

Stress fractures have been seen primarily in the lower third of the fibula and the metatarsals (March fracture). The upper part of the fibula maybe affected, but this is rather rare. Symptoms are dull ache (increasing as activity continues), point tenderness, and possibly visible swelling or deformity.

History will reveal that there is a pain, sometimes disabling, over the lower third of the fibula. Overnight rest seems to relieve pain, but as soon as activity is started again, the pain is noticeable. As exercise is continued, the pain will become more intense immediately after exercise. Fast running, etc., will also be tolerable, but deceleration is very painful. This condition occurs more on board running than in any other sport. Distance running on turf has not produced this injury. Inspection will not show any condition that is alarming. Palpation will reveal a tender area directly over the lower third of the fibula.

The injury is usually treated as a strain of the lower leg. After this preliminary aid fails and pain persists, an X-ray is taken. Invariably the result of the film will be negative. Whirlpool baths, baking, etc., with gradation of exercise are then started, but if these treatments effect no change after two weeks or so have passed, a check film will show that there has been a fracture to the fibula.

During this time the athlete will continue to walk, etc., but athletic activities will have been stopped. Whirlpool baths, baking, etc., are continued and a later check film is made (approximately five weeks after the injury). When the fracture has fully healed, the athlete will be allowed to return to activity.

Strains. Strains of the lower leg are very common conditions seen in athletics. All sports present this type of injury. The more common type of strain is seen in the posterior aspect of the leg. The muscles involved are gastrocnemius, soleus, and plantaris. Symptoms are pain, tightness, loss of function, swelling, and disability. Strains of this muscle group are mainly attributed to improper warm-up. Very few result from indirect trauma, such as piling on.

Strains of the calf group are found in three locations: the heads of the gastrocnemius (deep in the space in back of the knee; the medial head is found on the inside of the leg, while the lateral is found on the outside of the leg), the belly of the muscles, and the attachment with the tendon Achilles. The location of the strain can be felt by gently palpating the full muscle and then locating the tight area, which will also demonstrate point tenderness.

History will reveal that the athlete felt a tightness in the back of his leg. He felt he could work it out, so he continued to force the muscle with the result that he felt something "pop" in the back of his leg. He may describe the pain as a deep pain or a superficial soreness right under the skin. Inspection will show some swelling and tightness of the calf group. Palpation will reveal that there is tightness on touching the group of muscles.

To test for function of this group of muscles, the athlete lies on his stomach, bends his knee to a right angle, and pushes his toes downward. This motion will reveal the range of motion present. Test his other leg in the same manner to establish normal function. When this test is performed in the early stages of the injury, pain will be very evident, and the athlete will rebel at the action.

Treatment in the acute stage consists of the immediate application of a compression wrap and the application of ice packs to the area, with the trainer's instructions to remain off the leg as much as possible and to keep the leg elevated higher than the rest of the body. On the next day, heat and mild massage may be used with exercises to the limit of tolerance.

In the severe strain of the calf group, the use of crutches or bed rest may be indicated, along with the use of ice for as long as 48 hours. After this time, mild heat may be applied.

Exercises for the calf group consist of flexion and extension of the foot. The easiest way to perform this exercise is to rise on the toes, hold for a count, and then drop slowly. Repeat until required number is reached (about 40 to start), gradually increasing to limit of tolerance. Walking and jogging are also very effective.

To stretch the calf group, use a piece of a 2 by 4 foot timber or a thick book; place forefoot on edge of book and then let heels drop to floor. The athlete can stabilize his balance by holding onto a chair or table. This exercise is repeated about ten times and should be done several times during the day. An improvision of this exercise may be done on the edge of a stair step by holding onto the banister and letting the heels drop, thus stretching the calf muscles.

The athlete may return to activity when all symptoms are gone and the full stretch is demonstrated.

Plantaris "pull." The plantaris muscle originates at the lateral condyle of the femur and inserts with the tendon Achilles. The belly of the plantaris is short and small; the tendon is the longest in the body. Its action is the extension of the foot. When injured, the athlete's history will be that he felt a definite "giving away," pain, and in some instances, an audible snap. The calf will swell and walking will be very painful. The diagnosis from the history is very conclusive; there has not been a bruise, etc., to the area, and consequently there must be a pull. The degree of pull cannot be established before 24 to 48 hours. In many instances of this injury, there is a complete rupture of this muscle, and it may be very disabling for a few days. Treatment consists of compression, ice packs, and elevation for the first 48 hours, and after this, the application of

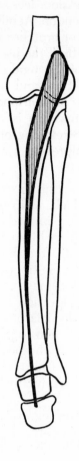

Plantaris muscle.

heat. Exercise may be started as soon as the athlete becomes comfortable. The wearing of a lift in the heel of the shoe will aid in recovery.

Pulled tendon Achilles. The tendon may "pull" from its attachment at the musculo tendinous junction or at its bony attachment. The pull at the muscle attachment is more common than the pull from its bony attachment at the calcaneus. Both conditions are very painful and disabling. In severe "pulls" or ruptures, the athlete will be in intense pain, and the loss of function will be noted. Inspection may reveal an indentation where the rupture has occurred.

Treatment for rupture of tendon is to send the athlete immediately to the hospital for surgical repair. The longer the delay, the more complicated the repair will be.

In the mild "pull" of the tendon, compression, ice, and elevation are started immediately. Strapping for tendon Achilles strain is very helpful. In the severe injury, the use of crutches is necessary. In the milder strain, when walking is permitted, the use of a ½-half lift in the heel will shorten the excursion of the tendon and lessen the strain. Tendons have very poor circulation, and the prognosis of a pull in the tendon is not good. The use of whirlpool baths, hot compresses, infrared heat, etc., plus mild massage is very helpful. Exercises may be started when tolerable. Stretching of the tendon after pain has subsided is very important to prevent a recurrence of the strain.

Contusions. The more common site of contusions of the lower leg is the anterior (front) part. By direct kick, whip block, etc., a bruise results on the shin. There may be immediate swelling (hematoma) or just plain pain. The athlete very often, when kicked on the shin, is able to continue to play, but after the contest the injury is painful. If the injury is directly over the tibia (shin bone), care should be taken to prevent serious bone damage. The immediate application of ice and compression and elevation are necessary. Daily checks should be made by the team physician to see that the injury is improving normally. It is not uncommon to see a cellulitis (infection) occur as late as many weeks after the occasion of the bruise. Proper padding is very necessary to prevent recurring bruise to the area. Heat and hot packs are very effective in the management of this injury.

Contusions to the posterior area of the lower leg, calf, and tendon are not so common as bruises to the shin bone or area. However, they are just as disabling and just as painful. Bleeding will be profuse in the injury to the calf muscles, and all precautions in the control of hemorrhage should be instituted. The immediate application of compression, ice, and elevation is very necessary. In severe contusions, bed rest or crutches may be indicated. If bleeding is profuse and a large hematoma results, the team physician may wish to aspirate. In the mild contusion the athlete may be able to resume full duty on the next day if a hot pack and a protective pad are applied. If the swelling and pain are still evident, the ice treatment may be continued another day, after which heat and mild exercises should be started. Disability in a mild contusion may extend only overnight. The severe type may last from two or three days to weeks.

Contusions to the tendons are seen but not too frequently. Treatment is essentially the same as for contusion of muscles of the lower leg. The severity of the bruise will determine the type of treatment and the amount of disability. Contusions of the tendon Achilles are very prolonged, as are those of the tendons of the peroneal group of the lower leg.

Injury to Peroneal Nerve. Contusion of the peroneal nerve, which is located superficially on the outside of the knee, presents a problem that has been seen from time to time in athletics. The pain may last from a few seconds to a few hours. There may also be an accompanying paralysis, but this is usually temporary. Treatment of this injury is rest and mild heat until normal condition obtains.

The more severe contusion of the peroneal nerve presents a more serious problem. When the numbness and loss of function (foot drop) appears, the team physician should be notified immediately and his orders carried out. Some of these cases respond to heat, etc., whereas others may require surgical intervention.

Tenosynovitis of the Tendon Achilles. Where there is a great deal of friction with other tissues, nature provides a membrane-lined sheath that gives off a liquid for lubricating the tendon. This sheath surrounds the tendon, keeping it supple and well lubricated. From overuse, pressure, or friction, the sheath becomes inflamed; this is then called *tenosynovitis*. Local tenderness is found on pressure, and a definite crepitus is felt when the foot is moved up and down. There may be swelling localized over the point of irritation, causing pressure on the tendon. This condition comes on rather slowly over a few days' time.

Treatment at this point is aimed at the absorption of the swelling. After a few days it is too late for ice, but compression and elevation can still be used. The application of an open-faced Gibney and a ½-inch lift in heel to shorten the excursion of the tendon will help. Heat indicated at this time may be of any type; excellent results are obtained with diathermy and ultrasonics. Activity may be started when the athlete is comfortable. This injury cannot be forced, and caution must be used because this injury is slow in responding and quite likely to linger if irritated.

SOME OF THE MUSCLES OF THE LEG

Thigh

Tensor fasciae latae, or tensor. This is a most peculiar muscle in that it has no bony attachments. It is small and lies to the front and side of the hip. The origin is just below the crest of the ilium,

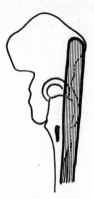

Tensor fasciae latae.

and its insertion is in the fascia of the thigh about one-quarter of the way down. The action is abducting the thigh, as well as assisting in flexion, and medial rotation of the thigh.

Vastus intermedius. The vastus intermedius muscle is a part of the quadriceps group and is situated on the front part of the thigh. Its origin is the anterior and lateral surfaces of the upper two-thirds of the shaft of the femur. Its insertion is in the rectus femoris tendon. This is a deep insertion at the base of the patella. The action is to extend the leg.

Vastus medialis (internus). A part of the group of extensor muscles of the leg, known as the quadriceps, is situated on the medial and front part of the thigh. Its origin is in the lower half of the intertrochanteric line, the medial lip of the linea aspera (a prominent ridge on the middle third of the femur), and the medial supracondylar ridge. Its insertion is the medial border of the quadriceps femoris tendon. Action is to extend the leg and draw the patella medially.

Vastus lateralis (externus). This is one of the four muscles composing the quadriceps group. Origin is the upper border of the intertrochantic line, greater trochanter, the linea aspera (a prominent ridge on the middle third of the femur), and the capsule of the hip joint. Its insertion is at the lateral border of the patella, forming a part of the quadriceps femoris tendon. Action is to extend the leg.

Rectus femoris. Rectus femoris is one of the four muscles in the quadriceps group. It is large and runs straight down the thigh. Its action resembles the triceps muscle of the arm. The straight head

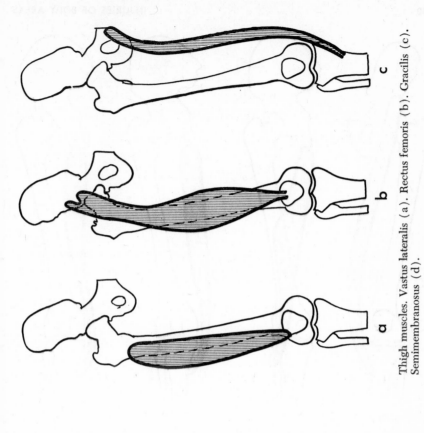

Thigh muscles. Vastus lateralis (a). Rectus femoris (b). Gracilis (c). Semimembranosus (d).

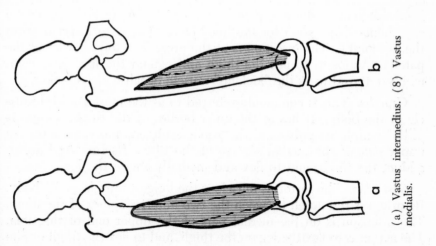

(a) Vastus intermedius. (8) Vastus medialis.

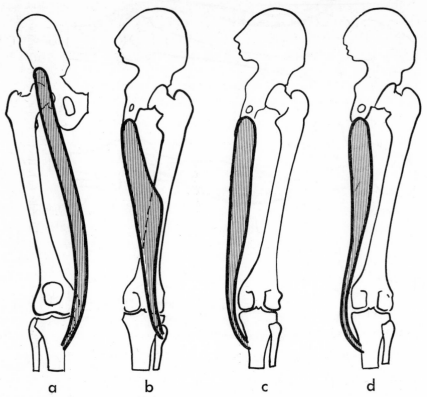

Thigh muscles. Sartorius (a). Biceps femoris (b). Semitendinosus (c).

originates at the anterior inferior spine of the ilium; the reflected head originates from a groove on the rim of the acetabulum (deep cup-shaped depression for the head of the femur to insert to form the hip joint). The insertion is at the proximal (top) border of the patella. Action is to flex the thigh and extend the leg. It is commonly referred to as the "kicking" muscle because of its action.

Gracilis. This is commonly referred to as the most graceful muscle of the body. It lies at the inner border of the thigh. Origin is at the symphysis pubis and the pelvic arch. Its insertion is on the upper part of the medial surface of the tibia. Its functions are to adduct the thigh, and to flex and medially rotate the leg.

Sartorius. The sartorius muscle is the longest muscle in the body. Its origin is the notch between the two anterior spines of the ilium. The insertion is on the medial part of the upper end of the tibia. The action is to flex the leg on the thigh, and to flex the thigh on the pelvis and rotate the thigh laterally.

Biceps femoris. The biceps femoris is similar to the biceps muscle in the arm. The origin of the long head is the tuberosity of the ischium; the origin of the short head is the lateral lip of the linea aspera (ridge of femur) and lateral supracondyle of the femur. The insertion is the head of the fibula and lateral condyle of the tibia. The action of the biceps is to extend the hip, rotate the hip outward, and to flex and rotate the knee joint outward.

Semitendinosus. A very close companion, its tendon, reaches halfway up the thigh. Its origin is the tuberosity of the ischium. The insertion is the front side of the inner tuberosity of the tibia along with the sartorius. The action is to extend the thigh, flex the leg, and rotate the leg medially when the knee is semiflexed.

Semimembranosus. This muscle lies alongside the semitendinosus and partly beneath it. The origin is the upper and lateral facet of the ischial tuberosity. The insertion is the inner half of the posterior surface of the inner tuberosity of the tibia. The action is to extend the thigh, flex the leg, and rotate the leg medially when the knee is semiflexed.

Lower Leg

Gastrocnemius. This muscle gives the rounded form to the calf of the leg. The origin is at two tendons on the back side of the condyles of the femur. The insertion is the back side of the calcaneus. The tendon is called the *tendon Achilles* and is very large. The action is to plantarflex the foot and flex the femur on the tibia.

Soleus. The soleus works with the gastrocnemius and is immediately below it on the calf of the leg. Its origin is the upper surface of the head of the fibula, the upper third of the fibula, middle third of the medial border of the tibia, and the tendinous arch between the tibia and the fibula. The insertion is at a common tendon with the gastrocnemius, which is the tendon Achilles at the calcaneus. The action is to plantarflex the foot and to stabilize the leg on the foot.

Popliteus. This is a very small and relatively unimportant muscle of the knee joint. It originates on the outer side of the lateral condyle of the femur. Its insertion is on the posterior surface of the tibia. The action of the popliteus is to flex and inwardly rotate the knee.

Tibialis anterior. This is a slender muscle on the outer side of the tibia on the front of the leg. The origin is the upper two-thirds of the outer surface of the tibia and a corresponding portion of the interosseus membrane. The insertion is the inner margins of the first cuneiform and the first metatarsal. The action is to invert the foot and also to dorsiflex the foot.

Tibialis posterior. This muscle is situated very deep on the back of the leg. The origin is the upper half of the interosseus membrane and the corresponding parts of the tibia and fibula. The insertion is the lower part of the navicular (scaphoid) and the first cuneiform bones. The action is to invert the foot and to plantarflex the foot.

Peroneus brevis. Brevis is a small member of the peroneus group of three muscles. It has its origin on the lower two-thirds of the fibula, and its insertion is on the lower side of the base of the fifth metatarsal. The action is to plantarflex the foot as well as evert it.

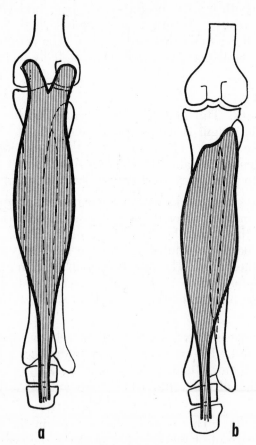

Lower leg muscles. Gastrocnemius (a). Soleus (b).

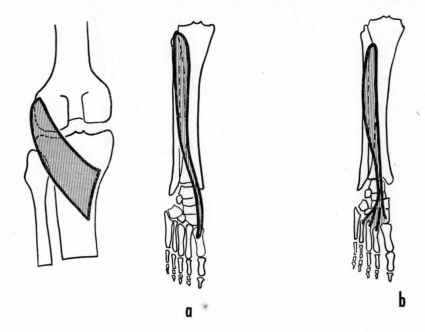

Popliteus.   Anterior tibialis (a). Posterior tibialis (b).

Peroneus longus. The longus is a very powerful muscle for its size and lies underneath the skin on the outer side of the leg next to the fibula. Its origin is the head and lateral two-thirds of the fibula and the lateral head of the tibia. The insertion is the outer side of the first cuneiform and the first metatarsal. The action is to dorsiflex the foot and to evert the foot. It is interesting to note that the soleus, gastrocnemius, and peroneus longus work together to form the triceps of the leg. The loss of the peroneus longus results in the athlete's having a flat foot.

Peroneus tertius. This is the third member of the peroneus family. However, this muscle is sometimes called the *fifth* tendon of the extensor digitorum longus. It originates on the lower anterior surface of the fibula. The insertion is the base of the fifth metatarsal. The action is to dorsiflex and evert the foot.

Extensor hallucis longus. This small muscle has its origin on the anterior surface of the fibula. Its insertion is at the base of the

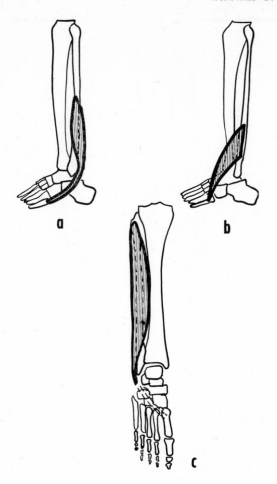

The peroneals. Peroneus brevis (a). Peroneus tertius (b). Peroneus longus (c).

second phalanx of the great toe, and its action is to extend the great toe.

Flexor hallucis longus. The flexor hallucis longus is situated on the lateral side of the fibula, from which it has its origin, and originates in the lower two-thirds of the fibula and the interosseus membrane. Its insertion is the under surface of the base of the second phalanx of the great toe. Its action is to flex the great toe and extend the ankle.

Extensor digitorum longus. This muscle is similar to the anterior tibialis and is situated on the front side of the leg. Its origin is the

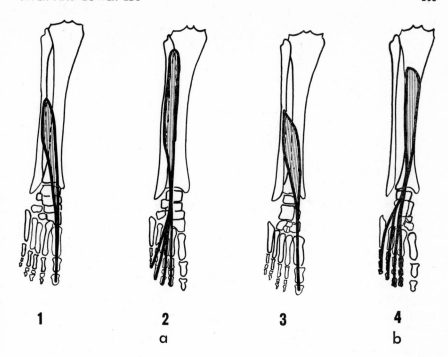

1   2   3   4
a   b

(a) Extensor hallucis longus (1). Extensor digitorum longus (2). Flexor hallucis longus (3). (b) Flexor digitorum longus (4).

lateral condyle of the tibia, the front of the fibula, and the interosseus membrane. Its insertion is the top of the bones of the foot (the outer toes). Its action is to extend the phalanges and to dorsiflex the foot.

Flexor digitorum longus. This muscle is situated in the back of the leg. Its origin is the posterior surface of the middle of the tibia, and its insertion is the plantar surface of the base of the outer four toes. Its action is to flex the phalanges and help plantarflex the foot.

Chapter 15

Knee

THE KNEE JOINT

Anatomy. The knee joint is a hinge joint, forming the articulation between the lower end of the femur and the upper end of the tibia. The fibula and the patella also complete the bone structure of the joint.

The lower end of the femur presents two condyles (rounded surfaces) which are projected downward. They are called the *medial* and *lateral* condyle, the medial being slightly longer and the lateral slightly broader. The deep notch between the condyles is called the *intercondyloid* notch. On each side of the condyles are found projections called *epicondyles,* the medial and lateral.

The tibia, the long bone on the medial side of the leg, has an upper portion called the *head,* which has two tuberosities, medial and lateral. The top has shallow depressions to bear the condyles of the femur (also the semilunar menisci, or cartilages). Between the depressions is the intercondyloid eminence. The tibial tubercle is a large, pronounced eminence in the front of the tibia just below the head.

The fibula is the long slender bone on the lateral side of the leg. The head articulates with the outer side of the tibia. The fibula does not enter into weight bearing but acts as an attachment for muscles, etc. It is on the head of the fibula that the lateral collateral ligament attaches.

The patella is roughly circular in outline and is situated in front of the knee joint within the tendon of the quadriceps. It is about 1½ inches in diameter and 1 inch thick. When the leg is extended, the patella is in front of the condyles of the femur; with the knee in flexion, it lies in the lower end of the femur in its notch. When kneeling, the weight of the body is not on the patella but on the tubercle of the tibia.

The medial meniscus and the medial collateral ligaments are the soft tissues of the knee joint that are most frequently involved in athletic injuries. The medial collateral ligament attaches at the medial epicondyle of the femur and the medial condyle of the tibia.

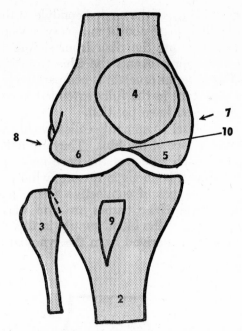

Important parts of the knee joint to be observed in all knee injuries. (1) Femur. (2) Tibia. (3) Fibula. (4) Patella. (5) Medial condyle. (6) Lateral condyle. (7) Medial epicondyle. (8) Lateral epicondyle. (9) Tibial tubercle. (10) Intercondylar notch.

It is a very strong ligament and is intimately connected with the capsule and the medial meniscus. Note that the meniscus is attached to the medial collateral ligament; this is not true of the lateral collateral ligament. The lateral collateral ligament extends from the lateral epicondyle of the femur to the proximal head of the fibula. This ligament is completely separate from the capsule of the joint. The medial collateral ligament is the stronger of the two. These ligaments are the major factors in stabilizing the knee joint.

The capsule is a strong but loose sac that completely surrounds the joint. It has its attachments on the femur, patella, and the upper borders of the tibia. The capsule is lined with a synovial membrane that gives off a liquid, known as *synovia,* for lubricating the joint.

Deep inside the knee joint are the cruciate ligaments, so-called because they cross one another. There are two cruciates: (1) The anterior ligament attaches on the front of the tibial floor and then extends backward and laterally to attach on the inner surface of the lateral condyle of the femur; (2) the posterior runs, not quite so oblique, a more direct course from the back of the tibial floor to the front of the lateral surface of the medial condyle of the femur. These ligaments are cordlike in structure and very strong. The anterior cruciate ligament prevents the tibia from sliding forward on the femur, and the posterior prevents the tibia from sliding backward on the femur. The anterior cruciate is comparatively loose, whereas the posterior is very taut in the fully extended knee. The opposite takes place in the flexed knee position.

The semilunar menisci (commonly called *cartilages*) are situated on the articulating surface of the tibia. They are half-moon in shape and are situated on each aspect of the knee joint, running front to back. They are fibrocartilaginous in texture, which means that they are composed of two types of connective tissue, namely, cartilage and fibrous tissue. Both these tissues are firm, elastic, and tough. There is some question of the blood supply in this tissue; the main source of nourishment is derived from the synovial fluid present in the joint.

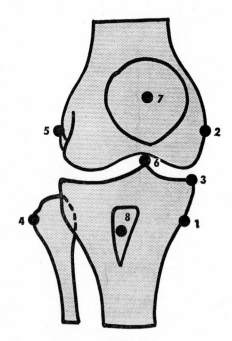

Common sites of injuries to the knee (not in order). (1) Attachment of the medial collateral ligament. (2) Femoral attachment of the medial collateral ligament. (3) Medial meniscus (cartilage) as it attaches to the medial collateral ligament. (4) Fibula attachment of the lateral collateral ligament. (5) Femoral attachment of lateral collateral ligament. (6) Cruciate ligaments. (7) Patella. (8) Tibial tubercle (attachment of patella tendon).

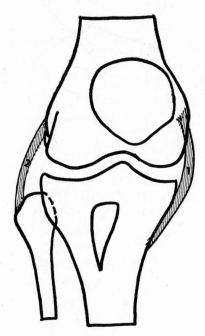

Medial and lateral collateral ligaments of the knee. (1) Medial collateral ligament. (2) Lateral collateral ligament.

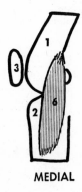 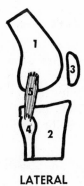

MEDIAL   **LATERAL**

Side view of the medial and lateral collateral ligaments of the knee. (1) Femur. (2) Tibia. (3) Patella. (4) Fibula. (5) Lateral collateral ligament. (6) Medial collateral ligament.

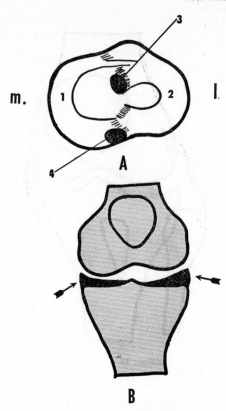

Menisci of the knee (cartilages). (a) Half-moon-shaped cartilage as it appears from
the top. (1) Medial meniscus. (2) Lateral meniscus. (3) Attachment of anterior
cruciate ligament. (4) Attachment of posterior cruciate ligament. (b) Relation of
menisci as seen from the front. Note thickness at joint margins (arrows).

These menisci are attached to the tibia by coronary ligaments
at the outer border. The rest of the menisci is not fastened to the
tibia, thus allowing for motion when the joint is used. The outer
border of the menisci is approximately ¼ inch thick and thins out
toward the middle of the joint, thus approximating the tibial femural
joint.

A fat pad is located just below the patella, which fills the space
when the patella is moved in knee flexion. The fat pad separates the
ligamentum patella from the joint capsule.

Bursae are found in the knee-joint area. These are sacs of fluid
that underlie moving tissues to prevent erosion and absorb shock.
Many of the bursae of the knee joint are continuations of the joint
capsule; many are independent.

Treatment of Injuries. All knee injuries cannot be treated alike. To assume so would be folly and not to the best interest of the athlete. If all were treated in the same way, examinations, etc., would not be necessary and each injury could be treated by "ear." The results of this type of procedure would be far from satisfactory. Functional tests included in a meticulous examination should be a part of the full coverage of the athlete. To ice, elevate, and compress all knee injuries routinely without proper examination is a simple and most convenient way to treat an injury, but without the benefit of a proper diagnosis, the injury may linger and linger until the knee becomes totally incapacitated.

Many athletes arrive at college with this type of history, and often the Department of Health surgeons cannot permit the student to participate in a sport, because of the laxity of ligaments in their knees. Treatments at this time to overcome the difficulty cannot be recommended. Without question, injuries to the knee may require surgical intervention, but to treat all knees with the thought that they will get well, whether surgery or other methods are used, is not true. This type of thinking does not go hand in hand with good medical coverage. The decision for surgery does not rest in the hands of the coach or trainer but with the orthopedic surgeon making the examination or with the surgeon affiliated with the school.

For the athlete to perform up to par, the best treatment should be made available to him. If 100 per cent results are not attained, the treatment has not been good. An athlete cannot do his best

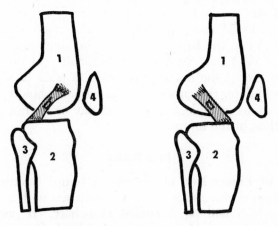

The anterior and posterior cruciate ligaments. (1) Femur. (2) Tibia. (3) Fibula. (4) Patella. Anterior cruciate ligament (a). Posterior cruciate ligament (b).

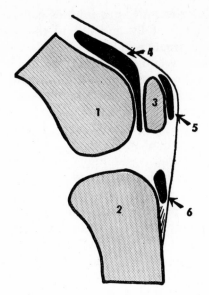

Bursae of the knee. (1) Femur. (2) Tibia. (3) Patella. (4) Suprapatella bursa. (5) Prepatella bursa. (6) Infrapatella bursa.

if he is not physically perfect, and if he is hurried back to work without fully recovering from the knee injury, he is not being treated justly. In spite of the urgings of the athlete, coach, or parents, permission to return to play should be given only when the treatment is completed, and not before. A recurring injury does not make the athlete or the attending personnel confident that the doctor has good judgment.

Treatments to be used are decided on as soon as possible and then carried out to the fullest; there are no short cuts. Very often the best treatment may be the most difficult and often the most inconvenient, but if the decision is made to treat in such manner, nothing should deter this procedure. Treatment should start as soon after the injury as possible, not the next day or so, but even on the field at the time of the injury.

FRACTURES

Fracture of Lower End of Femur. A femur fracture is a very rare injury in athletics and is not to be confused with an epiphyseal separation, which will be discussed elsewhere. It occurs usually from falling or jumping from a great height but may also be the result of a severe wrench. There is a history of severe injury and complete disability. Swelling is rapid and extensive. The swelling will cause a deformity of the lower end of the femur, confusing inspection. X-ray is essential to complete diagnosis.

Fractures of the lower end of the femur should be splinted with a full leg splint. A Thomas leg splint, if available, should be used. The athlete should be transported to the hospital as soon as possible for further treatment.

Fracture of Upper End of Tibia. A review of the anatomy of the upper end of the tibia shows the large end to be composed of cancellous bone (very porous and spongy in texture) which is forced to extend over the shaft of the tibia. The narrow portion of this junction is a potential fracture sight. These are uncommon in athletics. They occur as the result of a severe blow or a very severe outward torsion of the hip. The athlete will tell of a severe injury plus the loss of function of the knee and will not be able to bear weight on the leg. However, passive motion of the knee will be normal. Tenderness over the fracture sight and swelling (either local or general) will contribute to the diagnosis. X-ray will be necessary to establish the full extent of this injury. A full leg splint is recommended together with removal to a hospital for further treatment.

Fracture of Upper End of Fibula. Many times this is referred to as the "blind fracture" because it is not detected until calcium has formed and swelling noted. In some sprains of the ankle there will be other complications such as may occur in jumping from high places; the sprain of the ankle overshadows the upper end of the fibula. The fracture may also occur from a direct blow; swelling will occur and disability may or may not be present. Palpation may or may not suggest a fracture. X-ray must be used to make a final diagnosis. The athlete's knee should be wrapped with a compression bandage, and he should be supplied with crutches and then sent for medical treatment.

Fracture of Patella. Probably the most common fracture occurring in the knee area is that of the patella. The patella is in a very exposed position, and the nature of its function is such that it is subject to many strains and stresses. Most fractures occur from a violent wrenching of the patella over the condyles of the femur. The mechanics of the patella tendon and its association with the quadriceps cause a tension that may result in a transverse fracture of the patella. Falling on the knee usually results in landing on the tibial tubercle rather than the patella. With the close proximity of the patella to the knee joint, swelling into the joint will result. There will be a tear of the fibers of the quadriceps and the patella tendon and a loss of function in the knee joint. It is very easy when palpating to grasp the two fragments of the patella, and also to feel the space between the two fragments. X-ray is indicated to confirm diagnosis and rule out other bony pathology. The athlete should be placed in a posterior splint, crutches supplied, and sent to team physician.

DISLOCATION OF KNEE

Owing to the strong ligaments that surround the knee, this is a very rare injury. The broad ends of the tibia and femur make a good firm joint, and when the dislocation occurs, there is much damage to the soft tissues in the joint. There will be a complete tear of the cruciate ligaments, capsule, medial and lateral ligaments, and the attachments of the hamstring muscles. The types of dislocation are anterior, posterior, internal, external, or one that rotates on the femur. The anterior dislocation is the most common. The complete dislocation is very obvious; the incomplete is not so likely to be noticed because of the amount of swelling. The injury should be splinted and the athlete moved to hospital in an ambulance as soon as possible. Severe tearing of soft tissue may affect the blood and nerve supply to the lower leg and these should be checked thoroughly.

Patella. In reviewing the anatomy of the patella and its relation to the quadriceps muscles and the patella tendon, we find that the patella is almost in a state of suspension. The patella will move out of the notch and go to the outside of the knee or the inside. This dislocation is usually the result of a fall or a direct blow to the knee cap. Many have resulted from holding a blocking dummy by forcing the knee into the bag for stabilization. When contact is made, the bag and blocking force will produce a tension on the patella, forcing it in or out. There will be a complete loss of function of the joint and much swelling. The displaced patella will be obvious, and the flattening of the knee will be very apparent. The injury should not be reduced by the trainer, but the knee splinted with a posterior splint, crutches provided, and the athlete should be sent to team physician. The treatment after the reduction will be the same as for all soft tissue injuries of the knee.

Fibula. This dislocation is a very rare injury and is usually associated with another injury in the lower part of the leg. The dis-

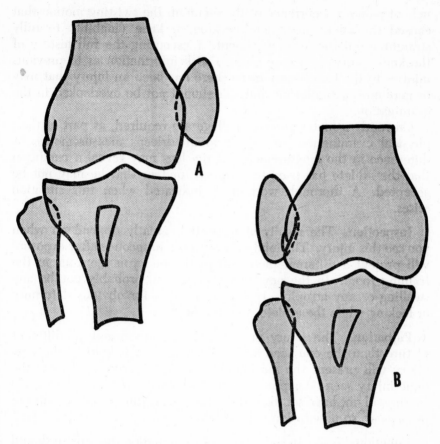

Dislocation of the patella. Medial dislocation (a). Lateral dislocation (b).

location may be forward, backward, outward, or upward. The diagnosis is made readily, as the bone is immediately below the skin. The immediate treatment consists of an elastic bandage applied snugly to the knee joint, crutches, and transportation to the team physician.

EXAMINATION OF KNEE JOINT

History. The athlete must give a complete recital of the incidents of the injury. Each detail must be noted and used. It is a good practice not to suggest symptoms, etc., during this part of the examination. The athlete will recite the degree of pain, the sharpness of pain on occurrence of the incident, the twisting motion that caused the involvement, and locking of knee (inability to fully straighten out the leg), if present. In securing the full history of the knee injury, it is very wise to seek information as to previous injuries to the knee. Very often there has been an injury that may or may not be significant, but this should not be overlooked in the examination.

Currently athletes entering college are required, as part of their physical examination, to submit to quadriceps measurements. A difference in the measurements of the legs may reveal a condition that the athlete has tried to suppress for fear that he may not be accepted. A thorough work-up is indicated when this situation arises.

Inspection. The results of inspection greatly depend on when you see this injury. The injury that you see in seconds after exposure will present a different picture than the one you see later in the training room. In the new injury there will probably not be any swelling or any atrophy. However, we look for obvious deformity or locking while the athlete is on the field.

Palpation. The injury on the field again presents a different picture than the one seen at a later time. On palpation, the new injury will present the maximum area of tenderness, whereas the same injury seen later presents a more diffused tenderness. Muscle spasm will not have set itself up at this time. Joint swelling will not be present, so no effusion will be felt.

Functional tests. In the process of examination the athlete should be flat on his back on a table high enough for the examiner to work on without discomfort.

1. *Flexion and extension.* Full flexion and full extension is the first condition noted. This test should be done with extreme caution. With the lower leg firmly held, bend the knee as far as it will go. Should you meet with opposition, make further inquiries as to why opposition is present (i.e., pain, tightness, or blocking). After this has been established, full extension is the next test.

As before, with leg under control, the lower leg is straightened as far as it will go. If leg is fully extended, this is normal; however, if opposition is felt, further questioning is indicated. The athlete will advise you that something is pulling or is tight in the back of the knee, or that he feels as though something inside the joint is blocking the knee.

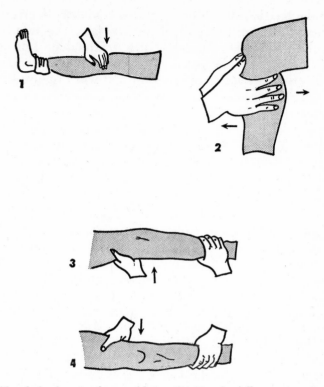

Position of hands for functional tests of knee. (1) Test for full extension. Arrow shows direction of pressure. (2) Test for cruciate instability. Arrow shows path of movements. (3) Test for lateral collateral ligament. Arrow shows pressure to outside of knee. (4) Test for medial collateral ligament. Arrow shows pressure used to open joint and stretch ligament.

2. *Lateral instability test.* Again, the athlete lies flat on his back. With the leg in full extension, grasp the ankle with one hand and place the other hand around the lower part of the posterior thigh. The leg then lies in a cradle-like support. By holding the thigh firm, gently pull the lower leg toward you; this will open the joint. Should motion be established, check the other knee in the same manner. (This is the test for stability of the medial collateral ligament; by reversing the procedure, the lateral ligament can be tested.)

Check the degree of instability in full extension. If there should be any motion in this test, there must be tearing of the ligament and a serious involvement of the joint. When this is found, the athlete should be referred to the orthopedic surgeon for treatment.

After the test in full extension, flex the joint 20 degrees and examine the stability in this position. Should lateral motion be found, check with the other knee for comparison. The degree of pain with this motion should also be noted; very often a previous injury to the knee will result in a laxity of the joint and will disguise the immediate findings.

3. While the athlete is still supine, with leg in flexion of 90 degrees, and with the heel on the table, the ankle is held firmly in one hand. The other hand is fixed on the thigh just above the knee joint, and the ankle is then rotated inward and outward. This will cause a pain on one side or the other, depending on the side that is injured.

4. *Cruciate ligaments.* These are tested by flexing the leg and placing the athlete's ankle under your arm and locking it in place with your elbow. Both hands are then placed around the upper part of the lower leg, with the thumbs upward on the tibial tubercle. By pressing down, the posterior cruciate is tested. By pulling forward, the anterior cruciate is tested.

Tests 3 and 4 can also be made by having the athlete sit, with legs hanging over the edge of the table. In test 3, with the leg hanging down, the lower leg is turned inward or outward, and the same results will show up. In test 4, both hands are placed on the lower leg as before, and the lower leg is pushed back or forward in the examination.

The interpretation of these tests will be given in the discussion of the specific injury, in later sections of this chapter.

Interpretation of Functional Tests

1. *Flexion and extension.* The knee joint, being a hinge joint, has two motions in the normal range of activity. These two motions should be the first to be tested in the series. Flexion will demonstrate nothing particularly important on the early test; at a later date, when the hydraulics of the joint have been changed and motion spasm sets up, some changes will take place in the range of motion in flexion. When injured, the patella, located within the tendon of the quadriceps, will show up in this test, and the possibility of injury to this bone should not be overlooked.

The joint should be allowed to extend fully of its own accord (active) and should not be forced. Let the knee "hit bottom" on the active test. If the knee falls at less than a 180-degree angle, passive extension should be tried. Gently push down the knee so that the leg will straighten; if all is well, the knee will go down and stay down. If there is an involvement of the cartilage or cartilages, the knee will bounce back up again, falling from 15 to 30 degrees short of full extension.

Limitation of extension must be viewed with caution. This symptom immediately suggests that there is something inside the joint, blocking it and thus keeping it from full extension. Damage to the cartilages or one cartilage may be suspected with this symptom; however, lack of full extension may also be caused by pain, swelling, or muscle spasm. Differentiation between all symptoms must be analyzed. Locking, or the inability to fully extend the knee, has always been regarded as the trigger for the diagnosis of injury to a cartilage. We see many involvements of cartilage that do not lock the knee; foreign bodies (joint mice), pinched fat, etc., will also manifest themselves with locking. As in flexion, the symptoms of swelling, pain, and muscle spasm may also contribute to the inability to fully extend leg.

2. *Test for lateral instability*. With a solid hinge, there will not be any lateral motion. Lateral motion will indicate that the ligaments holding the joint together have been stretched or torn so that motion will be found. Lateral motion of a mild degree is normal in some athletes; comparison with other leg will help to establish the normal movement. The degree of lateral motion will establish the degree of injury; i.e., slight range of motion signifies a mild injury, whereas much lateral motion suggests a moderate to severe sprain, possibly with a tearing of the ligament.

Testing for instability should be done as soon as possible after the injury, preferably on the field. A difference of 30 minutes will be sufficient for the laxity of the joint to be obscured; very often an athlete seen on the field with lateral motion will not show evidence of this motion when he is moved to the training room and examined; time elapsing may be just minutes, but this is enough time for muscle spasm, etc., to set in. Abduction (away from body) of the tibia (lower leg) will indicate injury to the medial collateral ligament; adduction (toward body) of the tibia will indicate injury to the lateral collateral ligament.

3. *Anterior–posterior instability*. The riding forward or backward of the knee joint indicates laxity of the cruciate ligaments. Unfortunately, injuries to these ligaments are not readily seen; the symptoms are disguised by the conditions of the other tissues. When a knee is sprained severely enough to damage these ligaments (cruciates), the surrounding soft tissue of the joint will also be affected. When the anterior cruciate is injured (stretched or torn),

the tibia will ride forward; the backward motion of the tibia will indicate that the posterior cruciate is damaged.

4. *Internal derangement of knee.* Rotation of the tibia on the femur, with the knee flexed, will help in the diagnosis of internal derangement of the knee. By rotating the tibia inward, the medial condyle of the femur will be in closer approximation with the cartilage, and if injury is present, pain and limitation will be found. The motion that causes the injury is usually the opposite of the foregoing cause, i.e., the femur rotates on the tibia. With this type of distortion the cartilages as well as the cruciate ligaments may be injured.

MANAGEMENT OF KNEE INJURIES

Medial Collateral Ligament. This ligament attaches to the femur at the epicondyle and at the medial condyle of the tibia. It is a short, flat, and broad ligament that is interwoven in the capsule of the joint and is partly attached to the medial meniscus. Injuries to this ligament are the most common condition that will be seen in knee problems. Contact sports will produce many more than non-

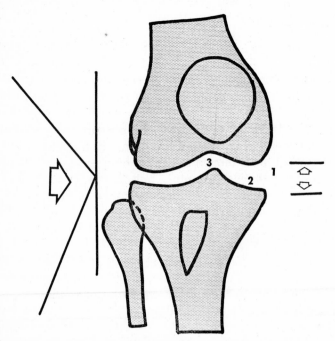

Arrow indicates force that results in injury to (1) medial collateral ligament, (2) medial meniscus, (3) cruciate ligaments.

contact sports, but contact is not necessarily needed to produce this injury. Stepping unevenly off a curb, squatting, or tripping can cause some form of this injury. In contact sports, the most common cause is a hit on the lateral aspect of the knee, with the foot planted on the ground. This motion causes the medial joint space to enlarge, thus stretching the medial collateral ligament. The degree of injury to this ligament will depend on the severity and direction of the blow and also the position of the knee and the foot at the time of injury. Invariably, with the stretching of the ligament, there will be a twisting motion at the same time. The degree of rotation will establish the degree of injury to the tissues inside the joint (cartilages and cruciate ligaments). Inasmuch as the ligament is interwoven with the capsule, we must assume that the capsule is also damaged. The ligaments are a collection of tough, white fibers that are compactly fitted together to form the cord or band. These ligaments are not very elastic and may become stretched. If the stretch is greater than normal, the result will be a tear. The tear may be at the attachments or in the body of the ligament itself. In a tear of the ligament, there will be a variation as to the number of fibers that are torn; the more that are torn, the more severe the injury, whereas the fewer torn, the simpler the injury.

Complete evaluation of the injury must be made. Listen to the athlete's story. He will tell you exactly what happened. Did he walk off the field without assistance? Does he have much pain? (Etc.) He will point with his finger or whole hand to the injured area. If he uses one finger, the injury will be very localized, whereas if he points with his hand, the injury will be diffuse. Inspect the knee joint, and compare it with the other knee. Check for normal landmarks: Hollows in and around joint will help to establish the extent of swelling in joint. Look for any abnormality. If swelling is present, note the degree and rapidity with which it develops. Feeling the area by palpating the joint will ascertain exactly the site of the injury. The area may or may not be swollen but feel for tightness of the soft tissues of the joint.

After these three steps have been taken, the functional tests should again be made. Examine for flexion and extension. Test for instability laterally and then for anterior–posteriorly. Rotation of the joint will also contribute to the evaluation of the injury.

The injury should be examined as soon as feasible, on the field if possible. The longer you wait, the more indeterminate your findings will be. A definite diagnosis of the knee should not be attempted until 24 to 48 hours have passed.

Injury to Medial Collateral Ligament

Mild injury to medial collateral ligament. From the above findings, you may be able to ascertain that the injury is a minor one and that the continuity of the ligament is intact. The degree of tear in mild injury will not impair the strength of the ligament, and lateral motion may not be found. In the mild injury, assume that there is a minor tear of the ligament, which will be tender; there may or may not be swelling, and there may or may not be much tenderness when you abduct the tibia (same motion that caused the damage). Treatment consists of compression, ice, and elevation. Preferred compression of the knee joint is with adhesive tape plus cotton and a snug elastic wrap. The use of the elastic wrap alone is not sufficient for proper compression.

The injury is reviewed the following day, functional tests are performed, and the degree of swelling and tenderness are checked. The negative findings (no tenderness, no swelling, no instability, and no locking) will confirm a mild injury, and the athlete may resume activity on a moderate scale. Activity should consist of quadriceps exercises, walking, and possibly jogging. The use of heat may not be necessary in this injury. Strapping or wrapping will depend on the findings. Use of a hot pack on this type of injury will be helpful and should be continued until all symptoms are gone.

Moderate injury to medial collateral ligament. Instead of a few fibers being torn, there will be a partial tear of the ligament in a moderate injury. There will be more pain, much tenderness over the site of the injury, more disability, localized swelling that will later diffuse, and much pain when repeating the motion that caused the initial damage.

The treatment will be much more comprehensive and prolonged. Immediate treatment consists of compression, ice, and elevation. For full compression, the use of elastic adhesive has been very effective. This tape is used in the same manner as regular tape; i.e., routine strapping. It is then reinforced with regular tape. If swelling is immediate, use sponge rubber over the joint after the tape has been applied. (A piece of ½ inch sponge rubber approximately 12 inches square with a hole about 2 inches in diameter is placed over the knee, with the hole encompassing the patella. This is held in place with the elastic bandage.) If swelling is not evident, use two strips of ½ inch felt 2 inches wide and about 1 foot long on either side of the patella. These strips of felt splints will be held in place by an elastic wrap.

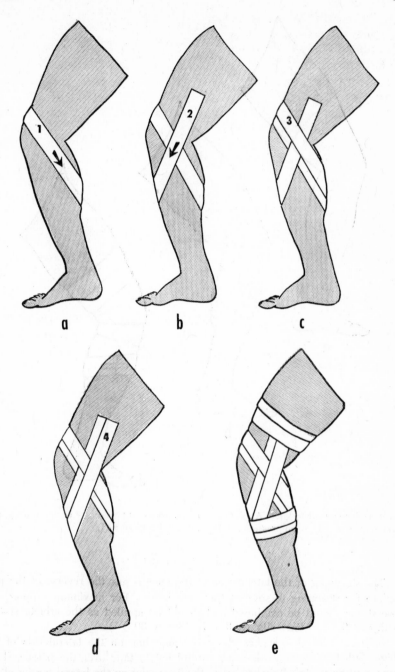

Strapping for medial collateral ligament injury (a), (b), (c), (d), show first layer of adhesive tape; (e) shows complete strapping with anchor strips.

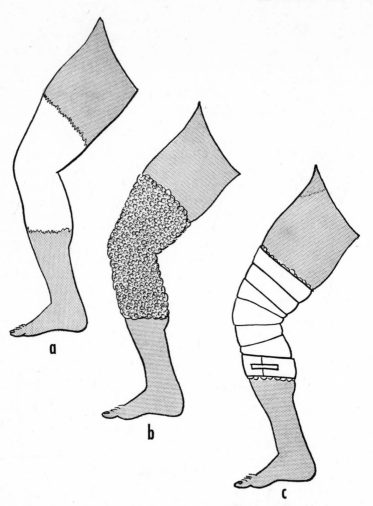

"Hot pack" applied to knee. Application of counterirritant to skin (a). Cotton applied over ointment (b). Compression wrap of elastic bandage (c).

KNEE STRAPPING I

The strapping of the lateral side of the knee is just the reverse of the procedure for strapping to support the medial side. For maximum support, the two straps should be combined and should be applied as the athlete stands, with foot flat and knee slightly flexed. (See p. 303)

Step 1. Starting 8 inches above the joint line on the lateral side of the thigh, pull tape downward, being careful not to tape over the patella (knee cap), and finish strip 8 inches below the knee joint on the lateral border of the calf.

Step 2. At 8 inches below the joint line on the lateral border of the calf, pull tape upward, bordering the patella, and cross strip 1 at the joint line. Finish strip 8 inches above the knee on the medial border of the thigh. (The patella should not be included in this strapping, as immobilization of the patella will limit motion of knee.)

Step 3. Strips 1 and 2 should be repeated as many times as needed for maximum support. Each additional strip should overlap the preceding one by at least three-quarters of the full width.

Step 4. Anchor strips must be applied to the upper and lower ends of the tape to prevent rolling and loosening. They should be applied snugly but not so tight that they will constrict. These strips should be applied at a diagonal so as to compensate for the contour of the leg.

The use of elastic adhesive for the strapping of knees has been a great advancement of the methods of support. Trainers find that elastic adhesive applied to the skin, with the regular adhesive applied over it, has eliminated much of the irritation when daily strappings are needed.

The use of elastic adhesive for the anchors has been very effective in the elimination of constriction and cramps of the calf. If additional strength is desired in the use of adhesive tape, folding the tape inwards about ½ inch for about 3 inches above and below the joint line will double the tape and make it difficult to tear. The application of an elastic bandage over this strapping will help the tape set. The elastic may be removed in about 30 minutes. (There is no harm done if the athlete leaves the wrap on while playing.)

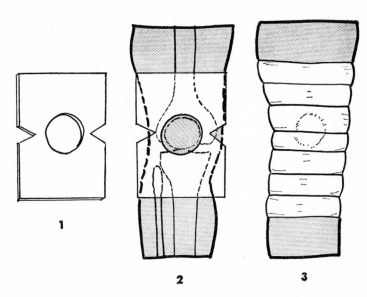

Compression wrap of knee. (1) Sponge rubber cut to form of knee. (2) Application of rubber to knee. (3) Compression wrap of elastic bandage applied very snugly over the rubber.

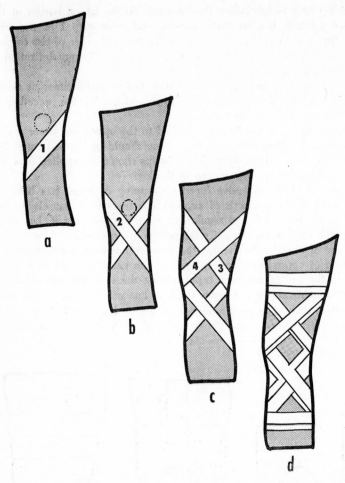

Full knee strapping. Strip 1 is applied (a). Strip 2 overlies strip 1 (b). Strips 3 and 4 are applied. Second and third layers added in the same order if needed. Elastic adhesive is indicated for the first two layers for maximum support (c). Complete strapping with anchor straps (d).

KNEE STRAPPING II

This is a complete strapping for knee injuries and may be changed as the condition warrants. For example, in injuries to the medial collateral ligaments, the lateral strips may be eliminated, and for strapping the lateral collateral ligaments, the medial strips may be excluded. Strapping is applied while the athlete is standing, with the knee flexed 15 degrees and the heel flat on the table.

To attain the proper angle of strapping, apply the cloth side of the tape to the area so that range of direction may be gauged before applying the adhesive side of tape to skin.

Step 1. Starting on the outside of the calf, 8 inches below the joint line, pull the tape upward. The tape should not include the patella (knee cap) but should border it as closely as possible. Tape then extends above the joint line 8 inches, ending on the back of the thigh.

Step 2. Starting on the inside of the calf, 8 inches below the joint line, pull tape upward, crossing strip 1 just below the patella. Cross the joint line and finish strip 8 inches above knee joint on the thigh.

Step 3. On the outside of thigh, 8 inches above joint line, pull tape downward, clear of patella, and cross the joint line, ending on the back of lower leg.

Step 4. Same as preceding step but in opposite direction. Tape is started on the inside of thigh and ended on outside of calf.

Repeat the above procedures, interweaving each strip of tape. The number of strips applied depends on the injury and the size of the athlete. The strength of the taping may be increased by folding back the tape along the joint line for about 3 inches above and below. Before applying the tape, fold back at least ½ inch and then apply pressure to set the strip of tape. This procedure may be applied to the last few layers of tape on the knee.

The use of elastic adhesive has been recommended for the taping of the knee, and we would urge that this be used, since it will strengthen the strapping and add to the comfort of the athlete who must be taped in this manner. Anchor strips are applied to the ends of the diagonal strips so that they will not pull loose or unravel when clothing is worn. These strips do not contribute to the support of the injury and should not be applied with pressure. Angles will have to be established to allow for contour of leg. The action of the calf and thigh muscles moving laterally must be allowed for when taping to prevent constriction and the resulting cramps.

Ice will diminish bleeding, and the less swelling as a result of hemorrhage, the better the response to treatment. If the damaged tissues are stretched over the swelling, less approximation will be had, and therefore a longer time for healing must be expected. When an injury occurs, greater stimulation to the area is immediate; therefore it is best to slow down metabolism. This also is accomplished by the use of cold packs. After the stimulated area is ready for normal pathology, heat and exercises may be started.

Rehabilitation program. The use of crutches for the first 48 hours will eliminate weight bearing and thus hasten recovery. This routine is carried out for at least 48 hours and sometimes longer. The early and vigorous treatment of this injury will retard progress. Too often swelling has been increased by the early application of heat or too early exercise programs. This degree of further injury must be prevented, as the tendency to incomplete recovery is high under these circumstances.

Heat applications and exercise are started at the same time. Progressive resistance exercises are started when tolerable, often on the fifth day. In the meantime quadriceps setting exercises, plus walking and jogging, will be programmed. In the recovery period, when running is indicated, the athlete walks 25 yards and then jogs 25 yards. This is done on a straight line, being careful to avoid the turns; as the range of motion increases and the knee loosens up, increase the distance to 50 yards for each exercise. After this, increase the running distance but let walking remain the same. After each work-out, a compression wrap is applied overnight and the next day the injury is reviewed. The degree of progress is noted, and if all is well, the same program of the day before is repeated. If there is an increase in swelling or symptoms that are new, the treatment has been too vigorous and must be slowed up.

Treatment at this time may indicate complete rest for a day or two and then a resumption of the original program. This injury will respond and will recover with good results and without any disability in the joint if it is not forced. The time of disability is from ten days to four weeks. This injury should be strapped with a protective strapping daily upon return to full duty until such time as full response is attained.

In the mild and severe injury where there is profuse swelling, the thought of aspiration is uppermost. (Aspiration is the drawing of fluid out of the joint by means of a hypodermic needle.) There are mixed opinions of this procedure. Many physicians feel that the act of aspiration will increase the trauma to the joint; others think that the sooner the aspiration, the better. Some physicians will aspirate once and only once, whereas others will aspirate whenever needed, maybe every other day. This is a procedure that must be done under the most aseptic of conditions and by a competent physician. The decision is his and only his; so, the decision to aspirate or not is out of the jurisdiction of the athletic trainer. The athletic surgeon at Yale will aspirate when needed, believing that the sooner the fluid is removed, the earlier the injury will respond to treatment.

Severe injury to medial collateral ligament. The incident causing this injury is the same as for the other injuries to the medial collateral ligament; namely, severe abduction of the lower leg plus rotation, forcing the ligament to go beyond its normal range. We must as-

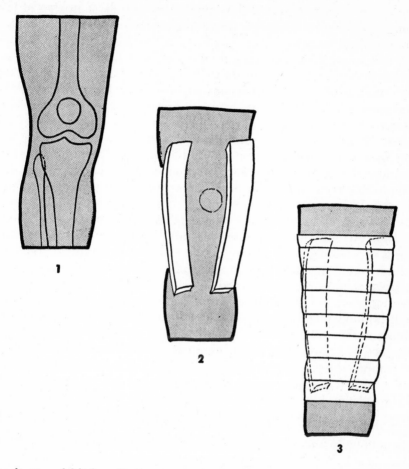

Application of felt for splinting an acute knee. (1) Anatomy of knee. (2) Location of felt strips for splinting. (3) Felt splints covered with elastic bandage for support and compression. Felt splinting is often used in conjunction with adhesive taping in an acute knee injury.

sume that in a severe injury, there will be damage to one or more ligaments and to the medial meniscus. The ligaments have been torn, and the cartilage may have been fractured and displaced. There will be much pain and localized swelling that will increase rapidly. Normal contours of the knee may be obliterated by the swelling. Abnormal motions will also be found laterally; the knee may seem as though there is nothing holding it together. On anterior and posterior motions, the tibia will move back and forth without much pressure. In this injury there may be a locking of the joint, which will indicate cartilage involvement. All severe injuries are routinely X-rayed; invariably there will not be any bony pathology in this injury, but abnormal motions may be confirmed.

Early examination of this injury is important; the longer the wait, the more disguised the symptoms will become. The rapid swelling and muscle spasm will in many cases prevent even a cursory examination if not seen immediately. The immediate treatment of this injury is compression, ice, elevation, and bed rest.

Conservative management would be the application of a plaster cylinder for a lengthy period of time, approximately six weeks. The newer approach is surgical exposure and suture repair of the damaged ligaments.

The rehabilitation time of this condition is a long and arduous period. Atrophy will be a serious problem. Quadriceps exercises are a very vital part of this program, starting with normal function without resistance and then progressing to the progressive resistance exercise regime. Complete recovery time will vary according to the method chosen. If conservative management is elected, the time will be longer and results will not be so effective. Surgical repair shortens the disability period and a more effective result will be attained. Both routines will extend over months rather than weeks, as compared to the minor injuries. Decision as to athletic eligibility must be based on the repair of the ligaments plus the condition of the quadriceps.

Lateral Collateral Ligament. Injury of this ligament is not so common as injury to the medial collateral ligament but is seen from time to time in athletics. The injury occurs in the opening of the joint on the lateral side of the knee and is caused by being hit on the inside of the knee, forcing the knee outwards. Severe wrenching of the knee will also effect this injury.

The lateral collateral ligament attaches to the lateral epicondyle of the femur and bridges the joint and attaches again at the head of the fibula. This ligament does not adhere to the lateral meniscus as does the medial collateral. It is not subject to the trauma as is the medial collateral, and consequently less of these than the medial are seen. The incidence is few and the injury is not so disabling as the medial. History, inspection, and palpation plus the functional tests must be used. There will be pain, some local swelling (which may or may not increase), and tenderness when the joint is adducted, the motion that caused the damage.

Treatment of lateral collateral injuries. In the mild sprain, where the fibers may be torn slightly but the strength of the ligament is not impaired, the treatment is the same as for the medial collateral ligament: immediate compression, ice, and elevation. Re-evaluation on the second day may or may not show anything different from the day before. There will not be any swelling, tenderness, disability, or instability. Strapping and exercise are indicated in this injury. There may not be any need for further treatment. A day or two of concentrated exercise, which includes much running, is the procedure used in this injury.

In the moderate sprain of the lateral collateral ligament, the application of ice may be carried out for another 24 hours. The use of crutches to eliminate weight bearing is also indicated. Felt splints combined in the original strapping will also enhance the treatment of this injury. Treatment is essentially the same as for moderate sprain of the medial collateral ligament.

In the severe sprain of the lateral collateral ligament, the use of a plaster cast may be indicated, as may the possibility of surgery for repair of the tear.

The rehabilitation of this injury is as important as for the medial collateral ligament, and it must be carried out in the same manner. A strong quadriceps group of muscles is a very important factor in reducing further injury or injuries to this ligament.

Hyperextension Strain of Knee. This is a rather common injury which manifests itself in tenderness over the back of the knee. Examination will reveal that there is tenderness over the attachments of the hamstring and the calf group of muscles directly in the fold of the knee joint. Early management is the same as for all acute knee injuries; i.e., ice, compression, and elevation. For adequate compression, adhesive strapping is very effective. After the immediate treatment has been performed, the application of heat and mild exercises are indicated. Disability varies with the degree of injury and the type of sport.

HYPEREXTENSION KNEE STRAPPING

Strapping should be applied with the athlete in a standing position. With the back of the knee facing the taper, the athlete is instructed to bend the knee slightly forward. Placing a block or wedge approximately 2 inches high under the heel will help to maintain this position. This position should be maintained until the strapping is completed. Before the application of tape, a piece of cotton, gauze, etc., should be placed in the space directly in back

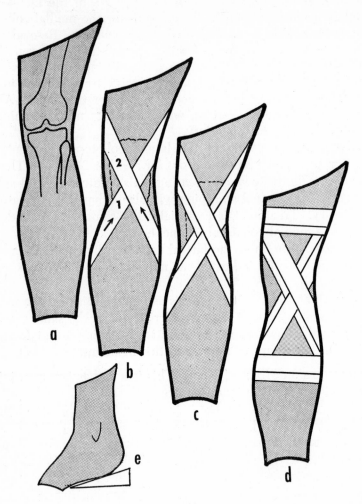

Strapping used for hyperextension of knee injuries. Anatomy of posterior aspect of knee (a). Strips 1 and 2 as applied to back of knee (b). Extra layers of adhesive as indicated (c). Complete strapping with anchor strips (d). This strapping is used many times in conjunction with the routine strapping of the knee. It is used very effectively for "pulls" of the hamstring tendons. (e) Shows wedge under heel for flexion of knee.

of the knee. This is a very sensitive area, and if tape is applied directly to the skin, an irritation will develop.

Step 1. Starting on the outside of the leg at a 60-degree angle, the tape is pulled upward, across the back of the knee, and ended on the inside of the thigh.

Step 2. This strip is applied in exactly the same manner, starting on the inside of the leg, pulling at the same angle, and crossing the first strip exactly in the center of the knee joint.

Step 3. The third strip is applied, overlapping strip 1 by almost three-quarters.

Step 4. The fourth strip is applied, overlapping strip 2 by three-quarters. The strapping, when completed, is a very complete X-shape.

The addition of more strips is optional and should depend on the severity of the injury and the size of the athlete. Anchor strips are applied above and below the X-taping for the purpose of securing the tape. It should not be applied tightly.

The use of elastic adhesive is recommended for the first four strips applied, followed by the use of regular tape over this.

Cruciate Ligaments. Review the anatomy of the cruciate ligaments and you will see that they are deep inside the knee, are very short, and are strong. Their function is to stabilize the knee in the anterior and posterior motion of the tibia. The anterior cruciate is the more common of the two to incur an injury.

The action of force in which the anterior cruciate ligament is injured is the hyperextension of the knee joint. In extension the anterior cruciate is very tight, and when forced into a motion beyond extension, the ligament will tear. Also, when there has been a severe injury to the medial collateral ligament (where the joint has been forced wide open), the anterior cruciate will tear as it assists in holding the joint approximated and helps to prevent abduction of the tibia. The anterior cruciate may also be injured by a severe wrench that causes external rotation of the tibia. When the cruciate is damaged, it must be assumed that there have been injuries to the medial collateral ligament and the meniscus on the medial side.

The posterior cruciate ligament is very tight when the knee is in flexion and may be torn when the knee joint is hyperflexed. A severe wrench of the knee may damage the posterior cruciate, but as a rule, both cruciates are torn when this action takes place. The posterior cruciate ligament is rarely injured by itself.

Treatment. The athlete will reveal that he has suffered a severe twisting of the knee or has been hit from behind. He will complain of much pain and loss of function, and that the "knee feels like it is giving out." Inspection will reveal much swelling. Compare with the other knee. Palpation will reveal tenderness all over the knee joint area; the cruciates cannot be palpated, but the other soft tissue structure should be. Tenderness over the medial collateral ligament attachments, lateral collateral attachments, etc., may reveal other damage to the knee.

Functional tests. The flexion and extension test should be carried out. If the leg hyperextends, both cruciates may be torn. (This test should be applied to the other leg as well; many persons are born with back knees that show this sign.)

To test anterior cruciate ligament stability, flex the knee; if the tibia moves forward, the anterior cruciate is stretching or torn. With the knee flexed, if the tibia rides backward, the posterior cruciate is damaged. If, in performing this test, you should find motion both forward and backward, then both ligaments are injured.

Rotation testing will reveal much in cruciate damage. With the knee flexed and the tibia rotated on the femur, there will be an abnormal amount of rotation as a result of cruciate damage. If there are complications, such as lateral instability, there will be a much greater range of rotation found.

X-ray will in all probability show nothing, but it should be employed routinely to rule out the possibility of any bony injury.

The actual treatment for cruciate tears are out of the jurisdiction of the trainer. However, immediate treatment should be aimed at the reduction of swelling and the control of hemorrhage in the joint. The use of a compression bandage, ice, and elevation should be routine until the athlete is seen by the team physician. In an injury as severe as tears of the cruciate ligaments, compression from the mid-lower leg to the upper part of the thigh is preferable. Ice is applied in ice bags to all surfaces of the knee. Elevate the foot at the back rather than under the knee joint itself.

The team physician may elect to place the knee in a full cast. This is the conservative approach and is prolonged treatment, usually for two months. The swelling may delay this procedure, and aspiration may or may not be carried out by the doctor. If the cast is applied immediately, it may have to be changed at a later date because of the absorption of swelling. The cast should be snug. After the cast is applied, the athlete will be on crutches, and exercises will be started for the elimination of as much atrophy as possible. Quadriceps-setting and leg-raising exercises are started when the cast hardens. The use of a small weight on the foot in leg raising may be added and increased when tolerable. After the cast has been removed, hot applications must be applied and exercises started to hasten the flexion of the knee. Massage is very effective for the promotion of recovery. Massage above and below the joint until tenderness is gone; then full massage over the joint itself may be instituted. Extensive progressive resistance exercises should be started after joint motion has been restored.

Orthopedists have used surgical repair immediately in this injury with excellent results. Consensus is that the longer the time elapsed from date of injury, the harder the repair and the less favorable the results.

The athlete must rely on good strong quadriceps to stabilize the knee when the cruciates are torn. If the lateral ligaments are intact, the knee will be a satisfactory one as a result of compensation strength of the quadriceps group.

Cartilage Injuries

Medial cartilage injuries. This is the most frequent type of internal derangement to the knee joint and is caused by a sudden, forceful internal rotation of the femur on the tibia and the abduction of the lower leg. In this action the condyle of the femur will grind into the cartilage, and the result will be a pinched cartilage which also may be torn. The cartilage may tear at the bony attachment, may split across or lengthwise, or may be wholly pulled from the floor of the tibia. The most common tear is the "bucket handle," which is almost impossible to reduce except by surgery. If the cartilage becomes displaced, it will lodge in the joint space, blocking the full extension of the knee. The sensation is that there is something blocking the joint, thus preventing full extension.

The typical position when standing is to place all the weight on the ball of the foot with the heel off the ground. Associated with this type of injury, the abduction of the leg will stretch or tear the medial collateral ligament to which the cartilage is attached. Damage to the cruciate ligaments is also a probability. In severe knee injuries, there is often other damage, and this must not be overlooked in the original treatment. In examining an internal derangement, we must not overlook the capsule; injury to this tissue will become readily evident, since the swelling of this injury is always rapid. It may start slowly but gain momentum in a short time.

History, inspection, and palpation in the diagnosis is very important. One of the basic facts will be that the leg "gives out," and the athlete has a peculiar feeling in the joint when this happens. There will be acute tenderness over the joint line. Active motion

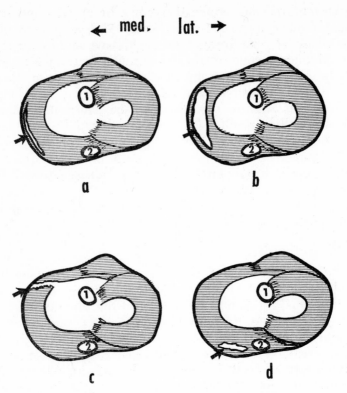

Variations of tears of the cartilages of the knee. Tear along medial border (a). Typical bucket handle tear (b). A complete tear on the anterior horn of the cartilage (c). Posterior tear of the cartilage (d).

will be very painful, whereas passive motion is not too aggravating. Extension may be limited to 15 to 30 degrees less than full extension. The floating patella will not be too demonstrable at this time because of the inability of the joint to reach full extension. Localized swelling will be found and will increase rapidly.

Functional tests are also carried out. These should be done as soon as the injury is seen (again, on the field), if possible. Testing of all functions will be necessary in this case, since sometimes the injury is diagnosed by the findings of negative signs in the other tissues. Limitation of extension is most characteristic of injury to the cartilage. When there is no locking, the diagnosis is difficult, as the cartilage is not displaced. In testing for abduction, should abnormal results be found, it is wise to suspect a tear of the cartilage without displacement.

McMurray's sign is a very valuable asset in the diagnosing of cartilage injuries. By placing the hand over the joint, a click will be felt when the tibia moves. The click may also be heard as well as felt. Motions of the tibia for this test include extension and rotation. The lack of extension on this sign should be noted and observed. X-ray will invariably be negative except when further study is carried out in addition to the routine examination; i.e., the injection of air into the joint, etc.

The immediate treatment of the involved cartilage is to reduce the dislocation. There are many ways to accomplish this. In recurring instances, the athlete knows his own particular manipulation well; if this is so, let him do it himself.

After the reduction, the treatment is aimed at the protection of the knee against increased trauma at this time. In the primary injury the use of a posterior molded splint to hold the knee in full extension is indicated, as are compression, ice, elevation, and complete bed rest. In elevating the leg, blankets, etc., must start at the heel and go back, being sure not to flex the leg at any time. The degree of swelling is noted; if profuse, the team physician may aspirate. Some team physicians may choose at this time to place the injury in a leg cylinder cast for a period of three to four weeks. This cast extends from the upper thigh to the ankle, for complete immobilization. (Many orthopedists will also include the foot in this cast.) The athlete can be up on crutches at this time but should not attempt weight bearing. Exercises such as quadriceps setting and hip flexion should be performed several times in the day. The less atrophy, the easier the rehabilitation period will be.

This procedure has been outlined as a means of treatment and is used by many physicians. There are those who do not believe that the torn cartilage will heal, and their treatment is completely symptomatic. After the cartilage dislocation has been reduced, the leg is wrapped in a compression wrap and ice and elevation are started. This will last from 24 to 48 hours, depending on the degree of disability. Under the heading of disability will be pain, loss of function, and the degree of swelling. If the swelling persists, aspiration may be attempted at this time. Opinions are divided on aspiration; some physicians will not aspirate, others will repeat aspirations over a few days' period. This is a decision that can be made only by the team physician. If this method is used, heat and exercise are started on the third day. The application of gentle massage above and below the knee will greatly enhance the recovery. The continued use of the compression wrap or elastic bandage alone must be carried out for at least one week. The recovery time in this injury will vary from a few days to months.

In the recurring type of cartilage displacement, the treatment is symptomatic. It will be necessary to reduce as soon as possible and apply a compression wrap, ice, and elevation. On the next day, the knee is re-examined. If there is no evidence of swelling or pain, the athlete may attempt to continue his work. In recurring injuries, the operative removal is indicated. Should there be reasons why this cannot be carried out, the intensive use of progressive resistance exercises and protective strappings may help to prevent further injuries.

Opinions are divided as to whether an athlete should continue to play with such a condition. However, this situation has to be handled on an individual basis. Certainly an athlete who has recurring dislocations that are painful and which cause much discomfort should be discouraged from continuing. On the other hand, the recurring injury that is easily handled (no swelling, pain, or loss of function) may allow him to finish out the season, but serious thought should be given to surgical treatment before continuing the following season.

Many athletes reduce the dislocations themselves, and you may never see them with a displaced cartilage. The more frequent the dislocation, the easier the unlocking becomes and the less symptoms are found. Cartilages are composed of fibrocartilage, the circulation of which is very poor, if it has any at all; therefore the decision to operate must be based on the fact that this lesion does not repair itself.

A sprain to the medial collateral ligament, which in the beginning seems very mild, may turn out to be a very troublesome cartilage injury. The tear may not be sufficient to give any outward sign, and after routine treatments, the knee seems normal. However, in the following season, minor sprains cause the damage to the cartilage to be more diagnostic, resulting in pain, disability, etc.

Lateral cartilage. This cartilage is subject to the same type of injury as the medial meniscus, but the incidence to this injury is about one in ten. The intent of the injury is the inversion action of the leg plus adduction. The condyle of the femur grinds into the cartilage and causes a tear, which in turn will cause a displacement. The lateral cartilage is not attached to the lateral ligament as the medial cartilage is. This injury, although not so common as the medial injury, is just as disabling, and the prognosis is just about the same.

In the case of history, pain and all other symptoms will be on the lateral side of the knee instead of the medial. In functional tests, reactions will be the same except for location. Maneuvers for reduction must be varied in some instances to allow for this change of location. Inspection and palpation are the same as for the medial cartilage. Treatment is exactly the same as for the medial cartilage.

Recurring dislocations to the lateral cartilage should be handled with the same attitude as that of the medial.

Joint Mice. *Joint mice* is a name given to foreign bodies in the joint proper. The cause is usually trauma; there is history of an injury to the knee, resulting in swelling, pain, etc. After symptoms subside, a momentary locking may take place; there will be immediate and sharp pain with this condition. By various and sundry motions of the leg, the condition is relieved. This may occur time and time again, and the athlete may not report this condition because it "goes away" in a few minutes. When the knee locks, and these maneuvers do not get response, the injury is reported.

X-ray will reveal the foreign body or bodies, and treatment by surgery is indicated. Foreign bodies allowed to remain in the joint may result in damage to other parts of the knee and may at a later date cause some concern and disability along with pain.

REDUCTION OF DISPLACED CARTILAGES

Method 1. Athlete lies flat on back; grab the ankle securely with one hand, and with the other hand and forearm encompass the thigh. Flex the knee joint several times to loosen the knee. Extend the knee with the help of the athlete, who kicks forcefully at the same time. If the cartilage is medial, the tibia may be abducted to open the joint. If the maneuver is successful, the leg will resume full extension. This may be repeated a few times. If failure results after a few times, further treatment will be necessary.

Method 2. Another method is to place the forearm under the knee joint and forcibly flex the knee over the forearm; this will open the joint and allow the displaced cartilage to resume normal position; then the leg is fully extended slowly. If the knee "hits bottom," the reduction is successful.

Method 3. Athlete may lie on table; flex knee to chest, place both locked hands around the lower leg, and forcibly hyperflex the knee. Again, if successful, the leg will fully extend. This maneuver may be done a few times, and if not successful, other arrangements should be made.

The use of a weight on the foot may enhance these methods, by the tiring and relaxing of the larger muscle of the thigh. The athlete sits on a table with leg hanging over the edge; place a weight (10 to 25 pounds) on the foot and swing lightly for a few minutes. Muscles will relax, and then manipulations may be tried.

Contusions. Contusions of the knee are very common, and we shall go into detail on a few of the more common injuries in this category. The muscles immediately overlying the joint are in a position to be injured very frequently. This injury is seen in all contact sports and is often caused by being "kneed," which in turn brings a very violent force to the tissues on top of bone, thus macerating the soft tissue against the hard structure of the bone. Fibers are torn and blood vessels ruptured. The swelling in this area is usually profuse. The swelling should be controlled as soon as possible. If it is permitted to remain, it will cause an irritation to the joint capsule, complicating the injury.

The treatment consists of minimizing the hemorrhage by the use of a compression bandage and the immediate application of ice with the leg in elevation. The athlete should not bear weight on the leg and should be supplied with crutches. This treatment is continuous for 48 hours, after which exercise should be permitted, starting with leg swinging over the end of a table and normal walking. If this exercise is tolerable, the athlete may be able to alternate jogging with the walking. Apply heat to this injury only after the effusion starts to absorb by natural processes.

This is a very hard injury to predict the prognosis and is treated symptomatically day by day. When full motion has returned and the swelling has subsided, the athlete may return to activity, protected by a sponge pad to prevent further injury.

Contusion of the joint capsule. Since the joint is enclosed in a capsule which is lined with a synovial membrane, we must surmise that the membrane will be injured as a result of a blow. Hemorrhage will result in the capsule. This condition may be mild or severe, depending on the injury and the immediate treatment. We have seen injuries that were slight on onset but which became progressively worse when the athlete was allowed to continue activity.

The athlete will report the "bump" on the knee, saying that it is not too bad and he feels as though he could continue. Should he be allowed to work, there will be an increase in the amount of fluid in the joint and the length of disability will be increased. It is folly to try to work out a joint injury. Such injuries will not respond to work and will be compounded into a long disability.

Apply a compression bandage to the knee immediately and then follow with ice and elevation. The use of a sponge-rubber doughnut or long pieces of felt applied to this area will effect better compression. The felt strips are approximately 12 inches long and 2 inches wide, placed on each side of the patella, and held in place with a snug elastic bandage. The use of crutches for the first 24

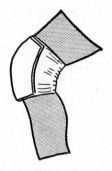

Foam rubber pad enclosed in elastic material. Worn to protect knee against direct contact.

hours will help shorten the disability. The procedure of aspiration in this injury is a decision for the team physician to make. It has helped lessen the disability time of the injury. Heat may be applied after the first 48 hours, and compression wraps are applied during the recovery period.

Many simple contusions occur in the knee joint area. Many manifest themselves in hematomas that may be aspirated and compressed without too much disability. The recurrence of this simple contusion is quite prevalent, and all precautions must be taken when the athlete resumes play. The use of knee pads of some soft material to absorb the blow must be made. The foam rubber pad and other new synthetic materials aid greatly in absorbing shock.

In the simple contusion we find that the use of ice and a compression bandage overnight is usually enough treatment. The compression is reapplied the next day, and the athlete is padded and sent back to activity without any further trouble.

Bone contusions (*bruises*). These are quite common in the knee joint area. Landing on the knees is encountered in all sports, and the bony structure which is close to the surface without the benefit of much padding is susceptible to bruising which is painful and in many cases self-limiting. It is in this injury that a complete history must be attained. The bony prominences that are bruised are the attachments for the ligamentous structure of the joint, and the establishment of a proper diagnosis is necessary before treatment should be started. Falling on the knee without twisting, etc., will be the typical history. There may or may not be swelling, and on palpation the bone will be very tender. This injury will heal slowly and recurs easily.

Treatment is designed for comfort of the athlete. The use of a compression bandage will help if it can be tolerated. The use of ice along with elevation will help lessen the pain and minimize swelling. The use of heat is indicated but should not be applied too early, since there is a tendency for heat to make the bone "ache."

Should this occur, continue the ice for another day. When heat is tolerable, use in daily treatments.

This injury must be protected at all times. The use of sponge rubber, ensolite, etc., is very effective for this type of padding. Hot packs used while in activity will greatly enhance the healing and give relief of pain. The length of disability depends on the injury, and in many instances no time will be lost.

Pinched Fat Pad. A mass of fat, located just back of the lower part of the patella between the patella tendons, fills the space between the condyles of the femur and the upper end of the tibia. Bruising, such as falling on a knee, will cause an irritation which in turn thickens the fat pad. Owing to its location, the symptoms are quite evident when the knee is in full extension. The inability to fully extend the knee may suggest a cartilage injury, but a complete history plus negative findings of a joint condition will lead to the diagnosis of a pinched fat pad.

Treatment consists of rest and heat for a few days. If the injury persists, partial removal of the pad may be indicated.

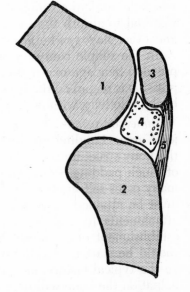

Location of fat pad. (1) Femur. (2) Tibia. (3) Patella. (4) Fat pad. (5) Patella tendon.

Bursitis. There are many bursae around the knee joint and these are subject to trauma. The prepatella, suprapatella, and the infrapatella are the bursae of the knee joint that are injured in athletics. If we review the anatomy of the joint and the location of the bursae, it will be easily understood why these injuries happen. Bursitis of

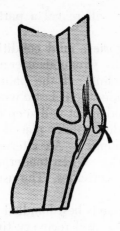

Typical swelling seen as a result of swelling in the prepatella bursa. Arrow indicates distended bursa.

the knee in athletics is usually caused by a series of minor bruises. The swelling is usually localized, i.e., if the swelling is over the patella, prepatella bursitis is suspected. The suprapatella bursa is involved when the swelling is generalized and the patella moves downward and forward. When the swelling is under the patella and the patella is pushed upward, the infrapatella bursa is involved. When the infrapatella is involved, this is usually called *housemaid's knee*.

Treatment of bursitis, if acute, requires ice applications and a compression bandage. The sac is by nature a self-limiting area, i.e., when the sac fills, the swelling will be stopped. Use ice, however, since it has a tendency to lessen the pain and relieve some of the discomfort due to the rise in temperature of the bursa. Aspiration is indicated early, along with the compression wrap. Heat is used after 48 hours to hasten the absorption. Bursitis of the knee joint is not disqualifying to an athlete, and during activity, the knee should be padded to reduce the trauma to the area.

OSGOOD-SCHLATTER'S DISEASE

This is seen in prehigh school and high school athletics and seldom, if ever, on the college level. The athlete will complain of pain on the prominence of the tibia just below the joint line. The pain will be more intense in knee flexion and kneeling. In order to ease the pain, the athlete will walk stiff-legged. History will be pain, increasing on flexion.

Inspection will reveal an abnormal bump on the front part of the knee. It will not be a typical swelling but a protruding bone. Palpation will reveal much tenderness localized over the tibial tubercle.

Swelling may or may not be present. X-ray will reveal a partial tearing away of the tibial tubercle.

Treatment will be divided into two categories: mild condition where pain is present only when aggravated by strenuous exercise, bumping the prominence, or prolonged kneeling. If the pain is acute, bed rest is ordered until symptoms subside; then elastic wraps for support should be worn. A posterior molded splint will keep the knee in full extension (felt or padded wooden splints placed in back of knee and wrapped with elastic bandage). An alternate support is a full leg cast, applied for two weeks. When tenderness disappears, the athlete may assume his normal activities. The usual disability period extends three to six weeks.

A chronic and painful condition of this disease is best handled by operative procedures. Results are very effective and recovery time is short, usually three weeks to a month. Wearing of protective sponge-rubber knee pads should be compulsory for players in this condition.

MEASURING QUADRICEPS FOR ATROPHY

Atrophy of the quadriceps after an injury is usually visible to the eye. However, exact measurements should be taken for the records. Steel tape should be used because cloth tapes have a tendency to stretch, and therefore the measurements will be inac-

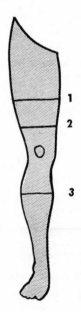

Location used for measuring the thigh for degrees of atrophy following injury. (1) Eight inches above the proximal pole of patella. (2) Three inches from pole of patella. (3) Eight inches from proximal pole of patella.

curàte. How to measure presents quite a controversial issue. However, we use the superior (top) border of the patella. Three measurements are taken: (1) Using the top of the patella, measure up the thigh 3 inches and 8 inches (leg in full exension on the table), marking the measurement with ink. This is also done on the good leg. (2) Using the same top of the patella, measure 8 inches below the knee, mark, and measure the calf circumference. These measurements (both legs) are filed and used for progressive checks.

In some literature the use of the patella is not recommended because of its inconsistency, especially in an injured leg. The swelling will disguise the location of the patella, and this in turn will throw the measurements off. Objectors to patella measurements prefer to use the anterior superior spine of the crest of the ilium. This is constant, and the measurements will be more accurate.

REHABILITATION OF KNEE

As we have noted previously, the knee is dependent on muscle support more than any other joint in the body. Firm quadriceps make for a very strong knee, and these muscles should not be overlooked in injury care. In all injuries to the knee, there will be atrophy. The degree will vary with the seriousness of the injury and the lack of use caused by the disability. To allow an athlete to return to activity without proper conditioning of the quadriceps group is inviting trouble. The use of supports, whether they be in the form of strappings or braces, will never take the place of good musculature around the joint. On the other hand, it would be folly to assume that the strengthening of the quadriceps is a guarantee that the knee will not be injured. However, we feel that there will be less incidences as a result of this program.

The question always arises, "Why won't normal activity, such as the regular practice programs, be enough for rehabilitation?" The answer is that if all previous activity has not prevented injury, how can it help to strengthen weakened muscles? Moreover, normal routine takes much longer. Resistance builds muscle, and the easiest and quickest way to restore the strength is by the use of weights. By using weights, a lot of work can be accomplished in a much shorter period of time and without the necessity of "knocking one's self out." Normal but strenuous work-outs will not produce the results derived from exercises directed to the one area.

Treatment by various methods of progressive resistance exercises, or just plain resistance exercises, has been very contributory to the successful return of the athlete to activity. There are many procedures, and the literature is loaded with the results of all. The consensus is that any method is good if the athlete (or patient) will work at it. The attitude of the individual is of uppermost importance in this type of a program. Breaking it down into plain words, it is "work, work, and more work" that produces the results. The ability of the trainer to carry out the team physician's orders is also of importance. Personality and approach is extremely important for a successful campaign against atrophy. Fortunately the athlete will have as his goal the desire to get well so that he may rejoin his team mates. Experience proves that the athlete with a goal will respond more favorably than the student without a goal. However, neither may realize that the exercise program is for the betterment of their condition.

Exercises (Without Resistance). Even though the knee is in an acute condition (second, third day, etc.), exercises can be performed that will help eliminate atrophy while not contributing to the recovery of the lesion. These exercises are also performed very early after surgery to the knee, usually on the second or third day. They may also be performed with the knee in a cast. This regime of exercise should be encouraged in all knee injuries that require immobilization by strapping, splinting, or bed rest. The three most important types of exercise are:

1. *Quadriceps setting.* With the leg in full extension, tighten the thigh so that the patella moves toward the pelvis; hold and then relax. Exercise should be done as often as possible, i.e., once every hour for a few minutes. This exercise may also be done in classes, movies, and while resting.

2. *Hip flexion.* With knee stiff, flex hip so that leg will be raised off the surface to a right angle; hold and then lower slowly. This may be done, as the quadriceps exercise, every hour for a few minutes.

3. *Abduction and adduction of hip.* With leg held stiff, move leg out to side with leg off the surface. Hold, and then return under control. Lower leg to surface and then repeat. This exercise is done in conjunction with exercises 1 and 2.

METHODS OF EXERCISE

Equipment

1. Boot made of aluminum or iron, with the cross-bar and clamps.
2. Plates (weights) varying from 2½ pounds up to 20 pounds. Total amount should be at least 100 pounds.

Assuming that a table will be available, this is not listed as necessary equipment. Proper supervision along with proper demonstration is necessary for maximum results.

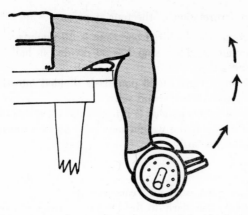

Progressive resistance exercise for quadriceps group of the thigh. Arrow shows course of path weight to be lifted. Full extension must be attained for maximum benefit.

Method 1

The most widely used method of rehabilitation of the quadriceps group is the De Lorme progressive resistive exercise program. This is a procedure involving the use of maximum resistance. To find the starting weight load has been a problem and very often takes valuable time of the trainer. However, the time should not be construed as wasted, for this program is very effective when applied properly.

Position. The athlete sits on the end of the table with a towel folded under his thigh. The boot with the proper weight is placed on the foot (the use of a shoe with a hard sole will enhance the stability of the boot). The leg hangs over the table and the exercise of extending the leg is started. The exercise is done slowly and deliberately to full extension; then hold for a count and lower leg slowly. Repeat. Three groups of ten repetitions each are used with the added weight in each set. A rest between each group will enhance the results. The arms may be folded across the chest or hands may grip the table for balance.

The leg must be locked in full extension for maximum results. If the leg cannot be fully extended and locked, the weight is too heavy, and a lighter weight should be substituted.

Step 1. After warming up the leg with very light weights or other leg exercises, the maximum load that the athlete can lift at one time is considered his top weight. (Attempting to find this weight load without a warm-up is unfair and not considered accurate.)

Step 2. The maximum weight load established is divided in half, and this weight is lifted ten times. Rest.

Step 3. The weight load in step 1 is divided into three-quarters, and this is lifted ten times. Rest.

Step 4. The maximum weight load in step 1 is now lifted ten times.

Mathematical interpretation of the four steps is:

Step 1. Maximum weight lifted one time is 36 pounds.

Step 2. Maximum weight in step 1 is 36 divided in half, or 18 pounds to be lifted in the first set.

Step 3. Maximum weight of 36 pounds is divided into three-quarters, or 27 pounds, to be lifted in the second set.

Step 4. The original 36 pounds is lifted in the third set. A slight variance may occur at this step and the weight may have to be reduced until exercise can be performed satisfactorily.

Method 2

This method has been used for years and has had excellent results. The •exercises are performed similarly to the De Lorme exercises, but the weight is constant. The maximum weight load is established for one lift, 5 to 7 pounds are deducted, and the athlete lifts this load 40 times in groups of ten. As the strength returns, the groups are increased to 20 at a time, and finally going to 40 at one sitting. When this stage is reached, weight is added at the rate of 2 pounds every work-out. This program is carried out on a three-day week plan: work one day and rest the next. Progress is noted and checked every two weeks. This program eliminates the changing of weights between each group, and the athlete can concentrate on one weight and become proficient in the performance.

Along with flexion and extension of the leg, we also add hip flexion and adduction and abduction exercises. These exercises are performed 20 times each, with a lighter weight.

Hip flexion is performed with the athlete on his back and a 10-pound weight on his foot; the leg is lifted to a right angle, held momentarily, and then lowered slowly. This exercise is repeated in groups of 5 to a total of 4 groups, or 20 lifts.

In adduction and abduction with the same weight as above, the leg is lifted 10 inches off the table and the leg is moved to the side, held, and then returned to starting position. The leg is then lowered to the table and the second repetition started. A total of 20 exercises is done, one at a time, with as much rest between as needed. These movements exercise all the muscles of the thigh as well as the quadriceps group.

The number of bouts per week in the progressive resistance program varies with the experience of the trainer and the team physician. There has been some evidence that three times a week with a day of rest between each bout has proved to be the most effective procedure. However, other reports say that a five-day week is the answer. There is no fixed procedure.

Supplementary exercises for knee. When the athlete is ready, supplementing the exercise program with running, bicycle riding, etc., is important. In early running, it is necessary that the athlete run on a flat surface and that he avoid running the turns until ready. Instruction as to distance and speed of running is also important. Start jogging on a straight line for about 25 yards, alternating this with the same amount of walking. As the athlete improves, the distances are lengthened to 50 yards and then to 100 yards. After this plateau has been reached, the running will increase in distance, but the walking will remain at 100 yards. Full circling of the field will be reached rather readily with this program. When normal action of knee has been attained, full-speed running straight ahead is encouraged. Full-speed bursts for about 15 to 20 yards are intermingled with the regular running program.

After full speed has been accomplished, starts from a stance are the next step. These starts are started at half-speed, gradually working up to full speed. When this part of the program has been successfully completed, cutting is the next step. Running about one-quarter speed in the pattern of a snake with well-rounded turns is the start of the cutting program. As agility improves, the speed is increased, but the circumference of the circle remains the same. The next step is the sharpening of the curves, gradually working into planting the foot and reversing the field. No set time can be allotted for this part of the program, for it must be dealt with on a day to day basis.

Some athletes will progress rapidly, others will be very slow to reach the cutting stage. It is not fair to the athlete to send him back to activity if he has the strength but not the ability to change directions rapidly and positively. Running straight ahead is not too much of a problem in the rehabilitation program; however, cutting is of the utmost importance, and this must be done satisfactorily before full activity is resumed.

Musculature may be regained rapidly with resistance exercises, but the ability to use this musculature in all forms of running is extremely important. We have seen remarkable results in the training room but very poor results on the field; therefore both parts of the program are extremely important.

Post-operative Knee. The subsequent discussion describes a typical procedure in the rehabilitation of a post-operative knee. (It must be stated here that all cases cannot be handled alike. Specific changes will be made from time to time by the team physician. It is most important that his instructions be carried out to the fullest.)

In the second or third day after surgery, quadriceps setting and full leg raising is started. This is continued until the stitches are removed, usually seven to ten days.

Flexion and extension exercises then begin. The athlete will sit on a table and hang his leg over the edge. Gradual swinging will increase flexion. (Do not force this motion; exercises are done only with gravity as the resistance.)

At about the third week progressive resistance exercises are started. Full power may be regained in two to three months.

Full weight bearing is variable with the condition. Crutches are used for the first ten days without any weight bearing. Gradual weight bearing is started on the tenth day, and when full weight bearing is tolerable (usually within three weeks), the use of a cane may be substituted.

KNEE BENDS

In the literature there has been evidence to support the feelings of many people associated with athletics who believe that knee bends are harmful to the structure of the knee. Many think that this exercise does not improve the athlete in any way, but written statistical evidence is lacking. Recently there has been support of this theory. Deep knee bends will stretch the medial collateral ligament as much as 8 per cent and the lateral collateral ligament as much as 10 per cent. We feel that this exercise is detrimental and should not be used.

Chapter 16

Ankle and Foot

ANATOMY OF ANKLE AND FOOT

Ankle Joint. The ankle joint is a hinge joint and is made up of the tibia, fibula, and the talus. The tibia enlarges as it extends toward the ankle, and a projection known as the internal malleolus (ankle bone) is formed. This acts as the attachment for the strong ligaments of the ankle, holding it firmly. The lower end is concave, to allow for the rounded surface of the talus to articulate.

The fibula is on the lateral side and is subcutaneous at the lower third. It has a long projection, called the *external malleolus* (ankle bone), which also acts as the attachment for ligaments of the ankle. Both malleoli form an inverted U into which the talus is placed. The talus is directly under the two larger bones of the leg, and the weight of the body is transmitted to the talus in weight bearing. The talus then transmits the weight to the other bones of the foot and ankle area. This bone is almost square except for the rounded surface that fits into the hollow surface of the tibia.

The tibia and fibula are held together at the lower third by the interosseus membrane; the ankle joint is enclosed in a thin capsule.

Holding the joint stable, even though the bone structure is designed so as to be strong, are the lateral ligaments. The medial ligament is called the deltoid ligament (shaped like a Δ). This is a strong ligament that attaches onto several bones of the ankle. The lateral ligament is a weak ligament, very narrow and straight. It has several attachments, but the expanse is not so great as that of the medial ligament.

Movements of the ankle are (1) raising the foot upward, or dorsiflexion; (2) downward motion of the foot, or plantar flexion. There is no provision made for lateral motion in the ankle. The two large bones enclose the talus, thus making it impossible normally to move the ankle laterally.

In discussing the ankle the inclusion of the foot is most imperative. The main part of the foot is composed of seven bones, called the *tarsus*. These bones are the calcaneus, talus, navicular, and cuboid, the first, second and third cuneiform. The two largest

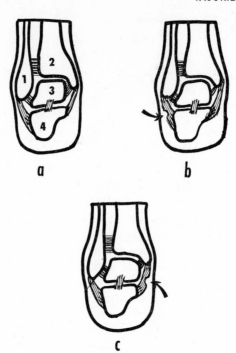

Section of ankle joint. (1) Fibula. (2) Tibia. (3) Talus. (4) Calcaneus. Arrow shows sprain of lateral ligament of ankle (b). Arrow shows sprain of the medial ligament of the ankle (c).

bones are the talus (sometimes called the *astaragalus*) and the calcaneus (sometimes called the *os calcis*, or heel bone). The talus articulates with the tibia on the top side and with the navicular on the front side, which in turn articulates with the cuneiform bone. The movements of the tarsus (namely, inversion, eversion, and rotation) have been given to us so that we may be able to walk on uneven surfaces. The width of the foot and the closeness to the ground compensates for the freedom of motion in the tarsus and metatarsus.

The five bones of the foot are called the *metatarsals*, and the bones of the toes are called the *phalanges*. The metatarsals correspond to the five bones of the hand, but they are bigger and stronger although similar in shape. The phalanges are shorter than those in the hand but are somewhat thicker.

Arches of the Foot. The longitudinal arch extends from the heel to the toes. The transverse arches are a series of arches running across the foot from one side to the other.

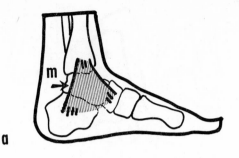

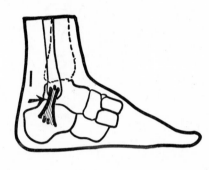

Major ligaments involved in the sprain of the ankle. Medial (inside) ligament (deltoid) of the ankle (a). Lateral (outside) ligament most frequently involved in sprains of the ankle (b).

FUNCTIONAL TESTS FOR ANKLE

1. *Flexion* (*dorsiflexion*). Raise the foot toward the knee. The lower leg is held firmly with one hand; the other grasps the foot and the toes are moved slowly toward the knee. These movements test normal dorsiflexion and also peroneal and tendon Achilles condition. The muscles involved are the tibialis anterior extensor digitorum longus, peroneus tertius, and extensor hallucis longus.

2. *Extension* (*plantar flexion*). Point toe downward, away from knee. Grasp ankle with one hand, encircle the foot with the other, and gently move toes down. These movements test for normal plantar flexion and stretching of other tissues which run over the ankle joint. The muscles involved are the gastrocneumius, tibialis posterior, flexor digitorum longus, soleus, flexor hallucis longus, and peroneus longus.

3. *Inversion*. Turn the foot inward with foot held firmly with one hand while the other encircles the lower leg; foot is gradually

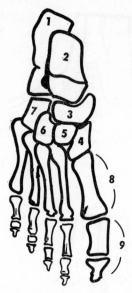

Bones of the foot. (1) Calcaneus. (2) Talus. (3) Navicular. (4), (5), and (6): First, second, and third cuneiforms. (7) Cuboid. (8) Metatarsals. (9) Phalanges.

turned in toward the mid-line. This tests for stability of lateral ligaments. The muscles involved are the tibialis anterior and posterior.

4. *Eversion.* Turn foot outward. Movements are the same as for inversion except that action is opposite. This test is for stability of deltoid ligament. The muscles involved are the peroneus longus, tertius, and brevis.

5: *Circumduction.* The foot and ankle make a free swinging circle on the lower leg, first to the inside and then in reverse to

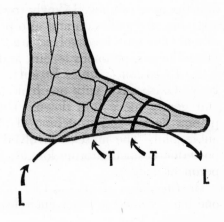

Arches of the foot. (L) indicates longitudinal arch. (T) designates the transverse arches of the foot.

outside turns. Even though the normal motions of the foot are flexion and extension, this test will reveal the looseness of the joint and will help in diagnosing various injuries to the foot and ankle.

ANKLE INJURIES

An ankle injury manifests itself considerably earlier than a knee injury, and many times it can be analyzed immediately after the injury. It is true, however, that the ankle may have many tender spots, but the "true injury" will be readily seen on proper examination. After spasm, pain and hemorrhage have set in, the diagnosis may be delayed because the symptoms are disguised as a result of these conditions. Therefore the sooner the examination is made, the more complete will be the diagnosis. Again it must be stressed that the injury should have immediate treatment, and any delay until the next day may result in a condition that will of necessity become a weakened and painful joint injury. Many complications can be avoided by the simple procedure of doing it *now* instead of tomorrow. The diagnosis of the first day must be checked and rechecked on succeeding days, and the condition of ligaments, etc., must be evaluated. Caution must be the watchword; gentle motion and palpation will give an accurate analysis. Treatment should be evaluated, and decisions as to changes should be made daily. To chart a course and then not deviate as a matter of principle is not the procedure for good treatment. Changed courses have good effect when indicated and will lead to good management of the athlete's problem.

The immediate examination must be complete and thorough. The mechanics of the injury are a great help in diagnosis of the injury. The location of tenderness will make it possible within a few minutes to ascertain if the injury is major or minor. Tenderness over the bone will indicate that the bone is damaged, and the bone injury should not be eliminated until X-ray has proved otherwise. Complete or partial ligament tears should also be suspected in serious ankle injury. The reason for the early examination is to observe the findings when the ankle is in a state of analgesia, which exists for a few minutes after the intent of the injury. Liberties may be taken at this time that may not be available after edema, muscle spasm, and swelling have taken place.

After the immediate examination, the injury will be classified in one of three categories: mild, moderate, or severe.

Fractures About the Ankle. The lower end of the tibia and fibula are the common sites of fractures in the ankle, the fibula more so than the tibia. Fractures are caused by direct blow, a fall, severe torsion, or by someone falling over an extended leg in pile-up.

The symptoms are pain, disability, and inability to bear weight. The important signs of a fracture in this area are deformity, tenderness, and disability. X-ray must be an integral part of examination for suspected fractures.

Tibia. Fractures of the shaft of the tibia are caused by direct blows, severe torsion of the leg with the foot immobile, and from leverage (such as a pile-up with foot anchored). The symptoms are pain, disability, and the inability to bear weight.

History will reveal the mechanics of the injury plus the athlete's story that he heard something snap or pop. Inspection will show tenderness over the bone; there may or may not be a displacement. Palpation will reveal pain over the fracture area. Feeling gently along the edges of the bone may show an interruption of the normal lines.

The leg should be splinted where the athlete lies, and he should not be moved without a splint. He should be transferred from the field on a stretcher. Treatment should be given by the team physician.

A fracture of the internal malleoli (of tibia) is seen rarely in athletics. A fracture that is not displaced is called a *sprain fracture*. However, a fracture with displacement must be treated as a fracture and not as a sprain.

History, inspection, and palpation will reveal a tender area with or without displacement over the internal malleoli.

Treatment consists of plaster cast, and in some instances a walking appliance is incorporated in the cast. Immobilization is for about four to six weeks, after which physical therapy for the purpose of normal ambulation is started. Heat and massage with exer-

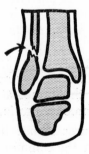

Potts' fracture of the distal portion of the fibula.

cise begins when the cast is removed. The use of an army-type high shoe is often prescribed for post-fracture recovery.

Fibula. Fibula fractures are rather common in athletics and may occur in the same manner as fractures of the tibia. The most common fracture of the fibula occurs in the lower third of the bone and is referred to as a *Potts' fracture.* This fracture is caused by violent eversion of the ankle joint. (The weakest point of the fibula is just above the ankle joint.)

History will reveal the mechanics of the injury, and there will be much pain and in some instances immediate swelling. The ability to bear weight should not obscure the possibility of a fractured fibula, as the tibia is the weight-bearing bone of the leg and thus allows for mobility.

Inspection may or may not reveal a deformity. Swelling may be quite evident in the area of the ankle and in some instances may manifest itself over the fracture site. By gently palpating the edges of the fibula, a change in contour of the bone can be felt.

Fractures of the fibula may be handled by a compression wrap and crutches. Immediate medical attention should be secured for proper disposition. Postponing medical attention may delay treatment, since the possibility of swelling may make the reduction considerably difficult. The best results are attained before swelling occurs.

Fortunately this type of fracture can be handled very well with the application of a cast for about a six-week period. The use of a walking cast is sometimes indicated. With the use of a walking cast, atrophy of the thigh, etc., is held to a minimum.

After removal from the cast, heat and massage plus exercise comprise the treatment indicated. The use of a high army shoe also enhances recovery in this injury.

Tarsus. Fractures of the small bones of the ankle, the tarsus, are not seen too often in athletics. The most direct cause of these fractures is a fall from a high place, landing on the heel of the foot. This activity does not enter into the normal routine of athletics, and so this type of injury is rare. However, a small fracture of one of the seven bones of the foot (tarsus) may be found in X-ray as the result of a sprain in the area. This is a condition that must be treated properly, as complications may arise in later life. In severe sprains, X-ray will pick up this injury. If discovered, treatment on the level of the orthopedic surgeon must be solicited.

The disability of fractures in this area is long, and usually the season will be lost to the athlete.

Foot Fractures

Fractures of the metatarsals. The long bones of the foot are quite susceptible to fractures, and these may occur in many ways. One of the most common causes of this injury is direct trauma, such as being stepped on by a cleated shoe or being piled on with foot in full extension. Running and jumping are also causes of this type of fracture. Many fractures of the metatarsals are missed, thus causing a disabling injury and prolonged disability. The fracture may involve one or more bones. Diagnosis is usually difficult because of the pain and swelling. Pain will involve the whole foot, later localizing over the site of the fracture. X-ray will confirm fracture.

History will reveal the incident, such as being stepped on, etc. Inspection will show swelling, and in some cases, a deformity. Palpation will reveal the degree of tenderness and exactly which metatarsal has been injured. By gently flexing and extending each toe, the exact location of injury can be ascertained. In suspected fracture sites, be gentle and do not attempt to reduce or manipulate any deformity seen.

In suspected fractures of the metatarsals, the athlete should be supplied with crutches and sent for further examination. X-ray is indicated, and the results of the X-ray will establish treatment. Cast immobilization is indicated, and the disability time varies from four to eight weeks.

The most common fracture of this type occurs in the fifth metatarsal and is commonly caused by being stepped on by a cleated or hard-soled shoe. Basketball, where rubber shoes are used, is a frequent contributor. However, the incident happens because the athlete lands on the outer border of foot with severe inversion of the ankle and foot, resulting in a spiral or transverse type of fracture to the fifth metatarsal. Cast immobilization is indicated, and disability extends over four to six weeks.

Fracture of phalanges. This is not a very common injury in athletics but is often caused in athletes by other activities such as walking barefooted and stubbing toes. One or more of the phalanges may be fractured. It is not a serious injury, but it usually disables. The bones of the toes are superficial and readily palpatable. Deformity and crepitus may be easily seen or felt.

Examination involves X-ray, and if a fracture is disclosed, a plaster cast or splint is indicated. Disability is from four to eight weeks.

Fracture of great toe. Fracture of the great toe is treated in the same manner as a fracture of the thumb. This is a very important member of the foot and its injury is very disabling. Fortunately it is not too common. Treatment consists of X-ray and plaster-cast or splint immobilization. Disability time extends from four to eight weeks.

Sprain fractures of the internal and external malleoli (ankle bones) is not uncommon in athletics. In lieu of a sprain, the ligament pulls a small portion of the bone away. Treatment varies with the degree of displacement. In mild sprain fractures (without displacement), they are handled as sprains of the ankle, using compression, ice, and elevation. Strapping is carried out for about six weeks. Weight bearing is allowed after the first week, and then the work load is increased to tolerance. Disability time varies with the individual and also with the degree of fracture.

Sprain fractures with displacement must be handled as regular fractures, with reduction, immobilization, etc.

March fracture. The March fracture is an unusual injury that may occur without apparent cause. It usually involves a transverse fracture of the shaft of the second or third metatarsal. The oncome is very slow, and in the beginning, the injury is not disabling. There will not be any specific history as to the cause of this pain. It is believed that constant and excessive exercise causes this condition. As the condition progresses, the pain increases as well as the amount of disability. In the beginning, there may not be any swelling, but as the condition persists, swelling will present itself on the top of the foot. Pain will be localized to the extent that the athlete will place his finger directly on the spot. These facts usually complete the history. Inspection may or may not reveal swelling, and palpation will elicit pain on the bone but no deformity or crepitus.

Treatment consists of X-ray for bony pathology. (Very often the early X-ray may reveal a negative plate, but on an X-ray taken approximately two to three weeks later, the fracture will be very evident. Callus will show up at this time.)

It is good policy to treat all possible March symptoms as fractures even though the X-ray may prove negative. Treatment is symptomatic and consists of rest and immobilization by means of a restrictive strapping and crutches or a light plaster cast. When symptoms subside, which is in about two to three weeks, a second film is taken. If again the X-ray is negative, then the athlete is permitted to participate in his sport on a controlled basis. If X-ray is positive at this time, the foot is then placed in a cast for the usual time (four to six weeks). After the cast is removed, whirlpools and strapping will suffice until full and normal motion has been regained.

Epiphyseal Injuries. The epiphysis affords points of attachments for muscles, forms joints, and helps to develop the length of the bones. At each end of the shaft of the bone, an epiphyseal line is seen. It is cartilage until bone growth ceases; then it becomes solid bone. Injuries to the epiphysis are found in the early years of the athlete. Prehigh school and some high school athletes may receive this type of an injury, but it is very rare in college athletics. The usual site is around the ankle area; namely, the lower ends of the tibia and fibula.

The cause of this injury is similar to the fracture mechanics. A severe wrenching of the leg, acute muscular action, and trauma may be contributing causes. Symptoms are pain, swelling, limitation of motion, and possibly a deformity.

Treatment is essentially the same as for a fracture, i.e., rest, immobilization, and avoidance of weight bearing. The use of a cast in the case of ankle involvements is quite common. Strapping, splinting, or braces may also be used.

DISLOCATIONS OF ANKLE

The dislocation of the ankle may be forward, backward, or sideways. The most common displacement of the foot is backward. The symptoms are pain, loss of function, and disability. On inspection, the abnormal condition is usually obvious. It is quite common to have a fracture accompany a dislocation in the ankle area.

Treatment consists of applying a splint and transporting by stretcher for final diagnosis and further management.

X-ray, reduction, and immobilization are usually the procedures carried out in this injury. After this phase of treatment, the athlete will be returned for rehabilitation. The use of whirlpool baths,

Dislocation of ankle (anterior), showing typical "step" symptom of dislocation.

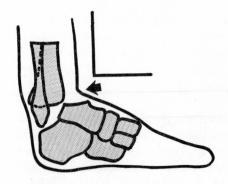

massage, and passive exercises is then started. Active exercises and weight bearing should begin as soon as possible.

After the cast has been removed, the use of protective strapping may be ordered. The open-faced Gibney is used until the swelling has subsided, and then routine strapping is applied. The wearing of a high army shoe is very effective, and in some cases they are used instead of adhesive strapping.

Dislocation of Phalanges. A dislocation of the toe is very obvious; the normal alignment is distorted and the typical step sign is noted. Treatment is early reduction and immobilization for approximately two weeks, after which heat, massage, and passive and active exercises should be started. The athlete may return to activity when full weight bearing and full range of motion is restored.

INJURIES AND TREATMENTS

Ankle Sprain. Perhaps the most common injury to the lower extremity in athletics is the ankle sprain. The causes may vary, from stepping in a hole, or an uneven surface to a severe wrenching suffered in a football pile-up. The degree of sprain will vary with the incident, and therefore we shall divide this injury into three categories: mild, moderate, and severe.

Mild sprain. In a mild sprain, with symptoms of mild pain, little or no swelling, and mild tenderness localized in the area of the lateral malleolus, assume that the lateral ligament has been stretched rather than torn. In such a case the athlete will be able to walk off the playing area and will complain of pain and slight disability. On examination there will be tenderness over the site of the sprain. The joint may or may not have any swelling.

The immediate treatment is to apply an open-faced Gibney strapping to the ankle and then to ice and elevate. Elevation consists of having the ankle higher than the body and thus allowing gravity to enhance the drainage from the injured area. Weight bearing is indicated in the mild sprain. After the first 24 hours, the ankle should be re-examined. In some instances the treatment rendered may not have been enough. However, if the swelling has increased and pain is still present, the same procedure should be continued. On the third day, the application of mild heat and light massage is applied to the area; restrap with routine strapping and encourage the athlete to exercise. Exercise should be active; walking and light jogging are excellent. Amount of walking and jogging may be increased as progress is made. This type of injury responds excellently to work, providing it is not too strenuous to start. Disability is usually three days to about a week.

Moderate sprain. In a moderate sprain there will be stretching of the ligaments and possibly some torn fibers. The tearing may be in the middle of the ligament or at the attachments. Bleeding into the joint will result along with the increase in synovial fluid. With the moderate sprain, damage to the capsule must be assumed. Immediate treatment is aimed at the control of hemorrhage in the area.

Moderate sprain of the ankle will have pain, some swelling, and inability to walk normally. With the moderate sprain, the athlete will attempt to walk with the foot out to the side; he can usually do this, but every once in a while the ankle will feel as though it were about to collapse. History will reveal the incident. Palpation will result in tenderness over the site of the injury, and in further palpation, pain will also be felt in other parts of the ankle as well as the acutely injured area. Inspection will show some swelling around the ankle joint, mainly below the ankle bone, but this may extend upward into the leg and also spread around to the front of the foot. Functional tests will probably show only tightness due to the swelling.

Immediate treatment consists of the application of the open-faced Gibney strapping, ice, and elevation. Crutches should be used for rest and easy ambulation. X-ray is routine in all moderate and severe ankle injuries.

In the moderate injury, continue the use of compression, ice, elevation, and crutch walking for at least 48 hours. On the third day, if injury is progressing (i.e., pain localized, swelling diminished, function recovered), start heat treatments and mild exercise. Massage above and below the injury may be used, but direct pressure on site of injury should be avoided for a few days. After treatment, the ankle should be strapped with the routine strapping and light weight bearing with crutches encouraged.

The increase of weight bearing should be rapid, and the athlete should be instructed to try this to the limit of tolerance. On the fourth day, treatment is the same, and full weight bearing starts without crutches. On the fifth day, active jogging and walking procedures should be started. The athlete walks 25 yards, jogs 25 yards. This is alternated and increased as the ankle loosens up. The athlete should not attempt to run any turns at this time. As the distances are increased, the speed also may be increased, that is, from a jog to striding and then to sprinting. When the athlete can run full speed straight ahead, start zigzagging slowly, gradually instituting cutting. When the athlete can change directions both ways and can cut in and out on his ankle, he is ready to go back to full work. To let an athlete play when he can run straight ahead but not change directions is only asking for trouble, for he will return shortly with a re-injury of the ankle.

When the tissues are torn, time is most important, and efforts to force this type of injury will result in much discomfort and an athlete who will not be so effective as a physically fit substitute.

The length of disability is usually two to three weeks in the moderate sprain. The use of adhesive strapping should be continued until the ankle has returned to normal.

Severe sprain. Severe sprain of the ankle will manifest itself with much swelling and complete loss of function. The athlete will not attempt to bear weight on the injured ankle. The pain will be very severe, and means to relieve pain will not be too successful (i.e., elevation, rest, etc.). A severe sprain will produce severe pain, and this is a characteristic incident in this injury; a fracture is usually not so painful as the severe sprain.

In a severe sprain we must assume that we have a tear of the ligament or ligaments of the ankle as well as much damage to the capsule and other soft tissue in the area. There will be much bleeding and an increase of fluid in the joint capsule. Immediate treatment is to control both conditions as much as possible.

The history will be dramatic, the incident will be severe, and in many cases the athlete will fall to the ground and will not move of his own accord and will not want to use the ankle in any way. Inspection will reveal much swelling; there may or may not be discoloration at this time. An obvious deformity resulting from the swelling will be seen. The swelling will be around the ankle joint, extending up into the leg and around the ankle to the opposite side. Palpation will reveal swelling and tenderness at any place touched. Early examination will reveal much laxity of the joint. The exact site of injury may not be known for about 24 to 48 hours. The athlete should be removed from the area by means of a stretcher; another examination in the training room should follow.

With severe injury, the use of compression, ice, and elevation should be started immediately. X-ray is indicated, along with bed rest. Severe swelling in an ankle will not absorb very rapidly, and the athlete should remain in bed until the swelling has completely disappeared. While the athlete is confined to the bed, continue ice treatments for at least four days; then heat can be started. An electric pad is very effective at this time. Motion of the foot and

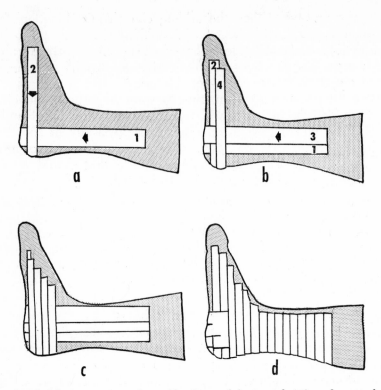

Open-faced Gibney strapping for ankle. Start of horizontal (1) and vertical (2) strips (a). Strips 3 and 4 are applied over strips 1 and 2 (b). Use as many vertical strips as are needed to enclose ankle (c). Complete strapping with front open (d).

ankle are encouraged, and the athlete should spend 10 minutes of every hour doing these exercises. When the swelling has shown a marked decrease, allow the athlete to attend classes on crutches, and start treatments. Again, heat and massage are used daily along with as much active and passive exercise as possible. We may at this time, depending on whether he can wear a shoe, allow some light weight bearing, with a crutch assist. The athlete must concentrate to make sure that he walks with the foot straight ahead rather than out to the side. (Turning the toe out is a very natural way for an athlete to walk with this injury, but as you can see, the ankle is not being used, the heel acts as the fulcrum, and there is no motion in the ankle joint; at this time some motion is needed in the area to help in the limitation of atrophy and scar tissue.) Experience has proved that ankles will recover faster if this type of walking is started immediately on ambulation.

ANKLE STRAPPING (OPEN-FACED GIBNEY)

The athlete sits on table with his foot at a right angle; leg should extend about 10 inches over the end of the table. If the athlete has trouble in holding his foot in this position, the use of a "rein" may help. With a gauze bandage hooked around the last three toes, the "rein" may be held by the athlete and pulled so that the ankle remains in the proper position for strapping.

Step 1. Start the tape approximately 6 inches above the internal malleoli (ankle bone); pull the tape around the heel, following close to and parallel to the tendon Achilles. The tape will end at about 6 inches above the external malleoli (ankle bone on outside of leg). Set tape by rubbing with palm of hand.

Step 2. Start at the base of the great toe, pull the tape around the heel and run it parallel with the bottom of the foot and as close as possible to the sole. Finish at the base of the little toe.

Step 3. Repeat step 1, overlapping at least halfway.

Step 4. Repeat step 2, starting about ¼ inch short of strip 2 and overlapping at least halfway.

Step 5. Repeat step 1; usually three vertical strips will suffice.

Step 6. Repeat the horizontal strips all the way up to the start of the vertical strips. Recess each one so that the front of the foot and ankle remains visible.

After the strap has been applied, 2-inch roller gauze may be used to set the tape. Caution must be observed so that the gauze is not applied too tightly, as this will defeat the purpose of the "open face."

The Gibney is a very versatile strapping and may be used routinely. However, it is most effective in acute injuries of the foot and ankle.

ROUTINE ANKLE STRAP WITH FIGURE EIGHT

This strapping is essentially the Gibney with variations and a reinforcement with a figure eight. The figure eight is applied over the Gibney. Caution should be observed, as the combination of the two straps can be very constricting. Where full extension of the ankle is needed, this strap may constrict and should not be used. It is applied with the athlete in a sitting position and the foot held at normal right angles.

Step 1. Using 1½-inch tape, start approximately 8 inches above the internal ankle bone. Fix tape, pull around the heel, and finish about 8 inches above the external ankle bone. Strip 1 should run as close to the tendon Achilles as possible and should be parallel to it. Smooth the tape with the palm of the hand or fingers.

Step 2. Overlap about halfway and repeat step 1. A third vertical strip may be needed to cover large ankles.

Step 3. The horizontal strip (1½-inch tape) starts on the inside of the ankle below the ankle bone and is pulled around the back of the ankle, ending on the top surface of the foot. Do not pull tape tight enough to irritate the tendon area of the ankle, as irritations in the form of blisters will result.

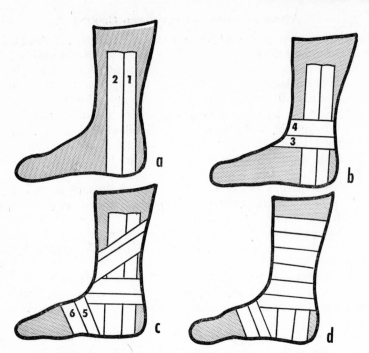

Routine strapping that includes a figure eight. Start with vertical strips 1 and 2 (a). Use as many as are needed to enclose ankle joint. Horizontal strips 3 and 4 applied (b). Figure eight, strips 5 and 6, over the vertical and horizontal strips (c). Complete strapping with anchor strips enclosing the full ankle (d). Detail of figure eight (e). Second strip of figure eight showing relation to first strip (f).

Step 4. Overlapping two-thirds, apply the second horizontal strip above strip 1. For extra support, these strips may overlap on the front part of the foot.

Step 5. The figure eight is applied over step 4. Start on the outside of the ankle at the beginning of the vertical strips, fix tape, and pull at an angle across the dorsal surface of the foot, under the arch and across the bottom of the foot. Inasmuch as we are supporting the lateral aspect of the ankle, the pull from here upward may be with some force, crossing the downward portion of this strip of tape. The tape will end on the inside of the ankle at the start of the vertical strips.

Step 6. The second figure eight will start below the first one and should overlap as much as necessary to make another figure eight. Keep wrinkle-free if possible.

A dry run may help attain the proper angle for the figure eight. This is done by reversing the tape and laying the cloth side on the ankle and trying the various positions that will be necessary to establish starting position and angle.

Step 7. Anchor strips are then applied in a circular manner, enclosing

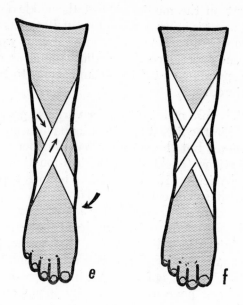

the full ankle strap with tape. Start from the bottom and work upward with the last strip covering all the ends of the tape.

Anchor strips on the foot are optional and one or two may be used. Caution should be observed when encircling the foot, since taping too tightly may result in loss of circulation and cramps.

The application of gauze next to the skin will lessen the irritation over the tendon area and the dorsum of the foot. If gauze is not used, small pads may be placed over the tendon and dorsal areas of the ankle to prevent blisters.

When the severe ankle sprain reaches a moderate stage, the same procedures should be carried out again.

The application of a plaster cast with a walking attachment has been advocated by many orthopedic surgeons for this type of injury. Although surgical intervention to repair torn tissue has been very successful, there are pro's and con's on these procedures, and both sides have proved their point beyond doubt. The decision as to procedure must be made by the team physician and not the trainer.

We have outlined the treatment for ankle sprains without stating which ligament is involved. With the mechanics of the ankle joint as we know them, we are dealing with the lateral ligament and the deltoid ligament on the medial side of the ankle (see page 133). The lateral ligament is injured at the rate of 10 to 1, so the incidence to medial sprains is rare. However, the treatment would be exactly the same. In our experience the medial sprain, as rare as it is, is very slow in responding to treatment and seems to be easily aggravated and reinjured.

Injections. The use of injections for various sprains of the ankle is recommended in the literature. Results have been very gratifying on many occasions, but the contrary has also been found. Hence, the use of injections (cocktails) is a decision that must be made by the team physician. If the decision to inject has been made, only the team physician can inject. To discuss the merits of this procedure is beyond the scope of this book. The reader will have to search the literature for the more recent findings.

Pain in an injury is indicative that that particular part of the body is not normal. To use novocain or other painkillers so that the athlete can participate is not wise. In blocking the pain sensation, the athlete will not have an opportunity to gauge the degree of activity that he can safely tolerate. When pain is present, the injury is not well, and to force the injury "to go" in this condition, even though the sensation of pain has been blocked, may lead to further damage of the tissues. It may also anaesthetize the area so much that other parts of the ankle may be injured and the athlete will not realize it. A physically fit substitute is a better candidate to play at this time than the partially injured regular who has been subjected to novocain injection so that he can play.

Shin Splints. In reviewing the muscles on the front of the leg (the tibialis anticus and posticus, and extensor digitorum longus and the extensor hallucis longus), we have the site of the injury known as "shin splints." The belief that this condition manifests itself in the tearing of these muscles from the bone, etc., has yet to be proved. The texture of surfaces, hard ground, and floors has been known to be a cause of this injury. It may be that poor mechanics of running is the underlying cause of this injury, and the end result is a simple muscle strain or sprain. In reviewing many cases of shin splints with athletes and coaches, plus innumerable trips to the areas to investigate this condition, we have come to the conclusion that running with the toes pointed out is the cause of

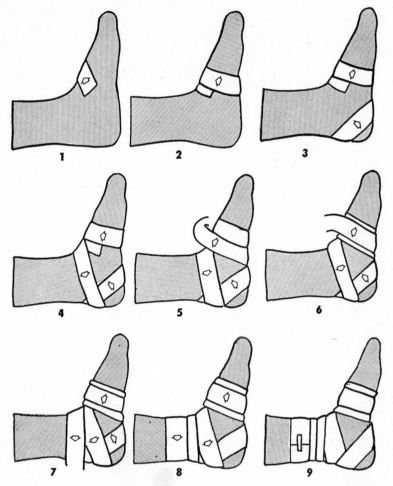

Ankle wrap with "heel lock." (1) Start on top of foot. (2) Completely circle foot. (3) Pull around heel. (4) Cross over ankle. (5) Go under arch. (6) Form heel lock on other side of heel. (7) Circle foot again. (8) Wrap around ankle just above the joint. (9) Repeat same and tape intact.

this condition. If caught early, the condition is immediately relieved by the exaggerated "pigeon-toed" walking. On the running surface, this same type of running helps to eliminate the pain and general soreness. A concentrated course in the mechanics of running will definitely eliminate this condition. In order to help alleviate this condition in the acute stage, apply an ankle wrap, using the heel lock along with instructions of toed-in running. This, to date, has been the finding, and the results have been excellent.

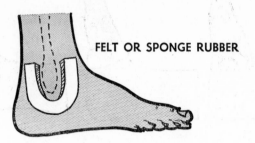

FELT OR SPONGE RUBBER

Horseshoe padding of felt or sponge to protect a contusion of the lateral ankle bone.

Contusions of the Ankle. The most common contusion of the ankle is one that occurs to either the external or internal malleoli. These bones are well pronounced and are quite easily bruised. Being kicked is the most common cause of this injury. Another common cause is the athlete's kicking himself as he runs. This occurs in slightly pigeon-toed runners. Another cause of this injury is hitting the hurdles with the ankle bone, a common injury that is painful but not very serious. The degree of disability depends on the extent of the blow. History will reveal the mechanics of the injury.

Inspection will reveal the site of the injury and also the degree of swelling. Palpation will cause more discomfort and therefore must be gentle.

Treatment consists of immediate compression and ice packs. The ice may be removed the next day and heat, if necessary, started. Infrared is very effective, as the damaged tissue is immediately below the surface of the skin. Protection must be supplied so that the injury will not be hit again. Sponge-rubber pads applied to the site will answer this need. Hurdlers may wear the pad during practice and eliminate it during meet. In football the use of low quarter shoes has contributed to the increase of this injury as of late. The use of the high-top shoe will prevent most of these conditions. The length of disability is from a day to three or four days.

Foot. The bones of the foot are in two groups, the medial and the lateral. The medial group, which bears most of the weight transferred from the tibia, is composed of the talus, scaphoid, the three cuneiforms, and the three metatarsal bones and their

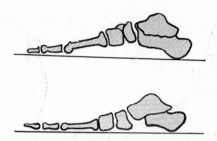

(Top) Normal arch of foot and bone structure. (Bottom) Bone structure of a depressed arch.

phalanges. The lateral group is made up of the calcaneus, cuboid, and the two lateral metatarsals and their phalanges.

In the mechanics of weight bearing, the weight is transferred to the talus from the tibia, backward to the heel, and downward and forward through the arches. Weight bearing is on the heel, head of the first metatarsal and outer border of the foot, and head of the fifth metatarsal. The motions of the foot are dorsiflexion (flexion), plantar flexion (extension), adduction and abduction, inversion (foot turned in toward mid-line), and eversion (foot turned outward). The muscles and tendons involved in these motions are the long muscles of the lower leg.

Longitudinal arch. The longitudinal arch consists of the medial and the lateral portions of the foot. The medial (inside) portion consists of the os calcis, talus, scaphoid, the three cuneiform bones, and the three metatarsals and their phalanges. The lateral portion consists of the os calcis, the cuboid, and the two metatarsals and their corresponding phalanges. The medial is higher than the lateral. The medial touches the ground at the calcaneus, and the lower portion of the metatarsal touches in front. The lateral portion is low and touches the ground at all times in weight bearing.

The talus is the keystone of the arch and receives the body weight and transmits it through the two portions of the arch. The longitudinal arch is supported by the long muscles of the leg and the short muscles of the foot; it is also strengthened by ligaments. Arches give elasticity through the ligaments. The ligaments are not so strong as muscles. Relaxation of muscles causes excessive activity of the ligaments, and they soon will "give out." Injuries to the longi-

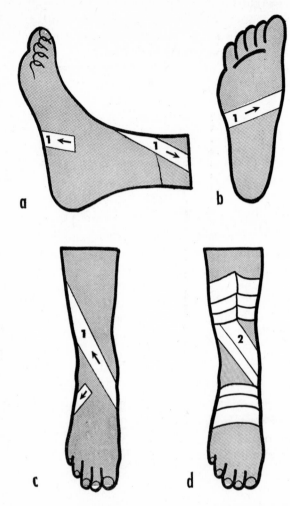

Longitudinal arch. The athlete sits on table with leg extended. With foot held in normal position, strip 1 is started on the outer edge of foot and pulled under the arch and up over the instep (a), (b), and (c). Strip 2 overlaps at least three-quarters of the way and is pulled in the same direction (d). The number of strips needed will be indicated by the length of the arch and the degree of support needed. Anchors are applied around the lower leg and foot. Anchors should not be applied tightly because they will constrict.

tudinal arch are caused by trauma (being stepped on, etc.), sprain, or a sudden stretch of the ligaments. The symptoms are pain, fatigue, rigidity, swelling, and a limp.

History will be very revealing. The athlete will have twinges of pain on weight bearing, which he can describe very vividly and can also point out exactly with his finger. Pain may be relieved when not weight bearing. Athlete will say that the foot feels as though it is "giving out from under him."

Inspection may or may not reveal any swelling. The foot will appear to be tight. Palpation will reveal point tenderness through the area of the arch and especially under the foot. The arch will be very tight, and any attempt to move the foot will result in rigidity.

Treatment consists of rest (preferably with foot elevated), strapping, heat, and massage. After the acute stage is over, exercises are indicated. Whirlpool baths are very effective, as are hot soaks. The use of contrast baths has been very effective in the acute treatment of a sprained arch. Contrast baths of about 4 minutes hot and 1 minute cold, alternated for 30 minutes, get good response from this injury.

Arch exercises. Exercises should always be performed in stockings or while barefooted.

1. Walk in an exaggerated "pigeon-toe."
2. Four-count exercise:
   a. Raise to ball of foot.
   b. Roll over to outer border.
   c. Back to ball of foot (inner border).
   d. Normal position.
3. Walk on outer border of foot, curling great toe in.
4. Sitting, place feet on edge of towel, curl towel up in toes with a firm grasp and release. Repeat until towel is under feet.
5. Pick up marbles with toes and move from one area to another.
6. Sit on chair with leg crossed, grasp foot with hand and fully extend foot, then forcibly pull foot inward and upward, finishing in normal position. This exercise will loosen foot and relieve pressure.

Metatarsal arch. The metatarsal arch is formed by the heads of the metatarsal bones of the foot and extends from one side of the foot to the other. The arch starts at the base of the great toe and curves upward at the second and third metatarsal, ending at the head of the fifth metatarsal. The arch affords stability, gives spring and resiliency to the foot, and also absorbs shock of weight bearing.

Good weight bearing consists of pressure on the first and fourth metatarsal, with the fifth combining with four to take all the weight of standing. If the arch is weak, the second and third metatarsal are called into action. This results in poor weight bearing and a bone bruise plus callous over the heads of these bones. Wearing too

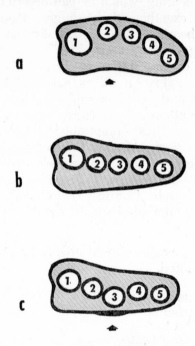

Metatarsal arch of the foot. Normal position of the heads of the metatarsal (a).
Depressed metatarsal arch (b). Depression of the third head of the metatarsal head
with callus formation (c).

short a shoe will also result in the change of mechanics of the
flexors of the toes. The flexors will shorten and thus cause an im-
balance between the two groups of muscles, the extensor and flexors.
The extensors will stretch and the arch will depress.

Causes, other than too short a shoe, are strain and trauma (constant pounding of the foot). Symptoms are pain, rigidity, callus,
sensitiveness over the bones, and spasm of muscles. History will
reveal much pain, with relief when weight bearing is stopped.
Inspection may or may not reveal swelling. Palpation, particularly
over the heads of the metatarsals, will reveal much tenderness, and
the tendons of the foot will be very spastic; the passive motions of
the foot will cause an increase of the pain.

Treatment is essentially rest until spasm subsides. Heat and
massage are very effective for the relief of pain. Strapping with a
felt pad or adhesive tape is indicated in the early stages, resorting
to correction of the shoe with the pad inserted in shoe for constant

wear. Exercises after acute pain subsides will help to postpone further acute conditions.

Exercises for metatarsal rehabilitation. Place towel on floor with foot at edge, curl towel up in toes with a firm grasp, and relax. This is carried out until the towel is completely under foot. Pick up marbles with toes and move from one pile to another.

Place opposite great toe on base of toe and trace the border of the tibia to the knee; rest and retrace pattern back to toe. (In acute conditions this exercise may cause a cramping of the arch. Caution in quick movements should be stressed.)

METATARSAL ARCH SUPPORT

This strapping is applied with the athlete sitting, with his foot held in the approximated position.

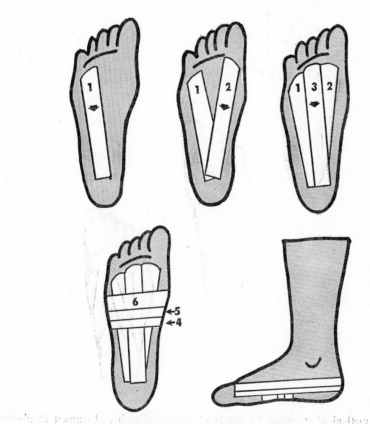

Strapping for metatarsal arch of foot.

Step 1. Cut the strip approximately 7 inches long (1½-inch tape) and curve the end that is applied to the arch. Start on the outside of the arch of the foot, just in back of the toes; press firmly on sole of foot and then pull toward the heel and anchor.

Step 2. Cut with end contoured for the ball of the foot and apply the same way as step 1 except on curve on the *inside* of the foot.

Step 3. Cut this strip with a full curve and apply down the middle of the foot, enclosing the full foot in tape.

Step 4. Taking a 7-inch piece of tape off the roll, start the tape in the middle of the foot and pull upward on both sides of the mid-line of the foot. This strip is applied to the bottom of the foot just in front of the heel.

Step 5: Same as step 4 but overlapping about one-quarter of the way; apply with the same amount of pressure.

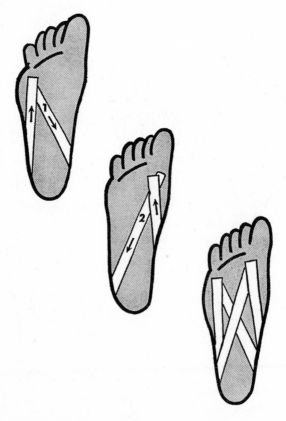

Alternate method of strapping for sprain of metatarsal arch and support of plantar ligament of foot.

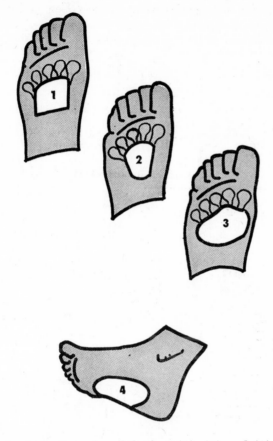

Various types of pads for the arches of the foot. (1), (2), and (3) are metatarsal pads; (4) is pad for longitudinal arch.

Step 6. Applied the same as strips 4 and 5. Three strips are sufficient unless athlete has a long foot.

Step 7. Starting at the base of the great toe and using 1-inch tape, pull the strip parallel with the bottom of the foot and encircle the heel, ending up at the base of the little toe.

Step 8. Apply this strip over strip 7, overlapping halfway. These are anchor strips to hold strips 4, 5, and 6 in place and to keep them from rolling when socks, etc., are worn.

Tendon Injuries. Muscles are attached to bone, etc., by tendons. Tendons are composed of dense fibrous tissue. Tendons are not elastic, and when stretched, they lose their power. When shortened,

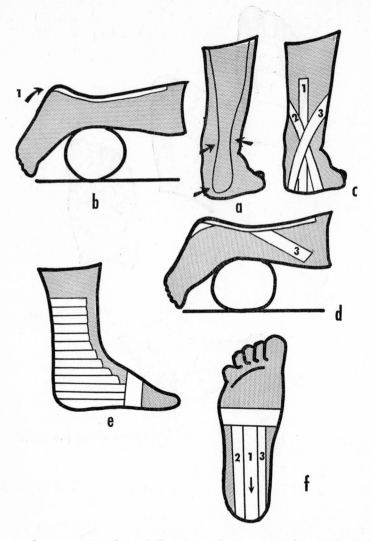

Strapping for injury to tendon Achilles. Areas of injury in tendon Achilles (a) and (c). Strip 1 applied from ball of foot and around heel, extending up to the junction of the tendon and the muscle (c). Pillow under foot (b). Strips 2 and 3 are applied diagonally from the foot across the tendon (c). Side view of strips 1 and 3 (d). Strapping reinforced with parallel strips to bottom of foot (e). Diagram of strips as they originate on the sole of the foot (f).

they gain power. The question of stretched tendons regaining their original length is quite controversial. The prevalent feeling is that they do not ever shorten again once they have been stretched.

Tendons are injured in a number of ways: sprains, strains, contusions, and various inflammations such as tenosynovitis and tendinitis. Symptoms are pain, tenderness, swelling, and limitation of motion.

Contusions of tendons. History will reveal that the athlete has been kicked, stepped on, or has dropped a heavy object on his foot. Inspection will reveal swelling around the area, and limitation of motion will be present along the course of the tendon. Palpation will reveal the exact tendon involved and the intensity of the swelling.

Treatment consists of compression, ice, and elevation. If the contusion is on the top of the foot, do not tape around the foot because constriction will result, and profuse swelling will be evident along with much pain of pressure. The use of crutches may be necessary during the first 24 hours. On the second day the same procedure may be followed if swelling and tenderness has not subsided. On the third day the application of a mild heat with exercise will enhance the progress. Weight bearing should be gradual. The athlete should not be permitted to resume activities without proper padding (usually over the shoe) to prevent recurrence.

Tendon Achilles sprain. History will reveal the twist or wrench that caused the injury. Inspection must be thorough, since tendons may possibly be pulled away from the bone or separated from the muscle to which they are attached. Tendons that are pulled away from bone or torn at the attachment of the muscle must be handled by the team physician, since the decision as to the possible surgical intervention must be made at the earliest possible moment. Palpation will reveal the tightness due to spasm, the amount of swelling in the area, and the possibility of a rupture of the tendon.

Treatment of ruptured tendons, etc., must be handled by the team physician. Sprains and strains are treated with ice, elevation, and compression.

The seriousness of the injury will decide whether weight bearing is indicated or not. Severe swelling in the foot, caused by a contusion or sprain, is best relieved by the use of crutches for the first 24 hours at least. If swelling subsides, the use of heat and massage plus exercise may be started. Response is slow in tendon injuries,

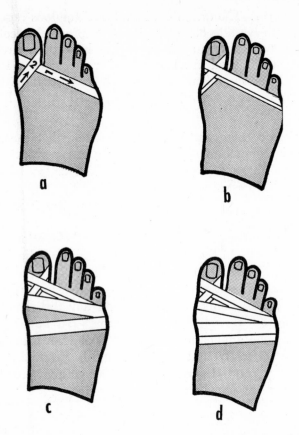

Strapping for sprain of great toe. Strips 1 and 2 cross over joint of toe (a). Additional layers of tape applied as needed (b). Support of foot included in toe strapping (c). Complete toe strapping (d).

and they should not be pushed. Proper early treatment will hasten absorption, and response to treatment of sprain or strain will be considerably better.

Tendon Achilles Strap

This strap is best applied with the athlete lying on his stomach. Place a pillow, etc., under the ankle of the leg affected. This will place the foot in the proper position, and the elevation will shorten the tendon Achilles so that it will be in the proper position for taping. (See p. 358)

Step 1. Use elastic tape; start under the foot, approximately in the middle of the long arch. Anchor the tape and then, with constant pressure, pull the tape over the heel and up the tendon Achilles for 8 inches.

Step 2. Start step 2 at the same area on the bottom of the foot and secure proper angle by practice; pull the tape across the heel and cross the tendon just above the bone. This strip will put pressure over the tendon where it is needed.

Step 3. On the opposite side of the heel, pull strip 3 over the same path as strip 2. This will cross over the tendon in the same position as strip 2.

Step 4. To hold the first three strips in place and to add further compression, the horizontal strips of the open-faced Gibney are used. Start at the base of the great toe and run parallel with the bottom of the foot; pull the tape around the heel and anchor at the base of the little toe. (This should be done with 1-inch tape only.)

Step 5. Overlapping halfway, the ensuing strips are to be added, completely encompassing the whole ankle. Anchor strip. To supplement the strapping further, a sponge-rubber heel can be used in the shoe. A piece of ½-inch sponge rubber can be used very effectively.

Sprain of Toes

Great toe. The great toe, owing to its location on the foot, is subject to many sprains. The mechanics of the injury are the same as for any sprain of a joint—abnormal motion. Forcing the toe to go beyond its normal limitations will cause a stretching of the ligaments and the capsule. Excessive pivoting will also cause a sprain to the great toe.

Treatment consists of strapping with a compression strap, ice packing and elevating. Whirlpool treatments are very effective in the treatment of this injury. Disability is from a few days to weeks.

Other toes. Again the mechanism is counter joint motion, forcing the toes to go beyond normal ranges. Kicking improperly or accidentally bumping into a leg of a chair will cause this injury.

Immediate treatment consists of strapping the toe to its neighbor and the application of ice packs to control hemorrhage. After the first 24 hours, whirlpool or hot soaks are very effective. Continue strapping until the athlete can tolerate full weight bearing. Disability lasts from a day to three or four.

Contusion of Foot. Bruises to the foot are primarily caused by being stepped on. If the athlete is stepped on by a cleated shoe, the bruise may be more painful than that of the basketball player who has been stepped on by someone wearing rubber shoes. The foot will be painful, and most of the bruises result in some degree of swelling. Disability may be limited, or the athlete may not be able to stand at all. Pain will be diffused for the first few hours and will localize to a specific point by the next day. History will reveal the incident.

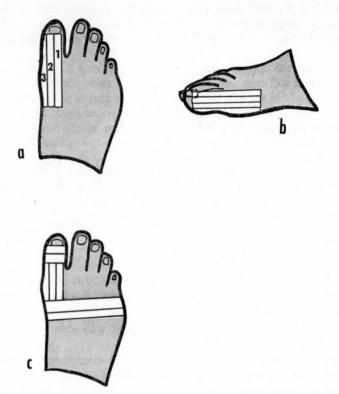

Alternate method of strapping great toes, sometimes called *bunion strapping*. Strips 1, 2, and 3 from the front of the toe extend over joint. Use as many as are needed to cover the joint completely (a). Side view of strips (b). Anchor strips applied to toe and foot for holding toe firm (c).

Examination of the bones of the foot should be made as soon as possible, and the tendons of the foot should also be observed. Swelling, which usually results in a few minutes, may disguise injury. Therefore the examination should be made as soon as possible. Inspection will reveal the "red" area where the blow was struck and also reveal swelling. Palpation will increase the tenderness, so should be very gentle.

Treatment consists of the immediate application of ice along with a compression strapping. (Care must be taken so as not to constrict by strapping too tightly.) Elevation will also be indicated. If there is any question of a possible fracture, the athlete should be given crutches to eliminate weight bearing. Examination the next day will reveal the extent of the swelling and the degree of injury. X-ray may be deemed necessary to rule out any bone injury. If swelling persists, the use of ice and compression should be continued along with crutch walking. On the third day heat and light exercise may be started.

Weight bearing with the crutches may be started at this time. The athlete is instructed to walk through the foot with most of the body weight supported by means of the crutches, gradually increasing the amount of weight bearing until full weight can be carried normally.

As soon as full weight bearing returns, the athlete will progress rapidly into jogging, running, etc. Cutting in and out may be delayed for a few days until all the soreness is gone. Wearing a toe pad will protect this area from further injury.

Disability varies with the degree of injury. Many athletes may return to activity the next day, while others may be disabled for three or four days to a week or longer.

GREAT TOE STRAPPING I

The athlete sits with his foot held at right angle and toe straight up in the air. (See p. 360)

Step 1. Use ½-inch tape; start under the great toe and pull the tape across the joint of the toe, ending on the outside of the foot.

Step 2. Starting from the opposite side of the toe and crossing strip 1 over the joint, continue around the foot and end on the outer border of the foot.

Step 3. Apply strip 3 the same as strip 1, overlapping at least halfway.

Step 4. Apply strip 4 the same as strip 2, overlapping at least halfway.

Step 5. Use 1-inch tape; encircle the foot. This tape is to be placed on the foot at an angle so as to conform with the change in contour of the foot. It should be continued until the front part of the foot is encased with tape.

GREAT TOE STRAPPING II

Apply this taping with the athlete sitting and his foot held at a right angle. Strips 1, 2, 3, and 4 are approximately 4 inches long and are pulled back from the toe to the foot. The degree of pull depends on the range of motion wanted in the great toe. A ½-inch tape is used for this strapping. (See p. 362)

An anchor strip is applied to the ends of the tape at the toe. 1-inch tape is used to anchor the strips on the foot. These strips should be applied snugly and should completely encircle the foot. They must be applied at an angle in order to conform to the shape of the foot.

Bursitis of Foot and Ankle. Bursae are sacs of fluid that underlie tissues, etc., to prevent friction. They are found between tendons and bone, between tendons and ligaments, etc., and are quite

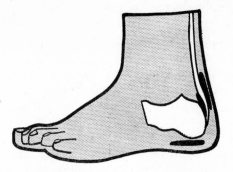

Bursae around the heel of the ankle. Darkened areas show bursae.

numerous around the foot and ankle. The bursa becomes inflamed and then swells, causing pain and limitation of motion. The chief cause of inflammation of a bursa is pressure, trauma, or excessive strain.

Diagnosis is made more by elimination than by any other method. Pain will be noticed first, followed by the disability. The history may or may not show a specific incident for diagnosis, but location and negative symptoms of sprain, etc., will help to diagnose this condition. The symptoms are tenderness and swelling (may be hard or soft). Heat, localized redness of skin, may be seen, or heat may be felt by placing hand or fingers over localized area. Limited motion, depending on the location and degree of inflammation,

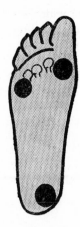

Tripod of foot. Weight bearing starts at the heel along the border of the foot and finally at the base of the great toe.

will exhibit loss of function. Pain is usually constant, and relief is not dramatic even with complete rest.

The cause is not easily determined because the athlete may not remember an injury, and since the condition may not become acute until some time after the incident, early treatment is not usually possible. However, excellent results are obtained from the use of ice to relieve pain and localized heat afterward, despite the necessity of delayed therapy. Strapping for immobilization is very helpful, along with felt pads for protection from further irritation. Diathermy, ultrasonic waves, and local mild heat are very effective.

Disability depends on the location and amount of tenderness; if athlete is able, there is no contraindication to continuing working out. If the treatments described above do not help the condition, and the injury becomes chronic, surgical removal of the bursa may be indicated.

Tenosynovitis of Tendon Achilles. This condition manifests itself in pain, disability, limping, and (on palpation) crepitus. Swelling will be localized over the tendon.

The tendon Achilles is enclosed in a tendon sheath that gives off a liquid (synovia) for lubricating the area between the sheath and the tendon. Irritation will cause symptoms of pain, swelling, and disability. Excessive activity, trauma, or strain (walking up a steep hill) will cause this irritation.

Inasmuch as this injury is not dramatic on onset, it is not usually seen immediately. The application of a compression strap, the open-face Gibney, is very effective, and a lift in the heel to lessen the excursion of the tendon is also effective. Whirlpool baths, diathermy, and ultrasonic waves are effective modalities in this injury. The complete absence of sports is also indicated. This injury is very slow to respond, and all efforts should be made to be sure that the injury is healed before the athlete returns to activity. The tendency to recur is quite prevalent in this condition. If seen early, three or four days of rest and treatment will be sufficient. However, if the injury is of a long duration (three or four days) before it is reported, the time will be greater, usually about two weeks.

Strapping may be eliminated when the athlete returns, but the use of a sponge in the heel should be continued for at least a month.

FLAT FOOT AND FOOT STRAIN

The size, shape, and contour of the feet do not indicate their strength and usefulness. There is no type of arch that may be considered normal. Some normal feet present a very low arch, whereas others present a very high arch. However, the foot that is abducted and everted (slew foot) is the type frequently seen with foot problems. Strains of the foot are rather common in athletics, and all sports contribute their share. Symptoms are pain, stiffness, and a certain degree of lameness. The point tenderness will be found over the bones of the foot, below the ankle bone, in the medial malleolus (inside ankle bone), and along the inner border of the foot. Cramps of the calf and bottom of the foot may also be noted.

If the condition is severe, bed rest is prescribed until pain and soreness subside. In the mild type, strapping with adhesive tape and heat treatments are very effective. The use of felt pads placed under the arch is also very effective. The athlete will have to get used to the padding, since it appears to add more pressure to the foot and feels strange. As soon as the felt molds to the foot, the athlete will be very comfortable. After the acute pain has subsided, exercises to strengthen the feet should be started. The continued use of the arch strapping may be indicated during the remainder of the playing season.

Flat Foot. Flat-foot conditions are not disqualifying in athletics. Some of the best runners that we have seen over the years have been extremely flat footed and very capable. This condition may be congenital or acquired. The congenital condition is not usually painful, whereas the acquired may have some tender areas that are readily relieved. The acquired condition may be of two types: the flexible type, which does not limit motion, or the rigid type, which is painful and disabling.

In the flexible type, where overweight is a problem, this should be handled first. Excessive weight will cause an aggravation of the flat foot by the tremendous demands put on it. Proper shoes and adequate conditioning of the athlete will also be necessary. In this condition, tolerance to work must be established. This is best accomplished by working for short times and gradually increasing the time as tolerance permits. Excessive strain will aggravate a flat-foot condition. Rigid flat-foot conditions are very hard to handle and should be placed in the hands of the team physician. We do not see too many of these conditions in athletics because they are not primarily athletic problems. However, manipulations, etc., are very helpful if performed by skilled hands.

Treatment of the acute flat-foot condition is very similar to that for strain of the foot. Strapping, heat, and exercises comprise the procedure. Exercise with the idea of overcoming flat-foot conditions is not very promising. Such exercises are intended to strengthen the feet and not to correct congenital condition. The use of felt pads as arch supports is recommended, as is the use of a permanent appliance for daily use. Proper shoes and walking habits are also necessary. Exercises are listed elsewhere for arch strength. Walking with the toes inward should be practiced by the athlete whenever possible, even to the extent of an exaggerated pigeon-toed stance. Excessive walking in this manner may lead to cramps of the foot, and therefore the athlete should be instructed to stop when he feels the cramp coming on.

NORMAL GAIT

The development of a normal gait after injury should be considered a very important part of the treatment of the ankle. If the normal gait cannot be regained, the athlete should be placed on crutches until he has achieved it. Walking with the toes to the side will not help repair an ankle; it leads to bad habits that may be difficult to overcome. Insist that the athlete walk with the toes straight ahead, and follow through with the normal roll of the foot. In this manner the damaged tissues will be strengthened; otherwise they will atrophy, and the result will be a more difficult rehabilitation problem. In the beginning, the athlete will have to work hard at this, since the normal tendency after an injury to the ankle is to evert the foot and walk with a stiff ankle. Walking will have to be slowed considerably to loosen gradually so that the ankle does not impede normal walking.

GENERAL FOOT CONDITIONS

Injury to Toenails. Injuries to toenails must include the subungual hematoma. This is a condition that results in blood under the nail. It is caused by being stepped on or by some other outside blow to the top of the toe. Blood "pools" under the nail cause much pressure and pain. Drilling a hole in the nail to release the blood will give immediate relief. A nail drill or a sharp knife blade (sterile) can be used for this.

Care must be taken to eliminate the possibility of infection. Sterile dressing must be applied daily, and if necessary, hot soaks to the toe will lessen the possibility of infection. The loss of the nail will result when a large subungual hematoma occurs. It is better to let nature run its course, by waiting for the nail to come off of its own accord. Strapping the nail down with adhesive tape to prevent sock irritation is necessary and should be used until the nail falls off.

Corns. Corns are caused by improperly fitting shoes. Friction causes an irritation to the skin, the skin in turn sets its protective mechanism in action, and the result is a callus and then a corn. Corns may be protected by adhesive felt cut in the form of a life saver to circle the area and keep pressure off the corn. By eliminating the pressure, the corn disappears. Cutting corns with a razor blade, etc., is risky and may lead to infection. Strong salicylic acid dressing will help to kill and soften the corn. Many of these preparations are available, and the team physician can prescribe the best preparation. Proper fitting of shoes will eliminate this condition. To cut off the corn and continue to use the same shoes will only produce another corn. Have the shoes stretched or use other shoes that fit properly.

Soft Corns. Soft corns usually occur between the fourth and fifth toes and are the result of too close approximation, resulting in a painful mass between the toes. Dampness, pressure, or overgrowth of bone will cause this condition. Treatment consists of drying well between the toes and applying a 10 per cent solution of silver nitrate daily. The toes should then be kept spread apart to allow for air to dry the area. The use of lambs' wool or felt to

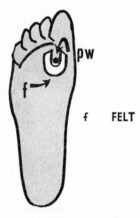

f   FELT

PLANTAR WART

Protection for plantar wart, shaped in the form of a horseshoe. Weight is borne on the felt rather than on the wart.

keep toes separated will help. Should this fail, the team physician will prescribe more effective treatments.

Plantar Warts. These are often described as being like an iceberg, where the visible part of the wart resembles a small seed wart and the bulk is below the surface. Paring off the surface may give some temporary relief, but the wart continues to become enlarged under the skin. The cause of these conditions is not completely known, but experience shows that irritation from improper shoes and faulty mechanics of the foot result in a plantar wart. The use of felt in the form of a horseshoe will relieve pain and in many instances will result in the disappearance of the wart. Use of the dessicants, such as used for corns, will also help. Keeping the wart soft with an oil also has some merit. If conservative methods do not give satisfactory results, electrocautery may be used by the team physician.

Calluses. Calluses are caused by friction and irritation. Causes vary from improperly fitting shoes to the type of activity the athlete participates in. The basketball player who must stop and start, change directions, etc., will be seen with calluses on the balls of his feet. Callus is necessary, to a degree, in this sport, but too much callus acts as a pebble in the shoe and is very irritating. If the callus is allowed to grow large, it will pull away from the skin and a very painful blister will result. The daily filing of the callus with an emery board will help to prevent the overproduction of the callus. The use of petroleum jelly or some other lubricant will help to soften the callus and lessen the pain. Felt pads on the ball of the foot will eliminate much of this trouble. A piece of $\frac{1}{16}$-inch adhesive felt, cut 2 inches by 3 inches, applied across the ball of the foot for practices and games, will lessen the degree of callus formed.

Ingrown Toenails. An ingrown toenail occurs when the nail grows into the soft tissues of the toe, on either side, or both. The nail digs into the soft tissue, and with each step taken, the irritation becomes an open wound. This wound is very susceptible to infection and results in a very painful and disabling condition. Causes are variable, from improper fitting of socks and shoes to improper nail hygiene (particularly improper cutting of the nails). When this condition starts, the use of hot soaks and the introduction of a wedge of cotton between the nail and the skin will prevent infection and will force the nail to grow normally. In cases of severe ingrown toenail, surgery may be indicated.

Heel. Injuries to the heel are very common in athletics, ranging from a simple bruise to a fracture of the heel. Fractures of the heel are very rare and can be detected by X-ray. Treatment consists of immobilization and rest. Disability caused by fractures of the heel is prolonged, and a season is usually lost with this injury.

Other conditions in the area of the heel involve the tendon Achilles and the bursae of the heel. Bone bruises are very common and present a very aggravating injury even though not serious. If the plantar surface of the bone is bruised, the athlete cannot walk. However, he soon finds that when he runs, there is no pain or discomfort. This is a very common injury on track, particularly with the jumpers and hurdlers. With the introduction of the heel cup (made of fiber glass), the number of heel bruises has lessened.

Treatment for bruised heel is rest and heat. The whirlpool is very effective for this injury. A heel pad made of ½-inch sponge rubber worn in the shoe will lessen the shock on the heel when walking.

Upper heel disability. Pain around the heel (upper portion) may be caused by the tendon Achilles or the bursae of the tendon. The condition may be due to pressure or constant strain in the area. Improper lacing of shoes (too tight) or wrinkles in socks, plus unevenness of counter of shoe, may be the source of the pressure over the heel. Treatment consists of rest and heat to the area. The use of a pad in the heel will lessen the excursion of the tendon and limit the strain at the attachment. Correction of the mechanical cause must be carried out.

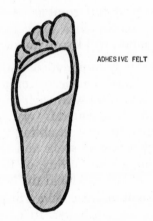

ADHESIVE FELT

Adhesive felt is placed on the ball of the foot to prevent friction. This is used extensively in basketball to eliminate blisters.

SIMPLE ORTHO DIRECTIONS FOR
HEEL CUP

Step 1. With athlete lying on stomach and foot in repose, draw an outline of the proposed appliance with a skin-marking pencil. For a complete heel cup, this outline should be approximately 3 inches long and 1½ inches in depth.

Step 2. Apply a thin coating of petroleum jelly and talc to the heel. This ensures easy removal of the plaster impression. Use quick-drying plaster-of-paris splints and make a cast of the entire heel surface. Wet a single strip of plaster splint and apply it to the body. Smooth it out flat with a rubbing action. Continue in this manner until the heel surface is covered. Apply a second layer at right angles to the first layer. Drying time is 15 minutes.

Step 3. If available, paint a coating of 50 per cent water glass (sodium silicate) solution on the inner impression surface to ensure separation of the stone model from the plaster impression. Mix artificial stone (100 parts powder to 22–25 parts water) for best results. Pour mixture into plaster cast. Insert tube or rod into center for ease of handling after drying. This is the model on which to build heel cup.

Step 4. Cut Ortho-Net No. 162* to pattern, outlining cutting margin with masking tape to prevent raveling when cutting and laminating. Four layers of cloth are sufficient for most heel cups.

Step 5. Draw an outline of the proposed appliance on the stone model with indelible pencil. This will transfer to laminate for trimming guide.

Step 6. Cover stone model with Ortho-Fre or petroleum jelly to facilitate removal of laminated appliance.

Step 7. *Wear rubber gloves* during this and all subsequent operations. Weigh or measure by volume four parts Ortho-Bond A and one part Ortho-Bond B. (For a heel cup, 100 grams of A to 25 grams of B is sufficient.) Use a paper cup or any disposable container for mixing resins. This saves a clean-up job.

Step 8. Apply a generous layer of the mixed liquid resin on the stone model. Place a first layer of cloth on the resin and work the resin up through the cloth. If any white spots appear, raise the cloth, add more resin, and again work up through the cloth to total wetting. Add resin and cloth in the above manner until the appliance is built to desired thickness. Ortho-Net may be cut and overlapped for fitting at heel base.

Step 9. Allow the assembly to remain at room temperature for 6 to 8 hours, or overnight. To speed up the cure, place the assembly under infrared heat lamps immediately upon completion of laminating procedure. Be sure lamps are 12 to 15 inches above laminate. Inspect in about 15 minutes. Excessive heat will discolor appliance. Cure is complete in about 1½ to 2 hours, when heat is used.

Step 10. Remove appliance from model by prying gently around edges with a screw driver or other suitable tool.

* Manufactured by Vernon-Benshoff Co., P.O. Box 1587, Pittsburgh 30, Pa.

Step 11. Trim appliance to size. Sand edges. Remove Ortho-Fre or petroleum jelly from inner surface and wash with soap and water.

Crutch Walking. To suggest that an athlete use crutches and then not tell him how to use them is obviously negligent. Proper fitting and instruction is very necessary. Adjustable crutches should be an integral part of every athletic set-up. To properly fit the crutches, there are two very effective ways:

1. Subtract 18 inches from the height of the athlete.
2. While the athlete is standing, measure from under the arms to 8 inches to the side of his foot.

Rubber tips as well as padding for the under arm area and hand grips should be part of the crutches.

The crutches are placed under the arm, held by the hands at the grip, and placed on the floor about 18 inches ahead of the body. The body is swung through, landing on the "good" leg. The crutches should be planted and stable on the ground before the body weight is transferred. If the crutches slip and the patient falls, many complications may aggravate a painful injury. Therefore care and safety must be practiced.

Appendix A

Sports Trainer's Equipment

Training Room and Equipment

The training room should be isolated from the locker room, if possible, but accessible to all athletes. It should be a special room and used only for the treatment of injuries. The room should be well lighted and ventilated (preferably an outside wall with windows) and painted with a light color to make the room bright and cheerful. Washable paints are very important to the cleanliness of the room. The floor should be of tile or a similar product for ease in cleaning. Extra electrical wall plugs and proper voltage facilities should be a part of the wiring set up. A sink for washing hands should be accessible. Drains for whirlpool and floor scouring should be included in the plans for a good training room.

A wall cabinet that can be locked is recommended. A refrigerator for ice is a very economical piece of equipment. (To buy ice every day is expensive and quite troublesome; also, the ice purchased the day before the need arises may not be available.) Waste cans for the disposal of used dressings, strappings, etc., should have covers.

Hooks on the wall or costumers are necessary for hanging clothes while treatments are given.

A desk or table with chair should be part of the equipment of the room together with a file cabinet for reports and the keeping of records.

A bench or chairs are necessary for those who may be waiting their turn; stools are also excellent for athletes who may be "baking" their shoulders or arms or who are taking whirlpool treatments.

Field Kit

The field kit is a very necessary piece of equipment to have on road trips. Many trainers work out of their pockets, but at times their pockets need replenishing and then the kit plays a very important role. The most common articles found in a trainer's kit are:

1. Thermometer (may be necessary while on trip or used on direction of team physician).
2. Scissors.
3. Eye cup and eye wash (to wash cinders, etc., from eye).
4. Sling (for arm and shoulder injuries).
5. Tourniquet (may be a piece of rubber tubing or a purchased tourniquet).
6. Alcohol, a very effective antiseptic or for a light rub.
7. Razor and blades, to prepare skin for taping, etc.
8. Safety pins, used in case of torn clothes and to hold sling in place.

9. Sterile pads wrapped in glassine bags.
10. Gauze roller bandage for holding dressings in place or to use under ankle strappings, etc.
11. Skin toughener, used before strapping with adhesive, may be tincture of benzoin or derivative.
12. Powder for massage or to prevent friction on feet, etc.
13. Ammonia capsules to aid in restoring unconscious athlete.
14. Aspirin, for relief of headache.
15. Oil of cloves to ease pain in tooth until dental care can be had.
16. Cotton, both sterile and unsterile; sterile for cleansing wounds and the unsterile for "hot packs."
17. Applicators for antiseptics, etc.
18. Elastic bandages for compression and support.
19. Petroleum jelly for ointment dressings.
20. Analgesic balm, counterirritant for use in "hot packs."
21. Surgical soap for cleaning wounds, such as cinder burns in track.
22. Salt tablets used in the prevention of dehydration.
23. Adhesive tape in various widths for strappings, etc.
24. Tongue depressors for use in applying ointments or splint to the fingers, etc.
25. Ice bag for the application of ice to acute injury.

The type of bag will depend on the individual and the amount of equipment to be carried. Metal bags are very popular and very durable and roomy. Plastic bottles are very light and will not break and are recommended for field kits. If the bag is of a good size, basswood splints may be placed on the bottom for accessibility.

Many small items can be carried in the bag. These will depend on the sport in season. For example, fingernail clippers should be available for wrestlers, and so on. A toe nail clipper will save wear and tear on scissors and is a very handy piece of equipment.

Various thicknesses of sponge rubber may also be needed for some sports, as will rosin for the ball-handling sports.

The field kit should be checked daily and replacements made when needed.

The phone numbers of the ambulance service, hospital, and members of the medical staff may be written on tape and applied to the inside of the field kit for reference in emergency.

TRAINING ROOM EQUIPMENT FOR THREE TYPES OF BUDGETS

Equipment and Uses	A*	B*	C*
Massage tables for treatments and taping. The size of the ideal training table is 23 inches wide, 6 feet 6 inches long by 30 inches high. The top should extend at least 3 inches over the frame at each end and should be padded and covered with canvas.	X	X	X
Diathermy machine. Excellent for treatment of sprains, pulled muscles, etc.	X	X	
Ultrasonics. Treatments as directed by team physician.	X		
Whirlpool bath. Excellent for heat and massage at the same time. Use in sprains, strains, etc.	X	(A)	
Heat lamps. Infrared, radiant heat. Use when you wish a surface heat.	X	(B)	(C)
Paraffin bath. Excellent for fingers and toes, ankles, knees, wrists, etc.	X	X	X
Scales and weight charts. Daily weights should be recorded before and after each practice.	X	X	X
Salt tablet dispenser. Use for the prevention of dehydration and heat exhaustion.	X	(D)	(E)
Field kit. Necessary for use outside the training room and on trips.	X	X	X
Ankle wraps. For the prevention of ankle injuries. These may be purchased in rolls, then cut to length.	X	X	X
Disinfectant. For lockers and training room floor. Training room should be cleaned every day.	X	X	X
Adhesive tape. Use for prevention and treatment of injuries.	X	X	X
Gauze. Use under strappings and to hold dressings.	X	X	X
Sterilized pads in individual bags. Handy for dressings.	X	X	X
Small dressings for minor cuts. Gauze and adhesive combinations.	X	X	X
Thermometer. When in doubt use, or call a physician.	X	X	X
Tweezers.	X		
Scissors.	X	X	X
Nail clippers. Long fingernails are dangerous. If one should break off, much pain may result. Cut nails short.	X		
Applicators (wood). Use to make swabs for application of medicants.	X	X	
Stretcher. Players who have been injured should not be dragged or lugged from the field.	X	X	X
Sponge rubber. Use to prevent and protect injuries. ¼, ½, ¾ inch thick.	X	X	X
Felt. Use to prevent and protect injuries.	X		

Col. A. For unlimited budget.
Col. B. For limited budget
Col. C. For small budget.

(A) Buckets may be filled with hot water, towels dipped into them and then placed on the injury.
(B) Heat lamps, large or small. Mild heat for a longer period of time is better than intense heat for a short period.
(C) Home-made heat lamps.
(D) Salt tablets.
(E) Salt tablets or a very liberal amount of table salt used at meals.
(F) Towels with ice.

Training Room Equipment for Three Types of Budgets (*cont'd*)

Equipment and Uses	A°	B°	C°
Heat pads. Electric three-way switch type. Use after hemorrhage has stopped. Chemical heat pads are very satisfactory and better to use on trips.	X	X	X
Ice bags. For immediate application of ice at the time of the injury.	X	X	(F)
Tongue blades. For examining the throat and to apply ointments.	X	X	
Epsom salts. Excellent for hot water treatment.	X	X	X
Tape remover. It is important that you use a fluid that is non-inflammable. Ether is highly inflammable. Carbon tetrachloride is very good.	X	X	X
Collodion. Use cotton and collodion for small dressings on the face.	X	X	X
Cotton. Use sterilized cotton for the cleansing of wounds. Use it also for the base of pressure wraps.	X	X	X
Corn and bunion pads. For relief of corns and bunions, and also for protection for small injuries. Use under tape.	X		
Rosin. Use on hands to prevent fumbling. Liquid or paste forms also available.	X	X	X
Elastic bandages. For compression over site of injury.	X		
Analgesic balm. Excellent for heat. Is a counterirritant. Use on bruises, contusions, sprains, pulled muscles, etc.	X	X	
Hot liniments. May be made by using mineral oil as a base, adding oil of wintergreen, etc.	X		
Lubricants for massage. Mineral oil, olive oil, cold cream, etc. Use as a lubricant only.	X		
Powders. Foot powder for sweating feet. For reduction of friction. Excellent in shoes and socks.	X		
Benzoin, compound tincture. Use to toughen skin, also as base for tape. Prevents tape rash.	X	X	X
General. Ammonia capsules for restorative. Aspirin for relief from headache and pains. Surgical soap for cleansing of wounds (very fine for removal of cinders after track injury). Oil of cloves for relief of toothache. Petroleum jelly, prevents dressings from adhering to wounds. Calamine lotion for prickly heat and other rashes. Ethyl chloride, an anesthetic for use in removal of splinters. Boric acid solution for washing eyes.	X		
Ointments. Whitfield's ointment for gym itch. Zinc ointment, soothing and healing.	X		
Butesin picrate. Antiseptic and anesthetic. Use on burns, especially lime burns.	X		
Antiseptics. Alcohol. Use recommended drugs only. See team physician.	X		
Adhesive felt. ⅛, 1⁄16. Padding for blisters, ball of feet and arches, etc.	X	X	
Crutches. Adjustable, for acute leg injuries.	X	X	X
Splints. Ready-made, such as Thomas rings for leg and arm; boards (1 x 4) in different lengths, padded with cotton, will work very well.	X	X	X
Elastic adhesive. For extra support and compression. Excellent for knee and rib strappings.	X	X	
Weights. For rehabilitation of knee, etc. Boot, bar, and discs. Total 100 pounds.	X	X	
Ankle wrap roller. To roll up ace bandages and ankle wraps.	X	X	

Appendix B

Trainer's Talk to Squads

At the beginning of each sports season, the trainer should outline the methods of operation and also the functions of the various services available. The following is an example of a talk to a football squad; it can be easily adapted for other sports.

Meal Schedule

During the early days of practice when double sessions are in order, meal schedules must be observed. Eating too close to practice presents a problem to the athlete; therefore he must adhere to time schedule. Breakfast is stressed and every athlete is awakened and sent to dining room to partake of this important meal. Breakfast is served at 7:30 A.M., lunch at 12:30 P.M., and the evening meal is set for 6:00 P.M.

Practice Schedules

The early practice is set at 9:30 A.M. and is over at 11:30 A.M. Afternoon sessions are held at 3:15 P.M. and end at 5:00 P.M. When classes begin and one practice a day is scheduled, it starts at 4:30 P.M. and ends at 6:25 P.M. Schedules of the practice sessions and their contents are always posted so that the athlete will know what is on the program and what is expected of him that day.

Physical Examinations

Time and place of examination is announced. All athletes are required to have a complete physical examination and a final review of findings is made by the team physician.

Medical Coverage

The introduction of the team physician and the athletic doctor is made, and the schedule of hours when he will be available at the Department of Health is announced. The team physician is on the field and available at all practices of the football squad.

Taping

Taping for protection, etc., is performed before the practice, and the athletes are advised of times that this must be done so that they will not be late for practices. The training room is open at all times so that this may be done.

Blisters

In early practices, especially after a very easy summer, blisters may present a problem. Foot powder is available in the locker rooms, and the athlete is advised to use this freely in his shoes and his socks. At the first sign of a blister, the athlete must let us know so that a protective pad can be applied. Do not wait until the blister is fully formed before seeking help. Athletes are advised to stop play and see trainer on the field at first sign of discomfort. Blisters are easier to prevent then they are to treat; early treatment also enhances recovery.

Salt Tablets

To replenish the salt that is lost through perspiration and to prevent heat exhaustion, salt tablet dispensers filled with 15 grain enteric-coated tablets are placed by all water fountains. Instructions as to the amount needed to replenish daily losses are announced. In individual cases the team physician will prescribe specific amounts to be taken. Routine prescription is two tablets after each work out with a glass of water.

Equipment

Equipment is issued and checked for fit, etc. Athletes must hang up this equipment after each work-out. Any equipment found on the benches or floor is picked up, and the athlete will have to draw equipment to replace that which has been returned to equipment room. Damage to equipment must be reported after each practice session so that repairs or replacements can be made. "White stuff" is placed in a bin and is issued on the "honor system." Soiled "white stuff" is laundered daily, and the athlete draws clean equipment every day. After use, the equipment is placed in a laundry bag which is located in accessible places in the locker room. Towels are placed by the shower room, and after use, they are to be placed in a hamper so that they may also be laundered. White stuff consists of socks, T-shirt, supporter, and underdrawers, and the athlete is responsible for placing the soiled equipment in the laundry bags supplied for this purpose.

Helmets are worn throughout the practice session; at no time is the athlete permitted to place helmet on ground. If his helmet is not on his head, it must be in his hand. The policy of taking the helmet off and placing on the ground in early practice increases the injury potential of a team mate stepping in helmet, thus injuring himself. By past experience this is a must with all football players at Yale because a very unnecessary injury was incurred by an athlete who stepped on a helmet and broke a leg, thus ending his athletic career. A similar incident occurred in basketball when an athlete stepped on a basketball that was adrift. All basketballs that are not in use must be placed on the rack or placed in a box provided for this purpose.

Weight Chart

It is very necessary to weigh out and in every day. Weigh in supporter only. A manager will be on hand to see that all athletes weigh and that the correct weights are marked on the chart. The weight chart is also used for attendance purposes.

Travel

A policy adopted at Yale a few years ago in reference to team travel states that the team goes as a unit and must return as one. "Staying over" in locations of play is not allowed. The coaches are charged with the responsibility of the safety, etc., of the athlete when he takes the athlete off the campus; therefore he must see that the athlete is returned to the campus and not allowed to remain at the site visited.

Missing Practice

There may be times when the athlete will be forced to miss practice for reasons other than illness or injury. The athlete is responsible to the coach for notifying him of absence from a practice. If at all possible, the athlete is requested to make other plans so that he will not miss the needed practice.

Leaving Field Without Permission

Do not leave the field without permission; the coaches must know where the athlete is at all times during the practice session. If the athlete is sent in by trainer, doctor, etc., this is reported to the coach so that the whereabouts of athlete will be known. Leaving practice early for any reason should be worked out in advance of practice so that arrangements can be made for a substitution.

Running While on Field

Time on the field is very short and the most must be made of the time available. Running between drills and different areas is required at all practices. Walking between drills only loses time and promotes a lazy athlete. Run, do not walk, from area to area.

Training Table

School policy requires the athlete to wear coat and tie to all meals. This is required at the training table as well as the school dining rooms. Conduct of athlete is very important at the table. Horseplay, etc., will not be tolerated in the dining room or at the training table.

Valuables

Do not bring valuables to the locker room. To do so is only inviting trouble. If it is necessary that valuables be brought to the area, be sure to put them in the valuables box. Manager will see that the box is placed under lock and key. Valuables will be picked up by the manager and he is responsible to see that they are returned to the athlete. Any valuables left in the box are brought to training table where they are claimed by the owner.

Drinking and Smoking

There is no place in the athletic program for an athlete who drinks or smokes. Both are harmful and are very detrimental to an athlete. Offenses will be dealt with severely.

Index

Abdomen, injuries of, 173, 174
  contusion of, 173
  ilium, crest of, 173
  pelvic girdle, 173
Abduction, 178
Abductor pollicis longus muscle, 233
Abrasions, treatment of, 77, 78
  face, 153
Abscess, 74
Acromioclavicular joint, injury of
  mild, 201
  moderate, 202, 203
  severe, 203–6
  strappings for, 197, 199, 206
Acromion process
  contusion, 210–12
  fracture, 192, 193
Active exercise, 139
Adam's apple, 157
Adduction, 178
Adductor brevis muscle, 188
Adductor longus muscle, 189
Adductor magnus muscle, 189
Adhesion, 62
Adhesive taping, 99–102; *see also* Strap-
    pings, adhesive
  fundamentals, 100
  preparations for, 101
  purposes of, 100
  removing, 101
  sensitivity to, 101
Ammonia inhalant, 99
Amnesia, 146
Amphetamines, use of, 94
Ankle
  anatomy of, 331, 332
  contusion of, 350
  dislocation of, 340, 341
  fractures of, 335, 336
  functional tests, 333–35
  sprains, 341–50
Appendicitis, 88, 89
Arches, foot, 332, 333
  exercises, 353
  longitudinal, 351, 352
  metatarsal, 353–55

Arm
  forearm, injuries of
    contusions, 228, 229
    fractures, 227, 228
  muscles of
    abductor pollicis longus, 233
    brachialis, 232
    extensor pollicis longus, 233
    flexor carpi radialis, 232
    flexor carpi ulnaris, 232, 233
    flexor pollicis longus, 233
    palmaris longus, 233
    pronator quadratus, 232
    pronator teres, 232
  upper, injuries of
    contusions, 226
    fractures (humerus), 225
    myositis ossificans, 226, 227
    strains, 225, 226
Arterial bleeding, 69, 70
  pressure points, 71
Arteries
  brachial, 71
  carotid, 71
  femoral, 71
  maxillary, 71
  subclavian, 71
  temporal, 71
Aspiration, 308
Athlete's foot, 84
Athletic injuries; *see* Injuries, athletic
Atlas, 158
Atrophy, 60
Axis, 158

Back
  injuries of, 161–67
    disqualification for athletics, 19
    functional tests for and interpreta-
      tion of, 163
    sprains, 161–67
  muscles of
    erector spinae, 186
    latissimis dorsi, 185, 186
    levator scapulae, 186
    rhomboids, 185, 214
    trapezius, 184, 185

Biceps brachii muscle, 220
  injury of, 220
Biceps femoris muscle, 279, 280
  injury of, 279, 280
Bleeding, types of, 69
  arterial, 69, 70
  capillary oozing, 69
  venous, 69
Blisters, 79, 80, 81
Boils, 75
Bone bruise, 61
Bone spur, 64
Brachial artery, 71
Brachialis muscle, 232
  injury of, 232
Brachioradialis muscle, 229, 230
  injury of, 229, 230
Brain, concussion of, 148–50
Broken teeth, 154, 155
Bursitis
  elbow, 242, 243
  foot and ankle, 363, 364, 365
  knee, 322, 323
  shoulder, 212, 213
  trochanter (hip), 177
Buttocks
  injury of, 168
  muscles of
    gluteus maximus, 187
    gluteus medius, 187
    gluteus minimus, 187

Calisthenics, 55, 56
Callus, 81, 82, 369
Calories, 30
  requirements of, 30
Capillary oozing, 69
Capsicum, 137
Capsule, joint, 121
Carbohydrates, 28
Carbuncles, 76
Carotid artery, 71
Cauliflower ear, 152
Cellulitis, 75
Charley horse, 125
Chewing gum, 92, 93
Chip fracture, 250
Cinder burns, 78
Circuit training, 46
Circulation, 122
Circumduction, 334
Clavicle, 190
Coccyx, injury of, 182
Cold applications, 126, 127
  ice bags, 127
  immersion, 127

Cold, common, 65
Collodion, 153
Coma, result of head injury, 147
Compression, 127
  bandage, 124
Concussion, brain, 148–50
Conditioning; see Physical conditioning
Conjunctivitis, 67
Consciousness, loss of, 146, 147, 148, 149
Contact lenses, 103
Contractures, 61
Contrast baths, 135, 136
Contusion of
  abdomen, 173
  ankle, 350, 359
  back, 167
  buttocks, 168
  chest, 173
  ear, 152
  elbow, 240, 241
  face, 150, 151, 152
  foot, 361, 362
  forearm, 228, 229
  head, 150, 151, 152
  heel, 62, 63, 64
  hip, 177
  ilium, crest of, 190
  kidney, 168, 169
  knee, 320, 321, 322
  lower leg, 275, 276
  neck, 157
  scrotum, 98
  shoulder, 210, 212
  thigh, 267–70
  throat, 157
  upper arm, 226
  wrist and hand, 255, 256, 257
Convulsion, result of head injury, 147
Coordination, 44
Corns, 368
Counterirritant, 137
Cramps, 95
Crepitus, 105
Crest of ilium, 173
  contusion of, 190
  strapping, 181
  treatment, 180
Cruciate ligaments of knee, 313–15
Crutch walking, 372
Cysts, 86
  pilonidal, 86
  sebaceous, 86

Deltoid muscle, 216, 217
  injury of, 216, 217
Dermatitis, groin, 85, 86

Dermis, 80
Diabetes, disqualification for athletics, 19
Diagnosis, steps in, 104, 105
Diaphragm, 184
Diathermy, 130, 131
Diet in athletics, 28–39
    calories, 30
        requirements, 30
    carbohydrates, 28
    crash diets, 38
    fats, 28
    food fads, 32
    gaining weight, 37
    menus, 34–36
    nutrition, 28–30
    pregame meal, 37
    proteins, 28
    reduction of weight, 37
Dislocations, 117–20
    acromioclavicular joint, 201–6
    ankle, 340–41
    compound, 120
    elbow, 237, 238
    factors in diagnosing, 118, 119
    fingers, 250
    hip, 175
    jaw, 145, 146
        reduction of, 145, 146
    knee, 294, 295
    neck, 155, 156
    phalanges (toes), 341
    shoulder, 194–201
    simple, 119, 120
    sternal clavicular, 206–8
    thumb, 250
    wrist, 249
Disorientation, result of head injury, 147
Disqualifications, physical, for athletics,
    17, 19, 20
Dizziness, 72

Ear, contusion of, 152
Eccymosis, 72
Elbow
    anatomy, 234–36
    bursitis, 242, 243
    contusion, 240, 241
    dislocation, 237, 238
    fractures, 237
    functional tests, 236, 237
    golfer's elbow, 243
    hyperextension, 239
    myositis ossificans, 243, 244
    sprain, 238, 239, 240
Endurance, 42, 43
Epidermis, 79

Epilepsy, disqualification for athletics, 19
Epiphysis, injuries of, 117, 340
Epistaxis, 154
Equipment, athletic, 102, 103
    contact lenses, 103
    mouthpieces, 103
Erector spinae muscle, 186
    injury of, 186
Erythema, 129
Eversion, 334
Exercise, 138, 139
    active, 139
    active assistive, 139
    active resistive, 139
    passive, 138
Extensor digitorum longus, 284
    injury of, 284
Extensor hallucis longus, 282
    injury of, 282
Extensor pollicis longus, 233
    injury of, 233
Eye
    conjunctivitis, 67
    foreign body in, 66
    lime in, 67
    pupil reaction, 147, 148, 149
    sty, 67

Face
    abrasions, 153
    fractures, 144
Faintness, 72
Faradic current, 133
Fat pad, pinched, 322
Fats, 28
Felt, adhesive, 81
Femoral artery, 71
Femur, 260–62
Fiberglass, 62
Fibrin, 62
Fibroblasts, 64
Fibrocartilage, 158
Fibula, 112
Fingers
    dislocations, 250
    fractures, 248–50
    mallet, 257, 258
    nails, 258, 259
        contusion, 258
Flat foot, 365–67
Flexion, 333
Flexor carpi radialis, 233
Flexor carpi ulnaris, 233
Flexor digitorum longus, 285
Flexor hallucis longus, 284
Flexor pollicis longus, 233

Folliculitis, 83
Food fads, 32
Foot
  anatomy, 350, 351
  arches
    exercises, 353–55
    longitudinal, 351, 352
    metatarsal, 353–55
  bone spur, 64
  calluses, 369
  contusions, 359, 361, 362
  corns, 368, 369
  crutch walking, 372
  dislocation of phalanges, 341
  flat, 365–67
  fractures
    great toe, 338, 339
    march, 339
    metatarsals, 338
    phalanges, 338
    sprain, 339
  heel bruise, 370
  ingrown toenails, 369
  normal gait, 367
  plantar warts, 368, 369
  sprain of toes, 361
  tendon injuries, 357–61
  toenail injuries, 367
Foot in axilla, 196
Forearm
  contusions, 228, 229
  fractures, 227, 228
Fractures
  acetablum, 176
  ankle, 335–36
  carpals, 247
  clavicle, 191
  colles, 246, 247
  elbow, 237
  face, 144
  femur (lower end), 292, 293
  fibula, 271, 272
  fibula (ankle), 337
  fibula (upper end), 293
  forearm
    radius, 227, 228
    ulna, 227, 228
  great toe, 338, 339
  handling of, 107, 108
  humerus, 193, 225
  ilium, crest of, 175
  jaw, 144
  march, 339
  metatarsals, 247, 248, 338
  neck, 155
  nose, 145

patella, 293, 294
pelvis, 174, 175
phalanges (fingers), 248, 249
phalanges (toes), 338
Pott's, 336
ribs, 170, 171
scapula, 191
  acromion process, 192, 193
  body, 191, 192
  corocoid process, 193
  glenoid fossa, 193
  spine, 192
spine
  compression, 160
  transverse processes, 160
splinting, 110-17
  arm, 114, 115
  fingers, 116
  foot and toes, 111
  leg, 112, 113, 114
  pelvis, 117
  spine, 110
sprain fracture (ankle), 339
sternum, 170
stress (lower leg), 272, 273
symptoms, 110
tarsus, 337, 338
thigh (femur), 260–62
thumb, 248
tibia
  lower end, 336, 337
  shaft, 271
  upper end, 293
types of, 108–9
  comminuted, 108
  compound, 108
  greenstick, 109
  impacted, 109
  simple, 109
Friction, 137
Functional tests for
  ankle, 333–35
  back (low), 163
  elbow, 236, 237
  groin, 178
  knee, 295–300
  shoulder, 200, 201
  thigh, 265, 266
Fungi, 84, 85
Furuncle, 75

Galvanism, 133
Ganglion, 88
Gastrocnemius muscle, 281
  injury of, 281
Gibney ankle strapping, 344

Gluteus maximus muscle, 187
Gluteus medius muscle, 187
Gluteus minimus muscle, 187
Golfer's elbow, 243
Gracilis muscle, 279
Grass drills, 47
Groin
    functional tests, 178
    muscles, 188–90
        adductor brevis, 188
        adductor longus, 188
        adductor magnus, 189, 190
        iliacus, 189
        psoas major, 189
    spica bandage for, 179
    strains, 177–79
    treatment, 178

Half time relaxation, 94, 95
Hamstring, 264
Hand; see also Fingers
    contusions, 255, 256
    fractures, 247, 248
    strapping, 253
    wounds, 257
Harness, shoulder, 204
Head
    concussion, 148–50
    headache, 65, 147–49
    injuries
        disqualification for athletics, 19
        symptoms of, 146, 147
Headache, 65
    result of injury, 147–49
Healing, 62
Heart, 17
Heat exhaustion, 86
Heat lamps, 128
    infrared, 128
    radiant heat, 128
Heat pads, 131, 132
Heat stroke, 86
Heel, 370
    bruise, 62, 63
    cup, 371
    strapping, 63, 64
Hematoma, 71, 72
Hemorrhage, 122
Hemorrhoids, 87
Hernia, 90
Hip, 175, 176
    bursitis, 177
    contusion, 177
    dislocation, 175
    fracture of acetablum, 176
    sprain, 176

Hip pointer, 180–82
History of an injury, 104
Hot packs, 136, 137
Housemaid's knee, 323
Humerus, 225
    contusion, 226
    fracture, 225
Hydrocollator, 134, 135
Hyperextension
    elbow, 239
        strapping, 241
    knee, 311
        strapping, 312
Hyperflexion, spine, 160
Hypertension, 17
Hypoglycemia, 33

Ice packs, 126, 127
Iliacus muscle, 189
Ilium, crest of, 173
    injury, 180
    strapping, 181
Infection, 73, 74, 75, 76
Infectious diseases, disqualification for
    athletics, 19
Inflammation, 75
Infrared, 128
Infraspinatus muscle, 218, 219
Injections, use of, 94
Injured athlete, moving an, 68, 69
Injuries, athletic, 104–25
    history, 104
    inspection, 104
    palpation, 104, 105
    prevention of, 6–9, 49–59
    types
        contusion, 125
        dislocation, 117
        fracture, 106
        sprains, 120–23
        strains, 123–25
Inoculation history, 17
Inspection, 104
Intelligence, low, disqualification for ath-
    letics, 20
Intercostal muscles, 172
Interval training, 45, 46
Inversion, 333

Jaw sprain, 150
Joint injury, disqualification for athletics,
    17
Joint mice, 319

Kidney, contusion, 168
Kneading, 137

Knee, 286–330
  anatomy, 286–290
  bursitis, 322, 323
  cartilage, injuries of, 315–19
    lateral, 318, 319
    medial, 315–18
  contusions, 320–22
  cruciate ligaments, 313–15
  dislocation, 294, 295
  fractures
    examination, 295–300
    femur (lower end), 292, 293
    fibula (upper end), 293
    patella, 293, 294
    tibia (upper end), 293
  hyperextension injury, 311
  joint mice, 319
  Osgood-Schlatter's disease, 323, 325
  pinched fat pad, 322
  quadriceps measuring, 324, 325
  rehabilitation, 325–330
  sprains, 302–311
    lateral ligament, 310, 311
    medial ligament, 302–10
Kocher's method, 195, 196
Kyphosis, 160

Lacerations, 78
  tongue, 153, 154
Laminae, 158
Lateral collateral ligaments
  ankle, 341–47
  knee, 310, 311
Latissimus dorsi muscle, 185, 186
  injury of, 185, 186
Leg, 260–85
  lower
    contusions, 275, 276
    fractures, 271, 272, 273
  muscles
    biceps femoris, 279, 280
    extensor digitorum longus, 284
    extensor hallucis longus, 282
    flexor digitorum longus, 284
    flexor hallucis longus, 285
    gastrocnemius, 281
    gracilis, 279
    peroneus brevis, 281
    peroneus longus, 281
    peroneus tertius, 281
    plantaris, 274
    popliteus, 281
    rectus femoris, 278
    sartorius, 279
    semimembranosus, 280, 281
    semitendinosus, 280

    soleus, 281
    tensor fascia latae, 277
    tibialis anterior, 281
    tibialis posterior, 281
    vastus intermedius, 277
    vastus lateralis, 277
    vastus medialis, 277
  peroneal nerve injury, 276
  plantaris pull, 273, 274
  strains, 273–75
  tendon Achilles, 275
    tenosynovitis of, 275
  upper leg
    contusions, 267–70
    fractures, 260–62
    functional tests, 265, 266
    myositis ossificans, 270, 271
    rehabilitation, 266, 267
    strains, 263–67
Letters, training, 50, 52, 53, 54
Levator scapulae muscle, 186
Ligaments, 120
Lime burns, 67, 68
  eye, 67
Longitudinal arch, 351, 352
Loose teeth, 154
Lordosis, 160
Lumbosacral sprain, 164–67
  strapping, 164
  symptoms, 164
  treatment, 164
Lymph nodes, 73
  lymphadenitis, 62, 73
  lymphangitis, 74

McMurray's sign, 317
Mallet finger, 257, 258
Mandible, 144
March fracture, 106
Massage, 137, 138
  effleurage , 137
  friction, 138
  petrissage, 138
Maxilla, 144
Maxillary artery, 71
Meals
  pregame, 37
  regularity, 31
Medial collateral ligaments
  ankle, 341–47
  knee, 300–10
Medical coverage, 20, 21, 23
  care of athletes, 24
  procedure, 25
  visiting teams, 24
Medical staff, 20

Meniscus, 288
Menus, training table, 34, 35, 36
Metatarsal arch, 353, 354, 355
Microwave, 131
Mouthpieces, 103
Movement of an injured athlete, 68, 69
Muscles, 41, 123
    pulled, 123, 124, 125
        belly, 124
        cramps, 95
        insertion, 124
        origin, 124
Myositis ossificans
    elbow, 243, 244
    thigh, 270, 271
    upper arm, 226, 227

National Athletic Trainers Association, 3
    athletic training program, 4, 5, 6
Nausea, 72, 88
Neck, 155–57
    contusion, 157
        throat, 157
    dislocation, 156
    fracture, 155
    sprain or strain, 156
Normal gait, 367
Nose bleed, 154
Nose fracture, 145
Novocain, 94
Nutrition, 28

Oblique muscles
    external, 183
    internal, 183, 184
Olecranon bursa, 242
Olecranon process, 236
Osgood-Schlatter's disease, 323, 324
Overload theory, 41
Oxygen, additional, 90
Oxygen debt, 47, 48

Palpation, 104, 105
Paraffin baths, 136
Paralysis, result of head injury, 147
Passive exercise, 138
Patella, 114
Pectoralis muscles
    major, 214, 215
    minor, 215, 216
Pelvic girdle, 173
Periosteum, 61
Periostitis, 61
Peripheral vision, 45
Peroneal nerve, injury of, 276
Peroneus brevis muscle, 281

Peroneus longus muscle, 281
Peroneus tertius, 282
Phalanx, 116
Physical conditioning, 40–59
    circuit training, 46
    endurance, 42, 43
    Fartlek, 46, 47
    grass drills, 47
    interval training, 45, 46
    oxygen debt, 47, 48
    second wind, 48, 49
    skills, 44, 45
    strength, 41, 42
    weight training, 45
Physical examination, 14
    case histories, 15
    disqualifications in, 17–20
    innoculation history, 17
Physical therapy, 126–40
    cold applications, 126, 127
    contrast baths, 135, 136
    diathermy, 130, 131
    exercise, 138, 139
    faradic and sinusoidal, 133
    galvanism, 133
    heat lamps, 128
    heat pads, 131, 132
    hot packs, 136, 137
    hydrocollator, 134, 135
    massage, 137, 138
    microwave, 131
    paraffin baths, 136
    steam baths, 136
    ultrasound, 132, 133
    ultraviolet, 129
    vibrators, 133
    whirlpool, 133, 134
Piles, 87, 88
Pilonidal cyst, 86
Pinched fat pad, 322
Plantar warts, 368, 369
Plantaris muscle, 274
Popliteus muscle, 281
Post-operative knee, 329, 330
Potassium permanganate, 85
Pott's fracture, 337
Pressure points, 71
Prevention of injury, 6–9
    calisthenics, 55, 56
    exercises, 51, 52, 53–55
    in-season program, 49–59
    pre-season, 49–59
Procaine, 94
Processes
    spinous, 158
    transverse, 158

Pronation, 235
Pronator quadratus muscle, 232
  teres muscle, 232
Proteins, 28
Psoas major muscle, 189
Pulse, 148, 149
Puncture wounds, 78
Pupil reaction, eye, 147–49

Quadriceps, 266, 268
  atrophy, 324
  measurements, 324, 325

Radius, 114, 227
Rami, 173
Rectus abdominus muscle, 183
Rectus femoris, 278
Rehabilitation of injury, 9, 10
  knee, 325, 330
    equipment, 326
    exercises, 326
    methods, 327, 328, 329
    post-operative, 329, 330
  shoulder, 222–24
  thigh, 266, 267
Removing adhesive tape, 101, 102
Repair, in healing, 62
Rhomboid muscles, 185, 214
Ribs, 169
Rigidity, result of head injury, 147

Sacroiliac, 164–67
Sacrum, 158
Salt tablets, 95, 96
Sartorius muscle, 279
Scalp wounds, 152, 153
Scapula, 190
Scoliosis, 160
Scrotum, contusion of, 98
Sebaceous cyst, 86
Second wind, 48, 49
Semilunar cartilages, injury of, 315–19
Semimembranosus muscle, 280, 281 ·
Semitendinosus muscle, 280
Serratus anterior muscle, 221
Shin splints, 348, 349
Shock, 72, 73
Shoulder, 190–224
  acromioclavicular dislocation
    mild, 201
    moderate, 202, 203
    severe, 203, 204, 205, 206
    strappings, 197, 199, 206
  anatomy, 190
  bursitis, 212, 213

contusions, 210, 212
  acromion process, 210–12
  soft tissues, 212
dislocations, 194–201
  chronic, 200
  reduction by foot in axilla, 196
  reduction by Kocher's method, 195,
    196
  strappings, 197, 198
  treatment, 196, 197
fractures
  acromion process, 192, 193
  clavicle, 191
  corocoid process, 193
  glenoid fossa, 193
  humerus, 193
  scapula, body of, 191, 192
  spine, 192
functional tests, 200, 201
sprain, 209, 210
sternoclavicular, 206–8
  strapping, 208
strains, 210
tenosynovitis (biceps), 213, 214
Shoulder harness, 204
Sinusoidal current, 133
Sitz bath, 88
Skills, 44, 45
Skin
  abrasions, 77, 78
  cinder burns, 78
  lacerations, 78
  puncture, 78
  ulcer, 79
Sleep, 90, 91,
Smoking, 38
Soleus muscle, 281
Spasm, of muscle, 124
Spine, 158–89
  atlas, 158
  axis, 158
  cervical vertebrae, 158
  contusions, 167
    buttocks, 168
    kidney, 168
  curves, 159, 160
  fibrocartilage, 158
  fractures, 160, 161
    compression, 160
    transverse processes, 160, 161
  laminae, 158
  lumbar vertebrae, 158
  sacrum, 158
  spinous processes, 158
  sprains, 161–67
  thoracic vertebrae, 158

transverse processes, 158
true vertebrae, 158
Spleen, injury of, 89, 90
Splinting, 110–17 ,
Sprains, 120–23
  ankle, 341–50
    mild, 341
    moderate, 342, 343
    severe, 343, 344
  back
    lumbosacral, 164–67
    mild, 161
    moderate, 162
    sacroiliac, 164–67
    severe, 162
  capsule, 120
  elbow, 238–40
  fingers, 254, 255
  groin, 177–79
  hemorrhage in, 122
  hip, 176
  jaw, 150
  ligaments, 120
  muscles, 120
  neck, 156
    collar for, 156
  sacroiliac, 164–67
    strapping, 166
    symptoms, 164
    treatment, 165
  shoulder, 209, 210
  thumb, 253, 254
  toe, great, 361
  toes, 361
  upper arm, 225, 226
  wrist and hand, 251, 252
Spur, bone, 64
Staleness, 93, 94
Steam baths, 136
  cabinet baths, 136
Sternum, 169, 190
Stiffness and soreness, 97
Stitch in side, 97, 98
Strains, 123–25
  belly muscle, 124
  insertion, 124
  origin, 124
  pulled muscles, 123–24
Strappings, adhesive
  acromioclavicular, 197, 199, 206
  ankle
    open-faced Gibney, 344
    routine, 345, 346
    wrap, 349
  back, low, 166
  elbow, hyperextended, 241, 242

finger, 255
groin, spica, 179
ilium, crest of, 181
knee, 303, 309
  hot pack, 304
  hyperextended, 312
shoulder
  cap, 198
  routine, 197
  severe, 206
sternoclavicular, 207, 208
tendon Achilles, 360
thigh, 269
thumb, 254
toe, great, 363
wrist and hand, 253
Strength, 41, 42
Stretcher, 111, 160
Stroking, 137
Sty, 67
Styloid process, 245
Subluxation, 194
Subscapularis muscle, 217
Supination, 235
Supinator muscle, 230
Swimming, as a conditioner, 93
Synovitis, 60
  synovial membrane, 121

Table, training, 31
Taping; see Adhesive taping; Strappings,
    adhesive
Teeth, 154, 155
  broken, 154, 155
  loose, 154
  protection of, 103
Temporal artery, 71
Tendon injuries
  ankle, 357–61
  contusions, 359
  tendon Achilles, 275
    tenosynovitis of, 365
Tenosynovitis
  biceps, long head, 213, 214
  tendon Achilles, 365
Tensor fasciae latae, 277
Teres major, 219
Teres minor, 217
Tetanus toxoid, 78
Therapy; see Physical therapy
Thigh
  contusions, 267–70
  fractures, 260–62
  muscles, 277–81
  myositis ossificans, 270, 271
  strains, 263–67

Thomas splint, 110, 112
Thorax
  contusions, 173
  fractures, 170, 171, 172
Tibia, 112
Tibialis anterior, 291
Tibialis posterior, 281
Timing, 44
Toenails
  care of, 82, 83
  ingrown, 369
  injuries, 367
Tongue, laceration of, 153, 154
Tourniquet, 72
Trainer
  duties, 3–10
  qualifications, 10–13
Trainer's equipment
  field kit, 373, 374
  for three types of budget, 375, 376
  training room, 373
Trainer s talk to squads, 377–79
  blisters, 377, 378
  drinking and smoking, 379
  equipment, 378
  leaving field without permission, 379
  meal schedule, 377
  medical coverage, 377
  missing practice, 379
  physical examinations, 377
  practice schedule, 377
  running while on field, 379
  salt tablets, 378
  taping, 377
  training table, 379
  travel, 379
  valuables, 379
  weight charts, 378
Training letters, 50, 52, 53, 54
Trapezius, 184, 185
Triceps muscle, 221, 222
Trunk, 169–73
  contusion of chest, 173
  fractures
    ribs, 170, 171, 172
    sternum, 170
  muscles of trunk, 172
  ribs, 169
    false, 169
    floating, 169
    true, 169
  sternum, 169
    body, 169
    manubrium, 169
    xiphoid appendix, 169
Tuberosity, 173

Ulcers, wound, 79
Ulna, 114, 227
Ultrasound, 132, 133
Ultraviolet, 128, 129
  carbon arc, 129
  cold quartz, 129
  erythema dose, 129
  mercury, 129
  quartz, 129
Umbilicus, 88
Unconsciousness, 68

Varicose veins, 87
Vastus intermedius muscle, 277
Vastus lateralis muscle, 277
Vastus medialis muscle, 277
Vegetarianism, 34
Venous bleeding, 69
Vibrators, 133
Vision, blurring of, 146
  peripheral, 45
Vomiting, result of head injury, 146, 147,
  148, 149

Warm up, 96, 97
Warts, 83
Water, 30
  on field, 38
Weight charts, 91, 92
Weight control, 37
  crash diets, 38
  gaining weight, 37
  reduction of, 37
Weight training, 45
Whirlpool baths, 133, 134
Whitfield's ointment, 85
Wind knocked out, 98
Wintergreen, oil of, 137
Wounds, 76
  abrasions, 77, 78
  butterflies, 76, 77
  cinder burns, 78
  dressings, 76
  hand, 257
  lacerations, 78
  puncture, 78
  scalp, 152, 153
  ulcers, 79
Wrist, 245–55
  anatomy, 245, 246
  contusions, 255
  dislocation, 249
  fractures, 246, 247
  sprains, 251, 252

Zygoma, 144
Zygomatic arch, 144